Human Physiology

Human Physiology

Dr. B.S. Yadav
Humaira B.

ADHYAYAN
Adhyayan Publishers & Distributors
New Delhi-110002

Published by
ADHYAYAN PUBLISHERS & DISTRIBUTORS
4378/4 B, 105, J.M.D. House, Murari Lal Street
Ansari Road, Darya Ganj, New Delhi-110002
Ph. : 011-23263018, 011-23277156, Fax : 011-23280028
E-mail : adhyayanpublishers@yahoo.com

Human Physiology

Edition : 2011
ISBN : 978-81-8435-242-9

Printed in India

Published by Harish Chandra Yadav for Adhyayan Publishers & Distributors, Laser Typesetting at Net Graphics and Printed at Tarun Offset Printers, Delhi.

Preface

The primary purpose of this book is to present the fundamental mechanism of physiology, as physiology is one of the most important and interesting aspects of the study of animal sciences but sufficient attention is not being paid, to its teaching in the Indian universities and colleges as compared to other branches. Since several years importance has been felt for the teaching of physiological processes, at the undergraduate levels so as to be of value to the students opting to the medical studies. For correct understanding of the physiology, fundamental knowledge of physiology is essential. Therefore, in the present book authors have made an attempt to provides the latest material for the students. The aim of this book is to provide the readers materials on the subject in a lucid and readable form so as to enable the students and teachers to understand the subject properly.

This book, the first of its own kind, is a modest effort to meet the challenging requirements of understanding physiological processes.

The book has been organised into 09 chapters, An extensive index has been provided. The text is profusely illustrated and accompanied by detailed legends, believe the book will serve as a suitable text and meet the requirement of students and provide them a solid foundation to understand the manifold phenomena of life.

The authors take this opportunity to express their sincere gratitude towards Honourable Samaj Shri Prashant Data Hiray, General Secretary, Mahatma Gandhi Vidyamandir, Malegaon Camp., for his encouragement and support provided time to time. We express our sincere thanks to respected Dr. Apoorva. P. Hiray. Co-ordinator, Mahatma Gandhi Vidyamandir Malegaon camp for generous support. Thanks are gratefully rendered to Shri Adavay, P. Hiray for support and encouragement. We are also thankful to the principal, M..S.G. College, Malegaon camp, for co-operation and suggestions. Thanks are gratefully rendered to our friends for their encouragement in production of this book. The Authors are very much thankful to the Adhyayan publishers and distributors for publishing this book.

Dr. B.S. Yadav
Humaira. B.

Authors

Contents

①

Nutrition and Digestion

Introduction

Humans are heterotrophs, organisms that cannot produce their own food. Heterotrophs must ingest or take in food. At least 95 per cent of the species of organism on earth, all animals, all fungi, and most protists and bacteria are heterotrophs. Food provides to the "other feeders" two things : (1) energy and (2) the raw materials to build the substance they need. The energy in food is described in units called calories or more properly kilocalories. The raw materials are called nutrients.

There are six classes of nutrients, carbohydrates, fats (lipids), proteins vitamins, minerals and water. These are the substances that make up most of your body. Assuming that you are a proper weight for your height, your body is made up of about 60 per cent water and about 20 per cent fat. The other 20 per cent is mostly protein, carbohydrate. Combinations of these two substances, and two major minerals found in your bones i.e. calcium and phosphorous. Other minerals and vitamins make-up less than 1 per cent of you.

Carbohydrates, lipids and proteins are organic (carbon containing) compounds and are used by the body as a source of energy or kilo-calories. They are referred in energy nutrients (proteins are not preferred energy source). In addition these three organic compound are used as building blocks for growth and repair as well as to produce other substances in body may need.

Body does not obtain energy from vitamins, minerals or water. Vitamins are organic molecules that perform functions such as helping body to form red blood cells and to unlock the energy in carbohydrates, fats and proteins. Although required in small amounts, each of the 13 different vitamins plays a vital role in the body. Many such as the B vitamins, are used for the synthesis of co-enzymes. Small molecules that help enzymes work. For example, niacin and riboflavin, two of the B vitamins are used to make the co-enzymes NAD and FAD which function in cellular respiration. The roles and interactions of some other vitamins such as vitamin C are not as well understood.

Minerals are inorganic substances and transported around the body as ions dissolved in the blood and other body fluids. Body uses a variety of minerals and they perform a variety of functions. Calcium, for example, does many jobs, including making up a part of the bones and teeth and helping blood to clot. Sodium plays a key role in regulating the fluid balance within the body. Magnesium is an important player in the process of releasing energy from carbohydrates, fats and proteins.

Water provides the medium in which all the body's reactions take place. Along with dissolved substances and suspended solids, it baths cells makes up much if the cytosol within cells and courses through arteries and veins. It even lubricates joints and cushions organs such as the brain and spinal cord.

To obtain these nutrients and energy from the food, body first digest the food. Digestion is a process in which food particles are broken down into small molecules that can be absorbed by the body. Digestion is also carried out mechanically in the mouth as food is crushed by the teeth and in the stomach as food is churned by the stomach's muscular wall. Digestion is carried out chemically in three ways: (1) by hydrochloric acid (HCl), which denatures or unfolds protein molecules and disrupts the protein glue that holds cell together, (2) by bile salts, which emulsify, or separate large lipid droplets into much smaller lipid droplets, and (3) by a variety of highly specific enzymes that help to cleave certain chemical bonds.

Enzymes are proteins that speed up the rate of chemical reactions in living things. The enzymes that help to digest the energy nutrients—proteins, carbohydrates and lipids are of three basic types.

1. **Proteases**—Which break down proteins to smaller polypeptides and amino acids.
2. **Amylases**—which break down starches and glycogen to sugars.
3. **Lipases**—Which break down the triglycerides in lipids to fatty acids and glycerol.

Where it begins—The Mouth

The water in the mouth is a secretion from a set of glands called salivary glands. Their secretion, saliva is a solution that consist primarily of water, mucous and digestive

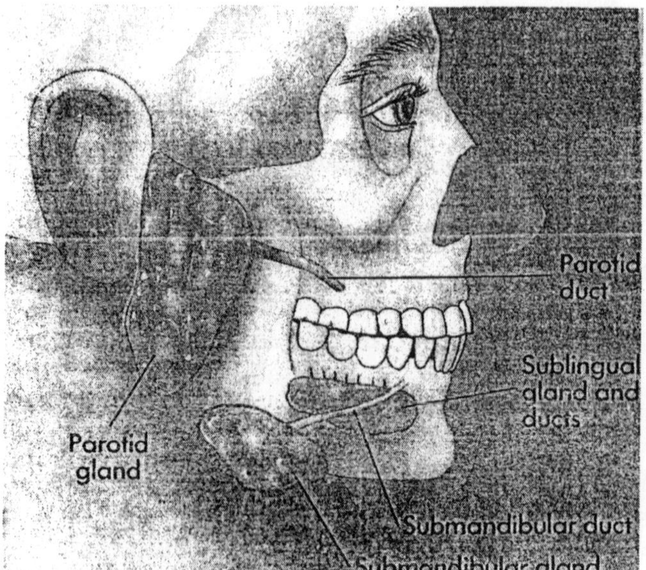

Fig. 1.1 : The salivary glands.

enzyme salivary amylase. Other susbstances can be found in smaller amounts such as antibodies and a bacteria killing enzymes.

Salivary amylase breaks down starch into molecules of the disaccharide maltose.

During this reaction the starch is broken down on the addition of water—a process called hydrolysis.

Starch + Water = Salivary amylase Maltose.

Enzymes that break down substances by hydrolysis are called hydrolyzing enzymes. Along with playing this role in digestion the saliva also moistures and lubricates food so that it is allowed easily and does not scratch the tissue of throat.

The secretions of salivary glands are controlled by the nervous system. Although the nervous system works to maintain a constant secretion of saliva in the mouth it speeds up the secretion when it is stimulated by the presence (or sometimes the sight smell or thought) of food. When food is in the mouth, nerve endings called chemoreceptors, which are sensitive to the presence of certain chemicals, Send a signal to the brain, which responds by stimulating the salivary glands.

Mechanical digestion begins when the teeth tear food apart into tiny pieces. In this way the surface area of the food is increased allowing the digestive enzymes to mix with

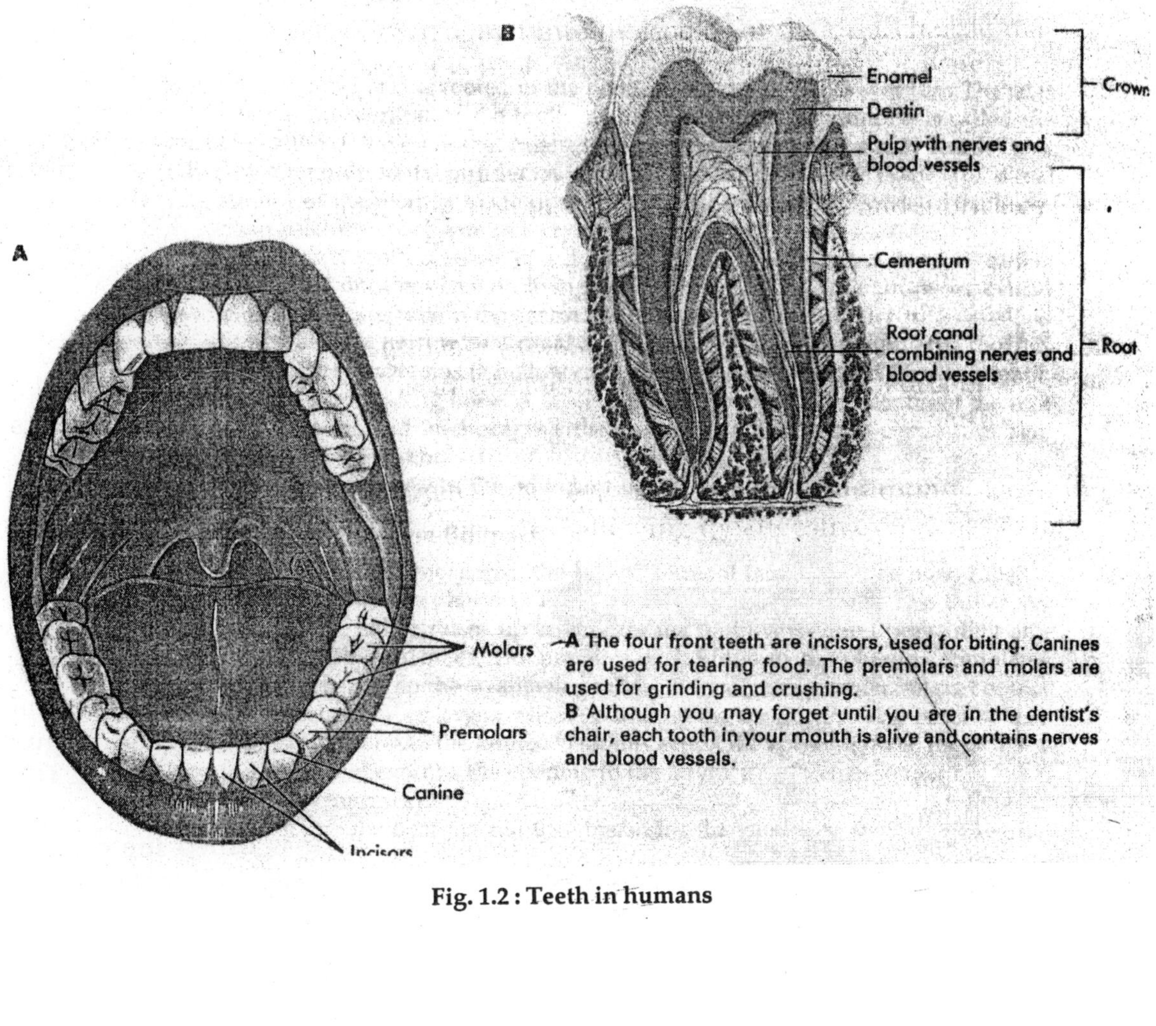

A The four front teeth are incisors, used for biting. Canines are used for tearing food. The premolars and molars are used for grinding and crushing.

B Although you may forget until you are in the dentist's chair, each tooth in your mouth is alive and contains nerves and blood vessels.

Fig. 1.2 : Teeth in humans

the food and break it down more quickly and completely. Human beings are omnivores. An omnivore eats both plant and animal foods. As a result human teeth are structurally intermediate between the pointed cutting teeth characteristic of carnivores or meat eaters and the flat, grinding teeth characteristic of herbivores or plant eaters.

In fact, the teeth of humans are like carnivores in the front and herbivores in the back. The four front teeth in the upper and lower jaws of humans are incisors. These teeth are sharp used for biting. On each side of incisors are pointed teeth called canines, which are used in tearing food. Behind each canine on each side of the mouth and along both top and bottom jaws are two premolars and three molars. In early childhood, human do not have these 32 adult teeth but only 20 "baby teeth". The first teeth are lost during childhood and are replaced by the 32 adult teeth.

Each tooth is alive and is rooted in the bone, of the upper and lower jaw. The jaws cover this bone, the portion of the tooth protruding above the gumline is called the crown. The portion of the tooth that extends into the bone is called the root. Inside lies a central nourishing pulp containing nerves, blood vessels and connective tissue. The actual chewing surface of the tooth is made up of enamel, the hardest substance in the body, which contain calcium phosphate in a crystalline term.

The bulk of each tooth consists of a mineralized substance called dentine, differs from bone in that it does not contain living cells. Instead cytoplasmic processes extend into the dentine form cells within the central pulp cavity. The pulp cavity receives blood vessels and nerves by a narrow root canal at the base or root of the tooth. The root sits within a bony socket or alveolus (a hollow cavity) collagen fibres extend from the dentine of the root to the surrounding bone. A layer of cementum covers the dentine of the root providing protection and anchoraging the periodontal ligaments cementum also resembles bone, but it is softer.

The neck of the tooth marks the boundary between the root and the crown.

The Journey of Food to the Stomach

As food is chewed and moistened, the tongue forms it into a ball like mass called a bolus and pushes it into the pharynx. The pharynx is the upper part of the throat. As this happens the soft palate raises up sealing off the nasal cavity and preventing any food from entering this chamber. The pressure of the food in the pharynx stimulates nerves in its walls that begin the swallowing reflex, an involuntary action. As part of this reflex action the voice box, or larynx, raises up to meet the epiglottis, a flap of tissue that fold back over the opening to the larynx. With this action the epiglottis, acts much like a trapdoor closing over the glottis, the opening to the larynx and trachea so that food will not go down the wrong way.

After passing into the pharynx and then bypassing the windpipe, the food enters the oesophagus, a food tube that connects the pharynx to the stomach. The oesophagus which is about 25 cm. long, pierces the diaphragm before it connects to the stomach. The diaphragm is a sheet like muscle that forms the floor of the chest cavity.

The oesophagus ends at the door of the stomach. This door is called the cardiac opening and is ringed by a circular muscle called the lower oesophageal sphincter. When the ring of muscle contracts, it closes the cardiac opening. When it relaxes it opens the stomach door.

The oesophagus does not take part in digestion but moving food down toward the stomach. The sets of longitudinal and circular muscles in its wall produce successive waves of contractions called peristalsis. The transports of food from pharynx to the stomach is called swallowing.

The Stomach

The lower oesophageal sphincter relaxes when food reaches it, allowing food to enter the stomach. The stomach is a muscular sac in which the food is collected and partially digested by hydrochloric acid and proteases.

The stomach and intestinal tract have the same basic structural plan. Their interiors are lined with a layer of tissue called the mucosa. The mucosa consists of epithelial cells, blood and lymph vessels and a layer of muscles. It covers a deeper layer of connective tissue the submucosa which is rich in blood vessels and nerves.

The inner surface of the stomach is dotted with gastric glands that extend from the epithelium but dip deeply into the mucosa. Two different kinds of cells in these glands secrete a gastric juice made up of hydrochloric acid and the protein pepsinogen. After the secretion of both the acid chemically interacts with the pepsinogen converting it to the protein—hydrolyzing enzyme pepsin. The hydrochloric acid also softens the connective tissue in foods denatures or unfolds large protein molecules and kills most bacteria that may have been ingested with the food. The pepsin digests only proteins breaking them down into short polypeptides, other epithelial cells are specialized for the secretion of mucous. This mucous produced in large quantities lubricates the stomach wall and protects the stomach from digesting itself.

The stomach controls the production of gastric juice by means of a digestive hormone called gastrin. Food stays in the stomach for approximately 2 to 6 hours. During this time the contraction of the muscular wall of the stomach churn the food, mixing it with the gastric juice and mucus. By the time, the food is ready to leave the stomach as a substance called chyme. The pyloric sphincter opens to allow the chyme to pass through.

The Small Intestine

Most of the digestion of food takes place in the small intestine within this organ. Starches and glycogen are broken down to sugars, proteins to amino acids and lipids to fatty acids and glycerol. These products of digestion then pass through the cells of the intestinal mucosa and diffuse into the blood in underlying blood vessels. The triglycerides move into the lymph in neighbouring lymphatic vessels.

All of this activity take place in the small intestine, the tube like portion of the digestive tract that begins at the pyloric sphincter and ends at its T-shaped junction with the large intestine. Although the small intestine is approximately 6 m. long only the first 25 cm. is actively involved in digestion. This initial portion of the small intestine is called the duodenum. The other portions of the small intestine, the jejunum and the ilium are highly specialized to aid in the absorption of the products of digestion by the blood and lymph.

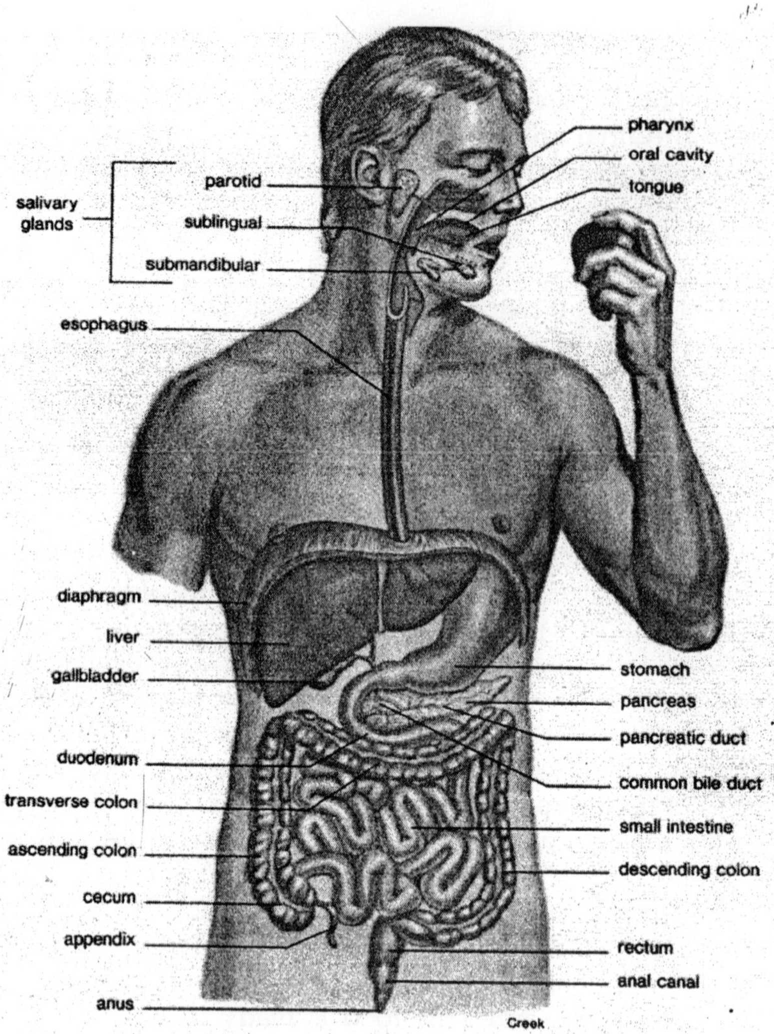

Fig.1-3 : The human digestive system

Accessory Organs that Help Digestion

Some of the enzymes necessary for digestion are secreted by the salivary glands, epithelial cells of stomach and epithelial cells of the duodenum. The others are secreted by the pancreas, lies behind the stomach, extending laterally from the duodenum, towards the spleen. It is an elongate pinkish gray organ with a length of 15 cm. The surface of the pancreas has a knobby texture and its tissue is soft and easily torn.

The pancreas is primarily an exocrine organ, producing digestive enzymes and buffers, pancreatic islets, which secrete insulin and glucagon account for only around 1 per cent of the cellular portion of the pancreas. The exocrine cells form the pancreatic acini. The ducts draining the acini carry secreted enzymes and buffers into the pancreatic duct, which carries these secretions to the duodenum. The pancreatic duct penetrates the duodenal wall with the common bile duct from the liver and gall bladder.

Pancreatic enzymes are broadly classified according to their targets. Lipases attack lipids, carbohydrases digest sugars and starches, and proteases break proteins.

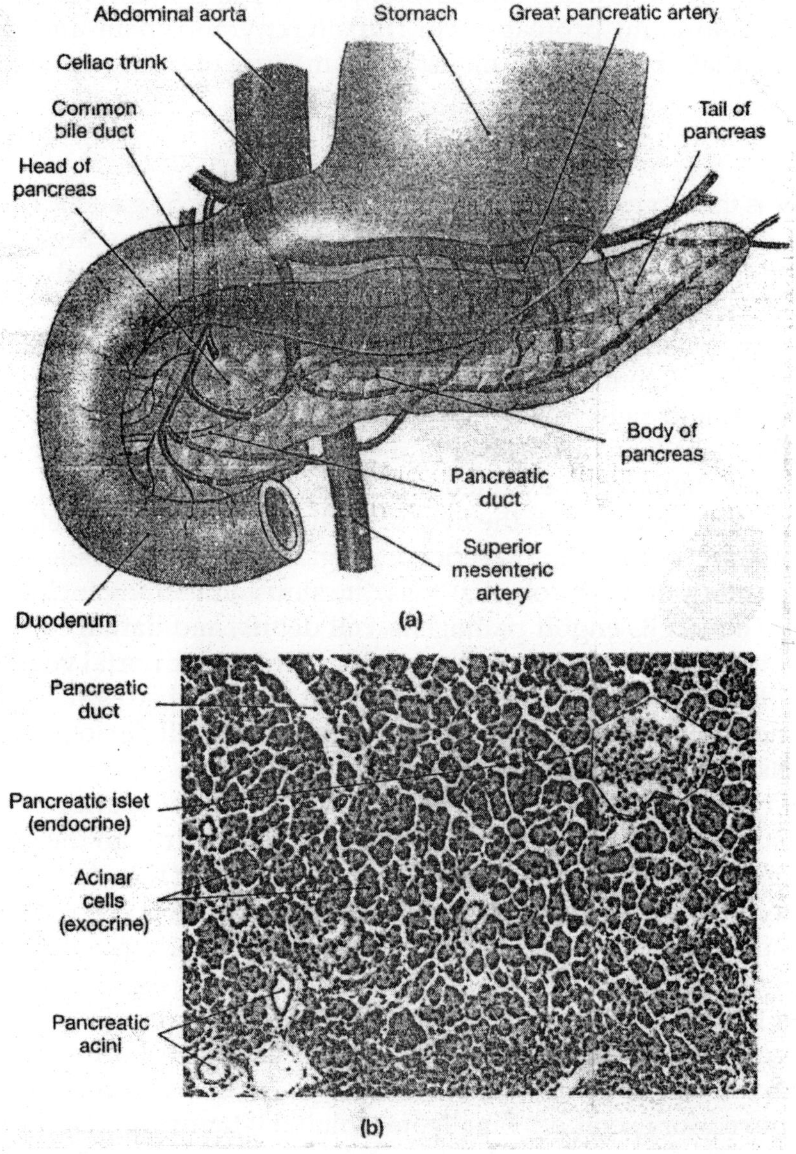

Fig.1.4 : The Pancreas
(a) Anatomy of Pancreas (b) A low power light micrograph of the pancreas

Control of Pancreatic Secretion

The pancreatic acini produce a watery pancreatic juice in response to hormonal instructions from the duodenum. When acid chyme arrives in the small intestine secretion is released. This secretion contains buffers primarily sodium bicarbonate that help bring the pH of the chyme under control. A different intestinal hormone cholecystokinin, controls the production and secretion of pancreatic enzymes. The specific enzymes involved are pancreatic amylase, Similar to salivary amylase pancreatic lipase, nucleases that break down nucleic acids and several proteolytic enzymes.

The most abundant proteases are trypsin, chymotrypsin and carboxypeptidase. Together they shatter complex proteins into a mixture of short peptide chains and amino acids.

The Liver

The liver is the largest visceral organ weighing about 1.5 kg and accounting for roughly 2.5 per cent of the total body weight. This large reddish brown organ provides essential metabolic and synthetic services that falls into the three general categories metabolic regulation, haematological regulation and bile production.

Liver is divided into four lobes two large (right and left) and two small (caudate and quadrate). A tough connective tissue fold the falciform ligament marks the division between the left and right lobes.

Under the right lobe of the liver is the gall-bladder, a muscular sac that stores and concentrates bile before it is excreted into the small intestine.

The basic functional unit of the liver is the liver lobules. Liver cells called hepatocytes within a lobule are arranged into a series of irregular plates. Sinusoids are highly permeable capillaries. In addition to endothelial cells, the sinusoidal lining includes large number of buffer cells. These cells engulf pathogens, cell debris, and damaged blood cells.

Blood enters the sinusoids from branches of the hepatic portal vein and hepatic artery, The liver cells absorb and secrete materials into the blood stream. Blood then leaves the sinusoids and enters the central vein. The central vein of all the lobules merge to form the hepatic veins that empty into the inferior vena cava.

Liver plays a vital role in metabolic regulation. In the heapatic portal system all blood leaving the absorptive areas of the digestive tract flows through the liver before reaching the general circulation. This routing enables the liver cells (1) to extract absorbed nutrients or toxins from the blood before it reaches the rest of the body, and (2) to monitor and adjust the circulating levels of organic nutrients. Excess are removed and stored and deficiencies are corrected by mobilizing stored reserves as synthesizing the necessary compounds for example, when blood glucose levels rise, the liver removes glucose and synthesizes glycogen. When blood glucose levels fall the liver breaks down glycogen and releases glucose into the circulation. Circulating toxins and metabolic waste products are also removed for excretion. Finally, fat soluble vitamins (A, D, K and E) are absorbed and stored.

Liver is the largest blood reservoir in the body. It performs hematological regulation. As blood passes by phagocytic cells in the liver remove aged or damaged red blood cells, debris and pathogens from the circulation. Liver cells synthesize the plasma proteins that determine the osmotic concentration of the blood, transport nutrients and establish the clotting and complement system.

Bile is synthesized in the liver and excreted into the lumen of the duodenum. Bile consists mostly of water, ions, bilirubin (a pigment derived from heamoglobin), cholesterol and bile salts. The water and ions help to dilute and buffer acids in chyme as it enters the small intestine. Bile salts are synthesized from cholesterol in the liver and are required for the normal digestion and absorption of fats.

Other functions such as maintenance of normal blood glucose, amino acid and fatty acid concentrations, synthesis and interconversion of nutrient types (e.g., transamination of amino acids or conversion of carbohyodrate to lipids) synthesis and release of cholesterol bound to transport proteins inactivation of toxins. Storage of iron reserves storage of fat soluble vitamins, synthesis of plasma proteins, synthesis of clotting factors synthesis of inactive hormone angiotensinogen, absorption and inactivation of lipid soluble drugs, etc., are performed by the liver. In such a way over 200 different functions have been consigned to the liver. Therefore, any condition that severely damages the liver represents a serious threat to life. The liver has ability to partially regenerate after injury but often liver function does not fully recover.

The Gallbladder

The gallbladder is muscular pear-shaped organ. It has two major functions, bile storage and bile modification. When filled to capacity, the gallbladder contains 40-70 ml of bile. As bile remains in the gallbladder, its composition gradually changes, water is absorbed and the bile salts and other components of bile become increasingly concentrated.

Most dietary lipids are not water soluble. Mechanical processing along the digestive tract creates large drops containing various lipids that are much too massive to be attacked by digestive enzymes. Bile salts break the drops apart in a process called emulsification which creates tiny emulsion droplets with a superficial coating of bile salts. The formation of tiny droplets increases the surface area available for enzymatic attack. In addition the layer of bile salts facilitates interaction between the lipids and lipid digesting enzymes provided by the pancreas.

The arrival of the intestinal hormone cholecystokinin or cck, in the circulating blood stimulates bile excretion, cholecystokinin relaxes the biliary sphincter, and contractions of the walls of the gallbladder then push bile into the small intestine. cck is released whenever chyme enters the intestine, but the amount secreted increases if the chyme contains large amounts of fat.

The Large Intestine

The horseshoe-shaped large intestine begins at the end of the ileum and ends at the anus. The principal functions of the large intestine include (1) the reabsorption of water and compaction of feaces, (2) the reabsorption of important vitamins liberated by bacterial action, and (3) the storing of faecal material prior to defeacation.

It can be divided into three major regions (1) the first portion of the large intestine cecum, (2) the largest portion colon, and (3) the part rectum.

The major functions of the large intestine include absorption and preparation of the feacal material for elimination.

The reabsorption of water is an important function of the large iritestine. Although roughly 1500 ml of watery material arrives in the colon each day. Some 1300 ml of water are reabsovbed from it and only about 200 ml of feaces are ejected.

In addition to reabsorpting water, the large intestine absorbs a variety of other substances from the chyme, Such as vitamins, bilirubin products, bile salts.

The rectal chamber is usually empty when one of those powerful peristaltic contractions forces feacal materials out of the colon. Movement of feaces through the anorectal canal requires relaxation of the internal anal sphincter but when it relaxes the external sphincter automatically clamps shut. Thus the actual release of feaces requires conscious effort to open the external sphincter voluntarily. If the commands do not arrive the peristaltic contractions cease until additional rectal expansion triggers the defeacation reflex a second time.

In addition to opening the external sphincter, consciously directed activities, such as tensing the abdominal muscles or making expiratory movements while closing the glottis elevate intra-abdominal pressures and help to force feacal materials out of the rectum. Such pressures also force blood into the network if veins causing them to stretch.

Digestion and Absorption

A typical meal contains a mixture of carbohydrates, proteins, lipids, water, electrolytes and vitamins. The digestive system handles each of these components differently. Large organic molecules must be broken down through digestion before absorption can occur. water, electrolytes and vitamins can be absorbed without preliminary processing.

The Processing and Absorption of Nutrients

Food contains large organic molecules many of them insoluble. The digestive system first breaks down the physical structure of ingested material and then disassembles the component molecules into smaller fragments. This produce small organic molecules that can be absorbed. Once absorbed these will be used by the body to generate ATP and to synthesize complex carbohydrates, proteins and lipids.

Foods are usually complex chains of simpler molecules. In a typical dietary carbohydrate, the basic molecules are simple sugars. In a protein, the building blocks are amino acids and in lipid they are usually fatty acids. Digestive enzymes break the bonds between the component molecules in a process called hydrolysis.

Digestive enzymes differ in respect to their specific targets. Carbohydrases break the bonds between sugars, proteinases split the linkages between amino acids, and lipases separate the fatty acids from glycerides.

Carbohydrate Digestion and Absorption

Carbohydrate digestion begins in the mouth through the action of salivary amylase. Amylase breaks down complex carbohydrates into small fragments producing a mixture primarily composed of disaccharides (two sugars) and trisaccharides (three sugars). Salivary amylase continues to digest the starches and glycogen in the meal for an hour or two before stomach acids render it inactive. In the duodenum, the remaining complex carbohydrates are broken down through the action of pancreatic amylase.

Epithelial Processing and Absorption

Before they are absorbed disaccharides and trisaccharides are fragmented into simple sugars by enzymes found on the surfaces of the intestinal microvilli. The intestinal epithelium then absorbs simple sugars. Simple sugars entering an intestinal cell diffuse through the cytoplasm and across the basement membrane to enter the interstitial fluid. They then enter the intestinal capillaries for delivery to the hepatic portal vein.

Lipid Digestion and Absorption

Triglycerides are the most abundant dietary lipids, which consists of three fatty acids attached to a single molecule of glycerol. Triglycerides and other dietary fats are relatively unaffected by conditions in the stomach and enter the duodenum in the form of large lipid drops. Bile salts emulsify these drops into tiny droplets that can be attacked by pancreatic lipase. This enzyme breaks the triglycerides apart and the lipids released interact with bile salts in the surrounding chyme to form small complexes called micelles. When a micelle contacts the intestinal epithelium, the enclosed lipids diffuse across the cell membrane and enter the cytoplasm. The intestinal cells use the arriving lipids to manufacture new triglycerides that are then coated with proteins. This step creates a soluble complex known as a chylomicron. The chylomicrons are secreted into the interstitial fluids, where they enter the intestinal lacteals through the large gaps between adjacent endothelial cells. From the lacteals they proceeds along the lymphatics, through the thorasic duct, and finally enter the circulation at the left subclavian vein.

Protein Digestion and Absorption

Proteins have very complex structures and several different techniques and used to disassemble them. The mechanical processing in the oral cavity increases the surface area of food exposed to gastric juices following ingestion. Placing the bolus into a strongly acid environment kills most pathogenic microorganisms, breaks down cell walls and provides the proper environment for the efforts of pepsin, the proteolytic enzyme secreted by chief cells of the stomach. Pepsin does not complete the process, but it does reduce the relatively huge proteins of the chyme into smaller polypeptide fragments.

After the acid bath has ended and the pH has risen in the duodenum, pancreatic enzymes come into play. Working together, each with its own specificities, trypsin, chymotrypsin, elastase and carbohydrase complete the disassembly of the fragments into a mixture of short peptide chains and individual amino acids. Enzymes on the surfaces of the microvilli complete the process by breaking the peptide chains into their component amino acids, and the amino acids are absorbed through carrier mediated transport. Carrier proteins at the inner surface of the cell then dump the absorbed amino acids into the interstitial fluid. Once within the interstitial fluids most of the amino acids diffuse into intestinal capillaries.

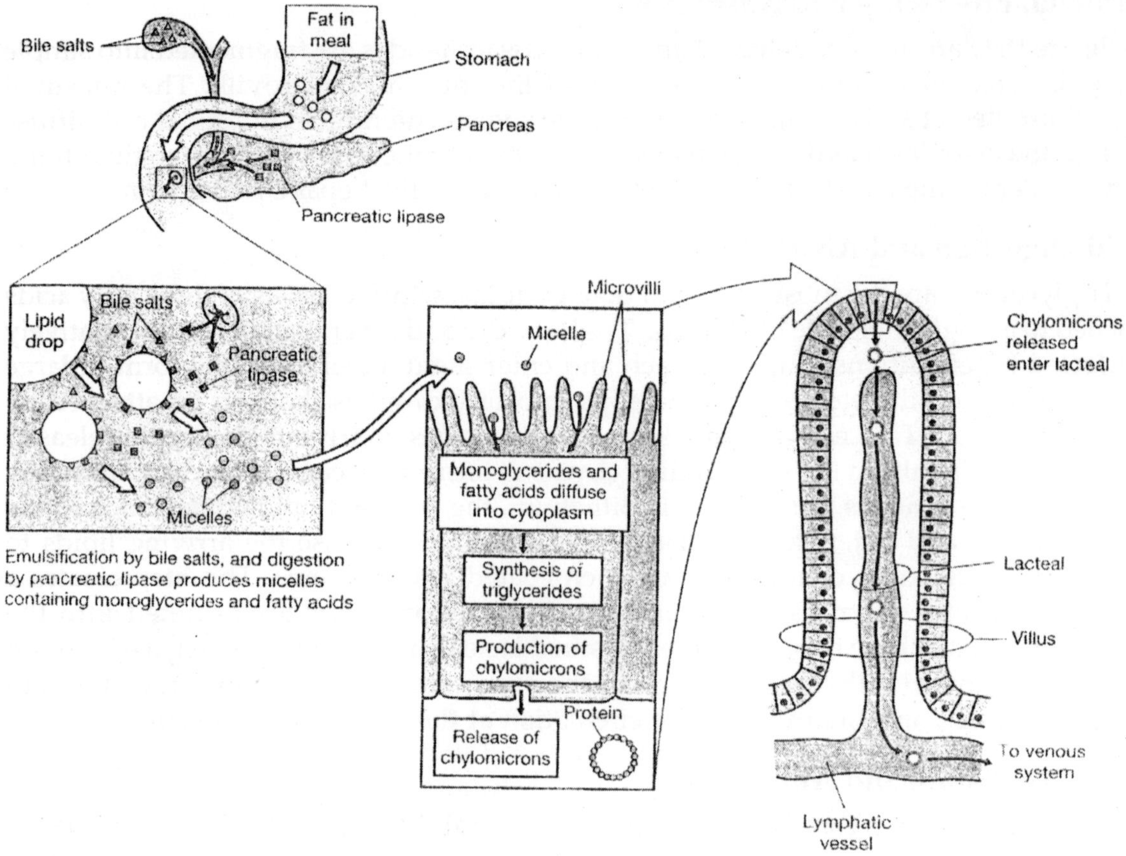

Fig.1.5 : The Absorption and Transport of Lipids

Water and Electrolyte Absorption

Each day 2-2.5 liters of water enter the digestive tract in the form of food or drink. The salivary, gastric, intestinal and accessory gland secretions provide another 6-7 liters. Out of that total, only about 150 ml are lost in the fecal waste. This water conservation occurs passively, following osmotic gradients, water always tends to flow into the solution containing the higher concentration of solutes.

The epithetial cells are continually absorbing dissolved nutrients, and ions, and these activities gradually lower the solute concentration of the intestinal contents. As the solute concentration decreases water moves into the surrounding tissues "following" the solutes and maintaining osmotic equilibrium. The absorption of sodium and chloride ions is the most important factor promoting water movement. Other ions absorbed in smaller quantities are calcium, potassium, magnesium, iodine, bicarbonate, and iron. Calcium absorption occur under hormonal control, requiring the presence of parathyroid hormone and calcitriol.

Absorption of Vitamins

Vitamins are organic compounds related to lipid and carbohydrates that are required in very small quantities. The nine water soluble vitamins function primarily as participants in enzymatic reactions. All but one, vitamin B12, are easily absorbed by the intestinal mucosa unless it has been bound to intrinsic factor, a protein secreted by the parietal cells of the stomach.

Fat soluble vitamins enter the duodenum in fat droplets, mixed with dietary lipids. They remain in association with those lipids when micelles form. The fat soluble vitamins are then absorbed from the micelles with the products of lipid digestion. One fat soluble vitamin, vitamin K, is also produced by bacterial action and absorbed in the colon.

Metabolism

Metabolism refers to all the chemical reactions of the body. Living cells are chemical factories using chemical reactions to break down organic molecules and to obtain energy, usually in the form of ATP. To carry out these processes, cells in the human body must obtain water, vitamins, ions and oxygen. Oxygen is absorbed at the lungs but all the other substances, usually called nutrients, are obtained by absorption at the digestive tract. The cardiovascular system distributes oxygen and nutrients to cells throughout the body.

The energy released inside a cell supports growth, cell division, contraction, secretion, and various other special functions that vary from cell to cell. Each tissue type contains different population of cells, and the energy and nutrient requirements of any two tissues (such as loose connective tissue and cardiac muscle) are quite different. Further more when cells, tissues, and organs change their nutrient requirements, thus our nutrient requirements vary from moment to moment (resting *versus* active) home to home (asleep *versus* awake) and year to year (growing child *versus* adult).

When organic nutrients, such as carbohydrates or lipids are abundant, energy reserves are built-up. Different tissues and organs are specialized to store excess nutrients, the storage of lipids in adipose tissue is one familiar example. The endocrine system with the assistance of the nervous system, adjusts and coordinates the metabolic activities of the body's tissues and controls the storage and release of nutrient reserves.

Cellular Metabolism

After the mechanical and chemical digestion of food. Simple sugars, amino acids and lipids are absorbed by the digestive tract and distributed by the blood stream. After diffusing into the intestinal fluid, these nutrients cross the cell membrane to join other nutrients already in the cytoplasm. All of the cell's metabolic operations rely on the resulting nutrient pool.

Catabolism breaks down organic molecules, releasing energy that can be used to synthesize ATP or other high energy compounds. Catabolism proceeds in a series of steps. In general preliminary processing occurs in the cytosol where enzymes break down large organic molecules into smaller fragments. For example, carbohydrates are broken down to short carbon chains triglycerides are split into fatty acids and glycerol and proteins are broken down to individual amino acids.

Relatively little ATP is formed during these initial steps. However, the simple molecules produced can be absorbed and processed by mitochondria and the mitochondrial steps release significant amounts of energy. As mitochondrial enzymes breaks the covalent bonds that hold these molecules together they capture roughly 40 per cent of the energy released. The captured energy is used to convert ADP to ATP, and the rest escapes as heat that warms the interior of the cell and the surrounding tissues.

Anabolism, the synthesis of new organic molecules, involves the formation of new chemical bonds. The ATP produced by mitochondria provides energy to support anabolism, as well as other cell functions.

Cells synthesize new organic components for three basic reasons.

1. To perform structural maintenance or repair : All cells must expend energy to perform ongoing maintenance and repairs, because most organic molecules and structures in the cell are temporary rather than permanent. Their removal and replacement are part of the process of metabolic turnover.

2. To support growth : Cells preparing for division enlarge and synthesize additional proteins and organelles.

3. To produce secretions : Secretary cells must synthesize their products and deliver them to the interstitial fluid.

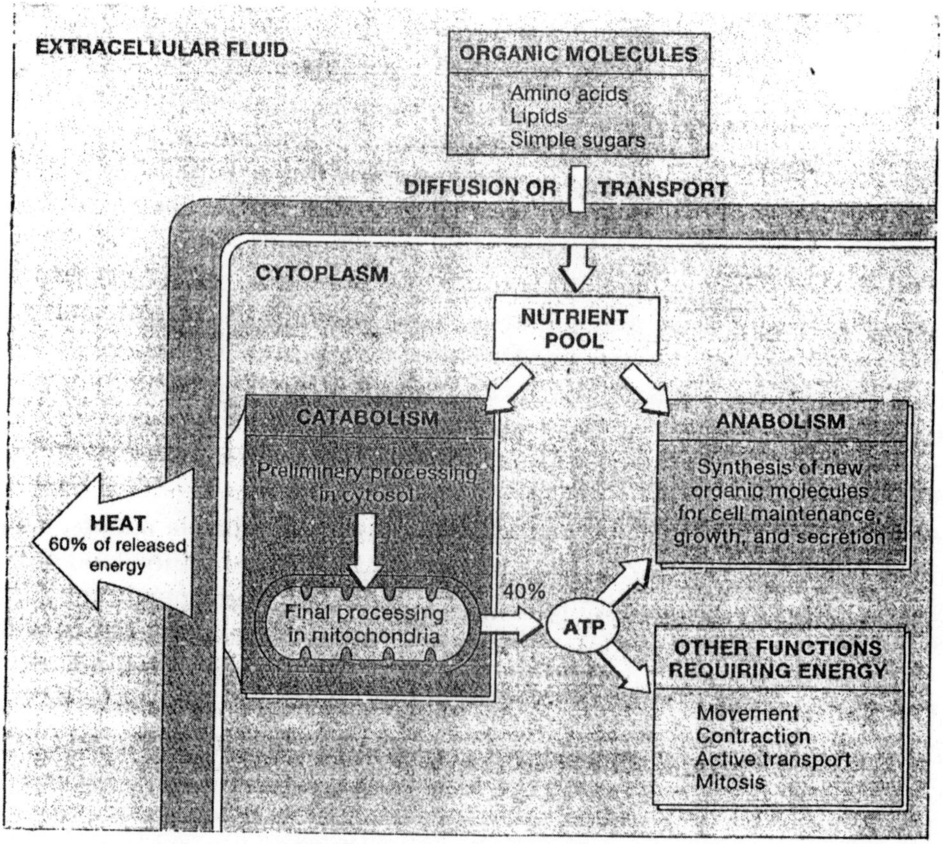

Fig.1.6 : Cellular Metabolism

The nutrient pool is the source for the organic molecules for both catabolism and anabolism. The cells tends to conserve the material also needed to build new compounds and breaks down the rest to provide ATP. The cell is continually replacing membranes, organelles, enzymes and structural proteins. These anabolic activities require more amino acids then lipids and relatively few carbohydrates. Catabolic activities tend to process these organic molecules in the reverse order. In general, a cell with excess carbohydrates, lipids and amino acids will break down carbohydrates first, lipids are a second choice and amino acids are seldom broken down.

Oxidation-Reduction Reaction and the Role of Coenzymes

The energy yielding (ATP yielding) reactions within cells are oxidation reactions. Oxidation was originally defined as the combination of oxygen with other elements. Examples are rusting of iron (the slow formation of iron oxide) and burning of wood and other fuels. In burning, oxygen combines rapidly with carbon, producing (in addition to carbon dioxide and water) an enormous amount of energy, which is liberated as heat and light. But when it was discovered that oxidation also occurs when hydrogen atoms are removed from compounds. So the definition was expanded to its current form: oxidation occurs by the gain of oxygen or the loss of hydrogen. When oxidation occurs, the oxidized substance always loses electrons as they move to a substance that more strongly attracts them.

This process can be explained by electron-attracting abilities of atoms. Because hydrogen is very electropositive, its one electron usually spends more time orbiting the other atoms of molecules that hydrogen helps to form. But when a hydrogen atom is removed its electron goes with it and the molecule as a whole loses that electron. Conversely, oxygen is very electron, hungry (electronegative), so when oxygen binds with other atoms the shared electrons spend more time in oxygen's vicinity. Again, the molecule as a whole loses electrons. Essentially, all oxidation of food fuels involves the step-by-step removal of pairs of hydrogen atoms from the substrate molecules, leaving only carbon dioxide (CO_2). Molecular oxygen (O_2) is the final electron acceptor. It combines with the removed hydrogen atoms at the very end of the process, to form water (H_2O).

Whenever one substance loses electrons (is oxidized), another substance gains them (is reduced). Thus, oxidation and reduction are coupled reactions known as oxidation-reduction (O-R) or redox, reactions. The key understanding about redox reactions is that "Oxidized" substances lose energy and "reduced" substances gain energy as energy-rich electrons are transferred from the first to the second. Thus, as food fuels are oxidized, their energy is transferred to a "bucket-brigade" of other molecules and ultimately to ADP to form energy rich ATP molecules.

Like all other chemical reactions in the body, oxidation-reduction reactions are catalyzed by enzymes. The enzymes that catalyze oxidation-reduction reactions by removing hydrogen are specifically called dehydrogenases, while those catalyzing the transfer of oxygen are oxidases. Most of these enzymes require the help of a specific coenzyme typically derived from one of the B vitamins. Although the enzymes catalyze the removal of hydrogen atoms to oxidize a substance, they cannot accept the hydrogen.

Their coenzymes act as reversible hydrogen acceptors, becoming reduced each time a substrate is oxidized. Two very important coenzymes of the oxidative pathways are nicotinamide adenine dinucleotide (NAD+) based on niacin, and flavin adenine dinucleotide (FAD) derived from riboflavin.

Mechanisms of ATP Synthesis

How do our cells capture some of the energy liberated during cellular respiration to make ATP molecules? There appear to be two mechanisms. Substrate-levels phosphorylation and oxidative phosphorylation.

Substrate-level phosphorylation occurs when high-energy phosphate groups are transferred directly from phosphorylated substrates to ADP. Essentially, it occurs because the high energy bonds attaching the phosphate groups to the substrates are even more unstable than those of ATP. ATP is synthesized by this route during one of the steps of glycolysis, and once during each turn of the Krebs cycle. The enzymes catalyzing substrate-level phosphorylations are located in both the cytoplasm and in the watery environment inside the mitochondria.

Oxidative phosphorylation is much more complicated but it also releases most of the energy that is captured in ATP bonds during cellular respiration. This process, which is carried out by electron transport proteins forming part of the cristae membranes in the mitochondria. In this case, some of the energy released during the oxidation of food fuels is used to pump hydrogen ions or protons (H^+) across the inner mitochondrial membrane into the intermembrane space. This creates a steep diffusion gradient for protons across the membrane. Then, when protons do flow back across the membrane, some of this gradient energy is captured and used to attach phosphate groups to ADP.

Carbohydrate Metabolism

Carbohydrates are important sources of energy. Most cells generate ATP and high energy compounds through the breakdown of carbohydrates, especially glucose. Glucose enters the tissue cells by diffusion. Immediately upon entry into the cell, glucose is phosphorylated to form glucose 6-phosphate by transfer of a phosphate group (PO_4^{3-}) to its sixth carbon during a reaction with ATP.

Glucose + ATP $\rightarrow$ glucose-6-phosphate + ADP

Because most body cells lack the enzymes needed to reverse this reaction, it traps glucose inside the cells. Since glucose-6-phosphate is different molecule from simple glucose, the reaction also keeps intracellular glucose level low, maintaining a diffusion gradient for glucose entry. Intestinal mucosal cells and liver cells have the enzymes needed to reverse this phosphorylation reaction. The catabolic and anabolic pathways for carbohydrates all begin with glucose-6-phosphate.

The breakdown occurs in a series of small steps and several of the steps release sufficient energy to support the conversion of ADP to ATP. During the complete catabolism of glucose, a typical cell gains 36 ATP.

$$C_6H_{12}O_6 + 6O_2 \rightarrow 6H_2O + 6CO_2 + 36ATP + heat$$

glucose oxygen water carbon dioxide

Glycolysis

Glycolysis is a series of chemical steps by which glucose is converted into two pyruvic acid molecules yielding, a net gain of 2ATP per glucose molecule. Glycolysis occurs in the cytosol of cells where its steps are catalyzed by specific soluble enzymes. Except for the first step during which glucose entering the cell is phosphorylated to glucose-6-phosphate, all of its steps are fully reversible. Glycolysis is an anaerobic process. Although this is sometimes mistakenly interpreted to mean that the pathway occurs only in the absence of oxygen this is not the case. The correct interpretation is that glycolysis does not used oxygen and occurs whether or not oxygen is present.

Glycolysis requires (1) glucose molecules, (2) appropriate cytoplasmic enzymes, (3) ATP and ADP, and (4) NAP, a coenzyme that removes hydrogen atoms during a complex reaction.

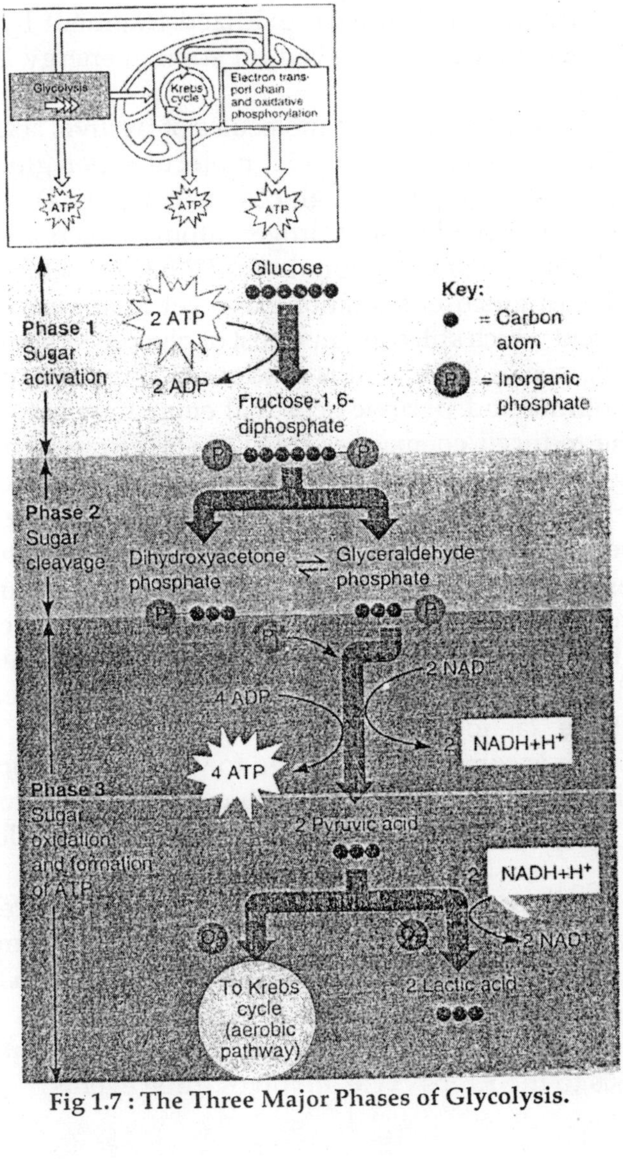

Fig 1.7 : The Three Major Phases of Glycolysis.

The basic steps in glycolysis are

1. **Sugar activation :** In phase 1 glucose is phosphorylated and converted to fructose-6-phosphate which is then phosphorylated again. These three steps yield fructose -1-6-diphosphate and use two ATP molecules. The two separate reactions of the sugar with ATP provide the activation energy needed to prime the later stages of the pathway hence this phase is sometimes referred to as the energy investment phase.

2. **Sugar Cleavage :** During phase 2, fructose-1-6-diphosphate is split into two 3-carbon fragments that exist as one of two isomers, glyceraldehyde 3-phosphate or dihydroxyacetone phosphate.

3. **Oxidation and ATP formation :** In phase 3 two major events happen. First the two 3-carbon fragments are oxidized by the removal of hydrogen, which is picked-up by NAD^+. Hence, some of glucose's energy is transferred to NAD^+. Second, inorganic phosphate groups (Pi) are attached to each oxidized fragment by high energy bond. Later as these terminal phosphates are cleaved off enough energy is captured to form a total of four ATP molecules.

The final products of glycolysis are two molecules of pyruvic acid and two molecules of reduced NAD^+ with a net gain of two ATP molecules per glucose molecule. Each pyruvic acid has the formula $C_3H_4O_3$, and glucose is $C_6H_{12}O_6$. Thus, between them the two pyruvic acid molecules have lost 4 hydrogen atoms which are now bound to two molecules of NAD^+. Although a small amount of ATP has been harvested the other end products (H_2O and CO_2) of glucose, oxidation have yet to appear.

The fate of pyruvic acid which still contains most of glucose's chemical energy, depends on the availability of oxygen at the time it is produced. There is a little supply of NAD^+, this glycolysis will continue and pyruvic acid will enter the next processing phase the Krebs cycle only if the reduced coenzymes ($NADH+H^+$) formed during glycolysis are relieved of the hydrogen acceptors. When oxygen is readily available this is not problem. $NADH+H^+$ simply delivers its burden of hydrogen atoms to the enzymes of the electron transport chain in the mitochondria which in turn deliver them to molecular oxygen forming water. When oxygen is not present in sufficient amounts, the $NADH+H^+$ produced during glycolysis unloads its hydrogen baggage back to pyruvic acid, thus reducing it. This addition of two hydrogen atoms to pyruvic acid yields lactic acid. Some of the lactic acid produced diffuses out of the cells and is transported to the liver. When oxygen is again available, lactic acid is oxidized back to pyruvic acid and enters the aerobic pathways. There it is completely oxidized to water and carbon dioxide. The liver may also convert lactic acid all the way back to glucose-6-phosphate and then store it as glycogen or free it of its phosphate and release it to the blood if blood sugar levels are low.

Krebs cycle : The Krebs cycle, named after its discover Hans Krebs (1937) is the next stage of glucose oxidation. The Krebs cycle occurs in the aqueous mitochondrial matrix and is fuelled largely by pyruvic acid produced during glycolysis and by fatty acids resulting from fat breakdown.

After pyruvic acid enters the mitochondria, it is converted into acetyl COA. This process, links glycolysis to the Krebs cycle, involves three events.

1. Decarboxylation : In which one of pyruvic acid's carbons is removed and released as carbon dioxide gas. CO_2 diffuses out of the cells into the blood to be expelled by the lungs.

2. Oxidation : By the removal of hydrogen atoms. The removed hydrogens are picked up by NAD^+.

3. Combining the resulting acetic acid with coenzyme A to produce the final product, acetyl coenzyme A or simply acetyl CoA. Coenzyme A is a sulfur containing coenzyme derived from pantothenic acid, a B vitamin.

Acetyl CoA is now ready to enter the Krebs cycle and be broken down completely by the mitochondrial enzymes. Coenzyme A shuttles the 2-carbon acetic acid to the enzyme that can condense it with a 4-carbon acid called oxaloacetic acid to produce the 6-carbon citric acid. Citric acid is the first substrate of the cycle and biochemists prefer to call the Krebs cycle the citric acid cycle.

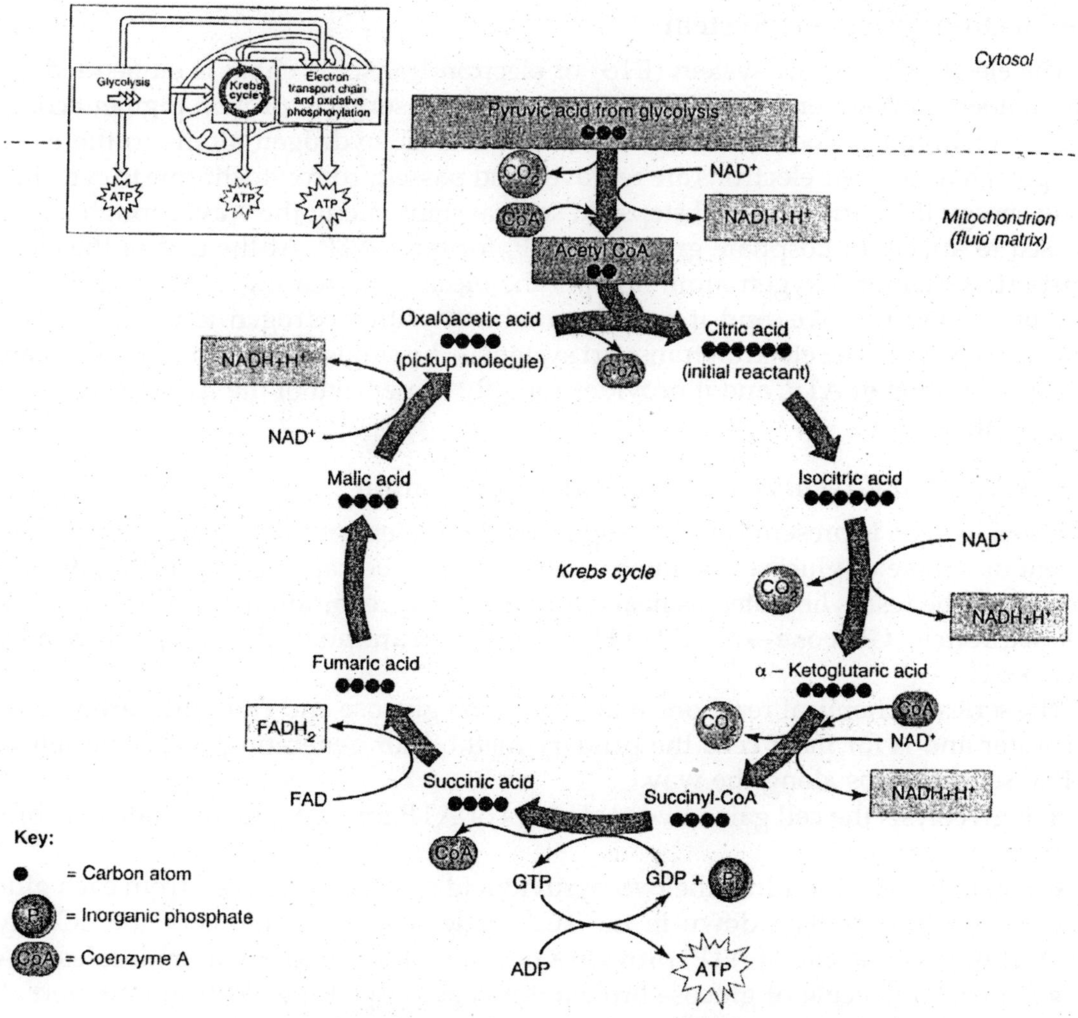

Fig. 1.8 : Simiplified Version of the Krebs Cycle.

As the cycle moves along through its eight successive steps, the atoms of citric acid are rearrange to produce different intermediate molecules, most caused Keto acids. The acetic acid that enters the cycle is broken apart carbon by carbon and is oxidized. Simultaneously generating $NADH+H^+$ and $FADH^2$. At the end of the cycle, acetic acid has been totally disposed of and oxaloacetic acid is regenerated. Because two decarboxylation and four oxidation events occur, the products of the Krebs cycle are two molecules of carbon dioxide and four molecules of reduced coenzyme. The addition of water at certain steps accounts for some of the released hydrogen. One molecule of ATP is formed during each turn of the cycle.

Now for the pyruvic acid molecules entering the mitochondria, a total of three carbon dioxides and five molecules of reduced coenzymes 1 $FADH_2$ and $4NADH+H^+$ are formed for each pyruvic acid. The products of glucose oxidation in the Krebs cycle are twice that, 6 CO_2, 10 molecules of reduced coenzymes and 2 ATP molecules.

The Electron Transport System

The electron transport system (ETS) or electron transport chain is embedded in the inner mitochondrial membrane. The ETS consists of a series of protein pigment complex called cytochromes. Coenzymes in the matrix deliver hydrogen atoms to the electron transport chain and the electrons are removed and passed from cytochrome to cytochrome losing energy in a series of small steps. At several steps, along the way, enough energy is released to attach a phosphate group to ADP, forming ATP. At the end of the electron transport system an oxygen atom accepts the electrons, creating an oxygen ion (O^{2-}). This ion is very reactive, and it quickly combines with hydrogen ions (H^+) to form a molecule of water. The electron transport system is the single most important mechanism for the generation of ATP, and it provides roughly 95 per cent of the ATP needed to keep our cells alive.

Energy Yield of Glycolysis and Cellular Respiration

When oxygen is present cellular respiration is efficient of the total 686 Kcal of energy present in 1 mole of glucose, as much as 262 Kcal can be captured in the bonds of ATP molecules. The rest is liberated as heat. During cellular respiration, most energy flows in this sequence, Glucose→$NADH+H^+$→elctron transport chain→proton motive force→ATP.

The series of chemical reactions that begin with glucose and end with carbon dioxide and water and is for most cells the primary method for generating ATP. The cell gains ATP at several steps along the way.

- In glycolysis the cell gains two molecules of ATP for each glucose molecule broken down to pyruvic acid.
- Inside the mitochondria, the two pyruvic acid molecules derived from each glucose molecule are fully broken down in the TCA cycle. Two revolutions of the TCA cycle, each yielding a molecule of ATP, provide a net gain of two additional molecules of ATP.
- For each molecule of glucose broken down activity at the electron transport chain will provide 32 molecules of ATP.

Summing up, for each glucose molecule processed a typical cell gains 36 molecules of ATP. All but two of them are produced by the mitochondria.

Glycogenesis and Glycogenolysis

Although most glucose is used to generate ATP molecules unlimited amounts of glucose do not result in unlimited ATP synthesis, because cells cannot store large amounts of ATP. When more glucose is available that can be immediately oxidized, rising intracellular ATP concentrations, inhibit glucose catabolism and initiate processes that store glucose as glycogen or fat.

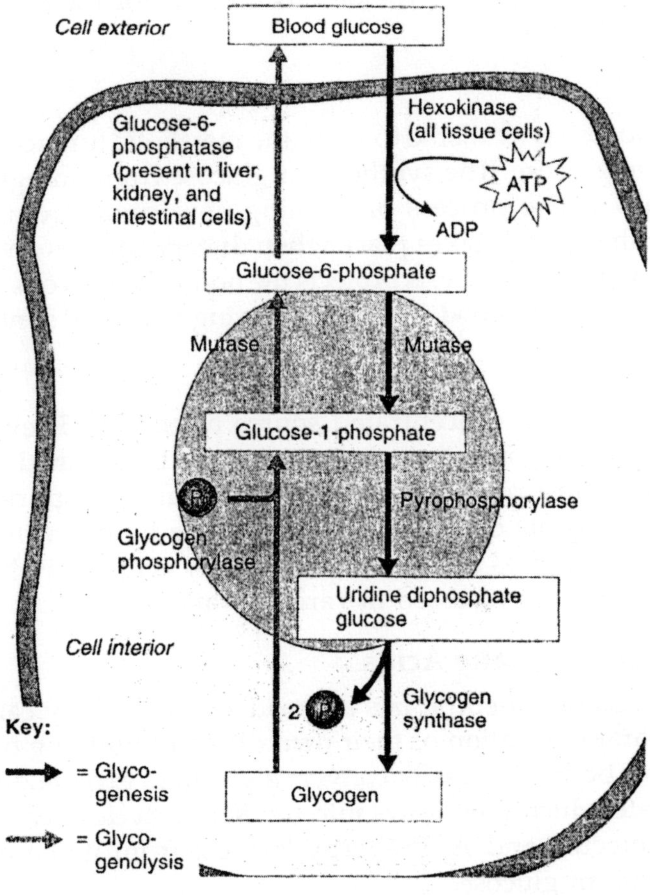

Fig. 1.9 : Glycogenesis and Glycogenolysis.

When glycolysis is "turned off" by high ATP levels, glucose molecules are combined in long chains to form glycogen. This process, called glycogenesis, begins when glucose entering cells is phosphorylated to glucose-6-phosphate and then converted into its isomer glucose-1-phosphate. The terminal phosphate group is cleaned off as the enzyme glycogen synthetase catalyzes the attachment of glucose to the growing glycogen chain. Liver and skeletal muscle cells are most active in glycogen synthesis and storage.

When blood levels of glucose drop, glycogen lysis or splitting occurs. This process is known as glycogenolysis. The enzyme glycogen phosphorylase overseas phosphorylation and cleavage of glycogen to release glucose-1-phosphate which is then converted to glucose-6-phosphate, a form that can enter the glycolytic pathway to be oxidized for energy.

In muscle cells and most other cells, the glucose-6-phosphate resulting from glycogenolysis is trapped because it cannot cross the cell membrane. However, hepatocytes contain glucose-6-phosphatase, a unique enzyme which removes the terminal phosphate, producing free glucose. Because glucose easily diffuses from the cell into the blood the liver can use its glycogen stores to provide blood sugar for the benefit of other organs when blood sugar levels drop.

Gluconeogenesis

When too little glucose is available to stoke the metabolic furnace glycerol and amino acids are converted to glucose. The synthesis of glucose from non-glucose precursors is called gluconeogenesis. The process of forming new sugar from non-carbohydrate molecules, occurs in the liver. It takes place when dietary sources and glucose levels are beginning to decline. Gluconeo-genesis protects the body, the nervous system in particular from damaging effects of low blood sugar by ensuring that ATP synthesis can continue.

Lipid Metabolism

Fats are the body's most concentrated source of energy. They contain very little water and the energy yield from fat catabolism is twice that gained from either glucose or protein breakdown. Most products of fat digestion are transported in lymph in the form of fatty protein droplets called chylomicrons. The lipids in the chylomicrons are hydrolyzed by plasma enzymes and the resulting fatty acids and glycerol are taken up by body cells where they are processed in various ways.

Oxidation of Glycerol and Fatty Acids

Of the various lipids only neutral fats are oxidized for energy catabolism of neutral fats involves the separate oxidation of their own different building blocks, glycerol and fatty acid chains. Most body cells easily convert glycerol to glyceraldehyde phosphate, a glycolysis intermediate which then flows into the Kreb's cycle. Glyceraldehyde is equal to half a glucose molecule and ATP energy harvest from its complete oxidation is approximately half that of glucose.

Beta oxidation, the initial phase of fatty acid oxidation occurs in the mitochondria. Many different types of reactions are involved, the net result of beta oxidation is that the fatty acid chains are broken apart into two carbon acetic acid fragments and reduced coenzymes are produced. Each acetic acid molecule is fused to coenzyme A, forming acetyl CoA. The term "beta-oxidation" reflects the fact that the carbon in the beta (third) position is oxidized during the process and cleavage if the fatty acid in each case occurs between the alpha and beta carbons. Acetyl CoA is then picked up by oxaloacetic acid and enters the aerobic pathways to be completely oxidized to carbon dioxide and water.

Lipogenesis and Lipolysis

When glycerol and fatty acids from dietary fats are not immediately needed for energy. They are recombined into triglycerides and stored. About 50 per cent ends up in subcutaneous tissue, the balance is stocked as other fat depots of the body. Triglyceride synthesis or lipogenesis, occurs when cellular ATP and glucose levels are high. Excess ATP leads to an accumulation of acetyl CoA and glyceraldehyde-phosphate, when these two metabolites are present in excess, they are channelled into triglyceride synthesis pathways. Acetyl CoA molecules are condensed together, forming fatty acid chains that grow two carbons at a time. Because acetyl CoA an intermediate in glucose catabolism is also the starting point for synthesis of fatty acids, glucose is easily converted into fat glyceral-dehyde phosphate is converted to glycerol, which is condensed with fatty acids to form triglycerides. Thus, even if the diet is fat poor excessive carbohydrate intake

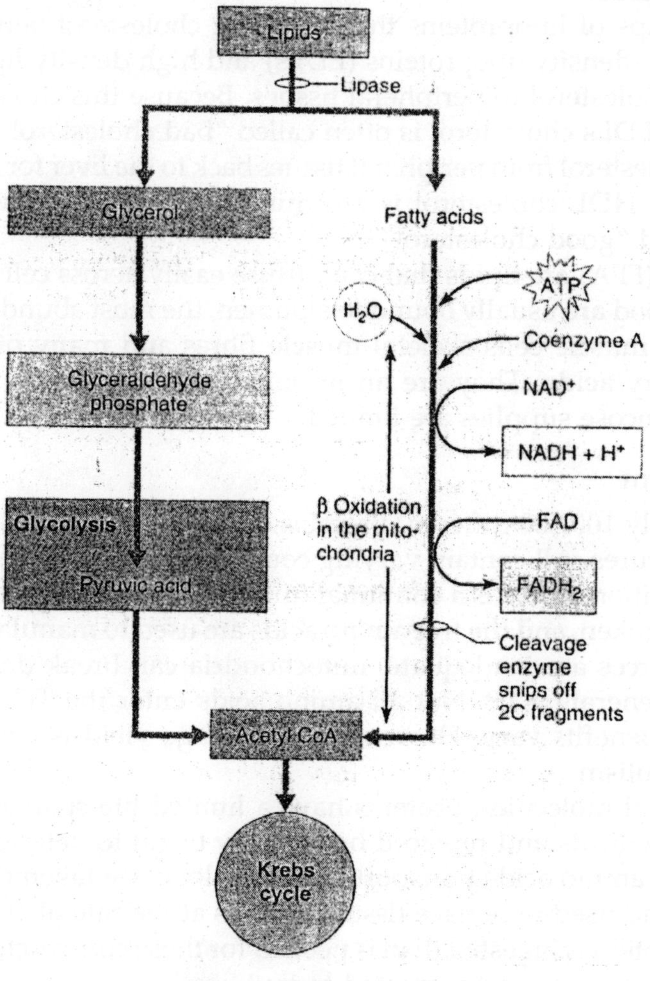

Fig. 1.10 Initial Phase of Lipid Oxidation.

provides all the raw materials needed to form neutral fats. When blood sugar is high lipogenesis is the major activity in adipose tissue and is also an important liver function.

Lipolysis, the breakdown of stored fats into glycerol and fatty acids. The fatty acids and glycerol products are released to the blood helping to ensure that body organs have continuous access to fat fuels for aerobic respiration. The fat burn occurs when carbohydrate intake is inadequate. Under such conditions, lypolysis is accelerated. When carbohydrates are deficient oxaloacetic acid is converted to glucose. Without oxaloacetic acid, fat oxidation is incomplete, acetyl CoA accumulates, and the liver converts acetyl CoA molecules to ketones bodies which are released into the blood. This conversion process is called ketogenesis.

Lipids circulate through the blood stream as lipoproteins and free fatty acids. Lipoproteins are lipid-protein complexes that contain large insoluble glycerides and cholesterol with a superficial coating dominated by phospholipids and proteins. The proteins and phospholipids make the entire complex soluble and the protein help regulate lipid absorption by cells.

Two major groups of lipoproteins that transport cholesterol between the liver and other tissues are low-density lipoproteins (LDLs) and high density lipoproteins (HDLs). The LDLs deliver cholesterol to peripheral tissues. Because this cholesterol may end up in arterial phaques LDLs cholesterol is often called "bad cholesterol". HDLs cholesterol transport excess cholesterol from peripheral tissues back to the liver for storage or excretion in the bile. Because HDL cholesterol is returning cholesterol that will not circulatory problems, it is called "good cholesterol".

Free fatty acids (FFA) are lipids that can diffuse easily across cell membranes. Those circulating in the blood are usually bound to albumen, the most abundant plasma protein. Liver cells, cardiac muscle cells skeletal muscle fibres and many other body cells can metabolize free fatty acids. They are an important energy source during periods of starvation, when glucose supplies are limited.

Protein Metabolism

There are roughly 100,000 different proteins, in the human body, with varied forms, functions and structures. All contain varying combinations of the same 204 amino acids. Under normal conditions there is a continual turnover of cellular proteins in the cytosol. Peptide bonds are broken, and the free amino acids are used to manufacture new proteins. If other energy sources are inadequate, mitochondria can break down amino acids in the TCA cycle to generate ATP. Not all amino acids enter the TCA cycle at the same point, so the ATP benefits vary. However, the average yield is comparable to that of carbohydrate catabolism.

Like all biological molecules, proteins have a limited life span and must be broken down to their amino acids and replaced before they begin to deteriorate.

Newly ingested amino acids transported in the blood are taken up by cells by active transport process and used to replace tissue proteins at the rate of about 100 grams each day. When more protein is ingested than is needed for these constructive purposes, amino acids are oxidized for energy or converted to fat.

Oxidation of Amino Acids

Before amino acids can be oxidized for energy. They must be deaminated that is their amine group (NH_2) must be removed. The resulting molecule is then converted to pyruvic acid or one of the keto acid intermediates in the Krebs cycle. The key molecule in these interconversion is glutamic acid, common non-essential amino acid.

The amino group may be removed by transamination or deamination. Transamination attaches the amino group of an amino acid to another carbon chain, creating a new amino acid. Transaminations enable a cell to synthesize many of the amino acids needed for protein synthesis cells of liver, skeletal muscles, heart, lung, kidney and brain which are active in protein synthesis, perform large numbers of transaminations.

Deamination is the removal of an amino group in a reaction that generates an ammonia molecule (NH_3). Ammonia is highly toxic even in low concentrations. Liver cells take the ammonia and convert it to urea, a harmless water soluble compound that is excreted in the urine. The carbon chain of some amino acids can be converted to pyruvic acid and then used for gluconeogenesis. Others are converted to ketone bodies.

Ketone bodies are not metabolized by the liver and they diffuse into the general circulation. The ketone bodies are used by other cells which reconvert them into acetyl-CoA for breakdown in the TCA cycle and the production of ATP. The increased production of ketone bodies that occurs during protein and lipid catabolism by the liver results in high ketone bodies concentrations in the body fluids, a condition called ketosis.

Amino Acids and Protein Synthesis

The human body can synthesize roughly half of the different amino acids needed to build proteins. There are 10 essential amino acids. Eight of them (isoleucine, leucine, lysine, threonine, tryptophan, phenylalanine, valine and methionine) cannot be synthesized at all, the other two (arginine and histidine) can be synthesized in amounts that are insufficient for growing children. The other amino acids which can be synthesized on demand, are called the non-essential amino acids.

Protein synthesis occurs on ribosomes, where cytoplasmic enzymes oversee the formation of peptide bonds linking the amino acids together into protein polymers. The amount and type of protein synthesized are controlled by hormones (growth hormone thyroxine, sex hormones and others). So protein anabolism, reflects the hormonal balance at each stage in the life cycle.

During the course of lifetime, cells synthesize 225-450 kg of proteins depending on body size. However, we do not need to consume anywhere because non-essential amino acids are easily formed by keto acids from the Krebs cycle and transferring amino groups to them by transamination. Most of these transformations occur in the liver. The liver also provides all non-essential amino acids needed to produce small amount of protein that the body synthesise each day. However, a complete set of amino acids must be present for protein synthesis to take place, so all of the essential amino acids must be provided by the diet. If some are not the rest are oxidized for energy even though they may be needed for anabolism. In such cases negative nitrogen balance always results because body protein is broken down to supply the essential amino acids needed.

Bioenergetics

When chemical bonds are broken energy is released. Inside cells, some of that energy may be captured as ATP but much of it is lost to the environment on heat.

In living cells organic molecules are oxidized to carbon dioxide and water. It is possible to examine the metabolic state of an individual and determine how many calories are being utilized. The result can be expressed as calories per hour, calories per day on calories per unit of body weight per day, but what is actually measured is the sum of total of all of the varied anabolic and catabolic processes occurring in the body. This value represents the metabolic rate of the individual at that time, i.e. the body's rate of energy output is called the metabolic rate. Many factors influence metabolic rate, it is usually measured under standardized conditions. The person is in a post-absorptive state (has not eaten for at least 12 hours) is reclining and is mentally and physically relaxed. The temperature of the room is a comfortable 20-25°C. The measurement obtained under these circumstances is called the basal metabolic rate (BMR) and reflects the energy the body needs to perform only its most essential activities. Such as breathing and maintaining resting levels of organ function. An average 70 kg. adult has a BMR of approximately 60-72 Kcal/h.

The factors that influence BMR include surface area, age, stress and hormones. If two people weigh the same the taller or thinner person will have a higher BMR than the shorter or fatty person. In general, the younger a person the higher the BMR. Children and adolescents require large amounts of energy for growth. In old age BMR declines as skeletal muscles begin to atrophy. Gender also plays a role. Metabolic rate is disproportionately higher in males than in females. Males typically have more muscles, which is very active metabolically even during rest. Fatty tissues present in greater relative amounts in females is metabolically sluggish compared to muscle.

Body temperature and metabolic rate rise and fall together. Fever resulting from infections and other factors results in higher metabolic rate. Stress, whether physical or emotional increases metabolic rate by mobilizing the sympathetic nervous system. Blood born non-epinephrine and epinephrine rise metabolic rate by stimulating fat catabolism.

The amount of thyroxine produced by the thyroid gland is the most important hormonal factor in determining BMR. Its direct effect on most body cells is to increase oxygen consumption, by accelerating the use of ATP to operate the sodium-potassium pump. As ATP reserves decline, cellular respiration accelerates. Thus more thyroxine produced the higher the BMR.

②

Respiration

Living cells need energy for maintenance, growth, defense, and replication our cells obtain that energy through aerobic respiration a process that required oxygen and produces carbon-dioxide. Therefore, the cells in the body must have a way to obtain oxygen and eliminate carbon dioxide.

The respiratory system consists of the nose, nasal cavity and sinuses the pharynx (throat), the larynx (voice box), the trachea (windpipe) and the bronchi and branchioles (conducting passages) and alveoli (exchange surfaces) of the lungs.

The Respiratory Tract

The respiratory tract consists of airways that carry air to and from the exchange surfaces of the lungs. The respiratory tract can be divided into a conducting portion and

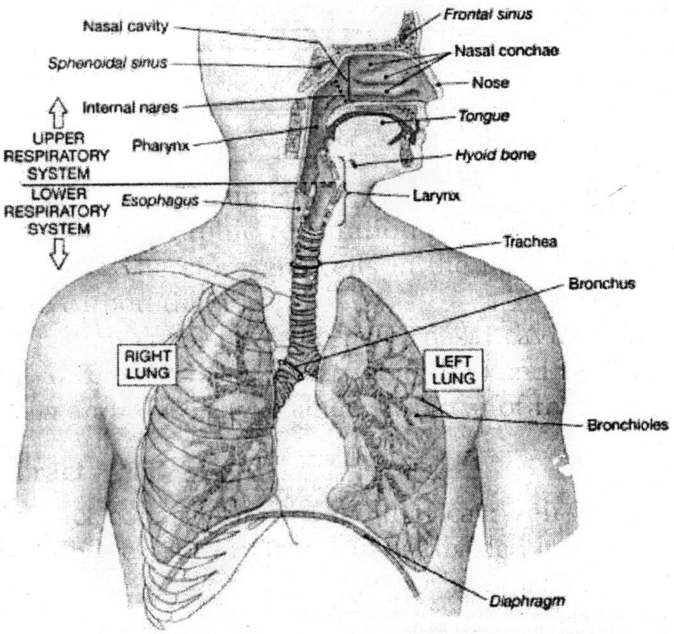

Fig. 2.1 : Components of the Respiratory System

a respiratory portion. The conducting portion begins at the entrance to the nasal cavity and continues through the pharynx, larynx, trachea, bronchi, and a larger bronchioles.

The respiratory portion includes the small tract and most delicate bronchioles and the alveoli that are the site of gas exchange.

In addition to delivering air to the lungs, the conducting passage ways filter, warm and humidity the air thereby protecting the alveoli from debris, pathogens and environmental extremes. By the time the air reaches the alveoli, most foreign particles and pathogens have been removed and the humidity and temperature are within acceptable limits.

The Nose

Air normally enters the respiratory system via the paired external noses (nostrils) that communicate with the nasal cavity. The vestibule is the portion of the nasal cavity

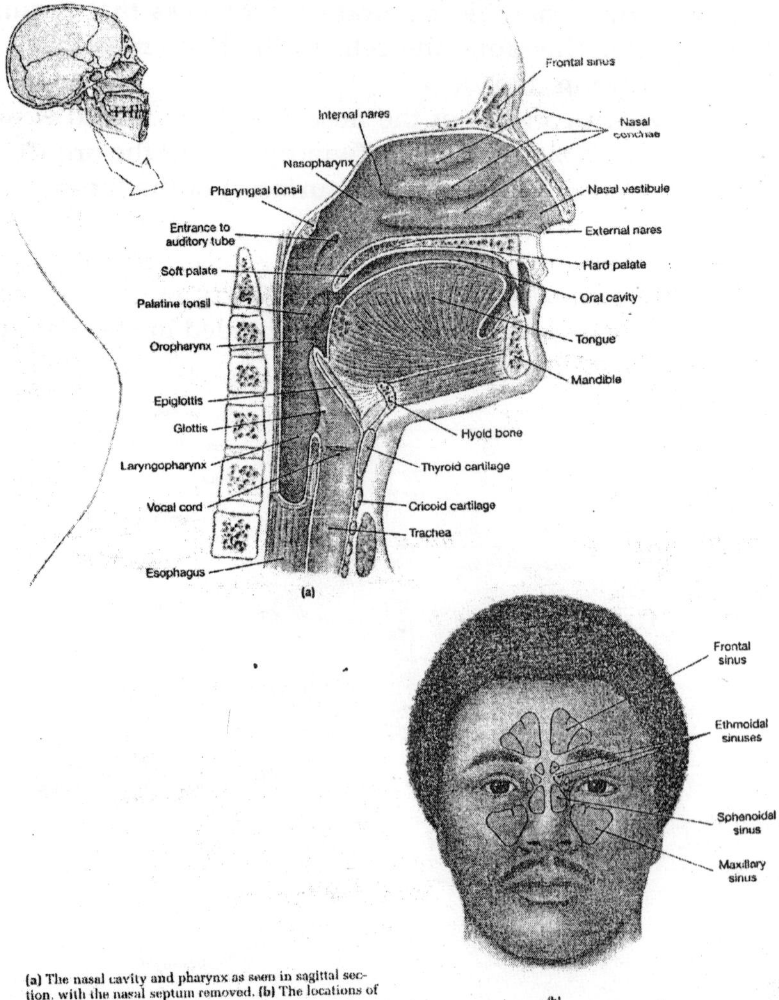

(a) The nasal cavity and pharynx as seen in sagittal section, with the nasal septum removed. (b) The locations of the paranasal sinuses.

Fig. 2.2 : The Nose, Nasal Cavity, and Pharynx

contained within the flexible tissues of the external nose. Here coarse hairs guard the nasal cavity from large airborne particles such as sand dust and insects.

The ciliated lining of the nasal cavity contains numerous goblet cells. The goblet cells and mucus cells produce mucus that baths the exposed surfaces of the nasal cavity, Cilia sweep that moves and any trapped debris or microorganisms toward the pharynx, where it can be swallowed and exposed to the acids and enzymes of stomach.

The Pharynx

The pharynx is a chamber shared by the digestive and respiratory systems that extends between the internal nares and the entrance to the larynx and oesophagus. The soft palate separates the nasopharynx from oropharynx. The oropharynx extends between the soft palate and the base of the tongue at the level of the hajoid bond. The palatine tonsils lie in the lateral walls of the oropharynx. Materials entering the digestive tract pass through both the oropharynx and laryngopharynx.

The Larynx

In coming air leaves the pharynx by passing through a narrow opening, the glottis which is surrounded and protected by the larynx. The elastic epiglottis projects above the glottis. During swallowing the epiglottis folds back over the glottis preventing the entry of liquids or solid food into the respiratory passageway.

The Vocal Cords and Sound Production

The vocal cords vibrate when air passes through the glottis. These vibrations generate sound waves. The pitch of the voice is regulated by the amount of tension in the vocal cords, which is controlled by skeletal muscles that change the position of the arytenoids. The volume depends on the force of the air movement. Further amplification and resonance occur within the pharynx, the oral cavity, the nasal cavity and the personal sinuses. The final production of distinct words, further depends on voluntary movements of tongue, lips and cheeks.

The Trachea

The trachea a "windpipe" is a tough flexible tube. It extends between the level of sixth cervical vertebra, where it attaches to the cricoid cartilage of the larynx, and that of the fifth thorasic vertebra where it branches to form a pair of primary branch.

The walls of the trachea are supported by about 20 tracheal cartilages. These C-shaped cartilages stiffen the tracheal walls and protect the airway. They also prevent its collapse or overexpansion as pressure change in the respiratory system.

The Bronchi

The tracheal branches within the media stinum, giving rise to the right and left primary bronchi. The histological organization of the primary bronchi resembles that of the trachea complete with cartilagenous C-shaped rings. The primary bronchi and their branches form the bronchial tree. As it enters, the lung, each primary bronchus give rise to secondary bronchi that enter the lobes of the lung. The secondary bronchi divide to form 9-10 tertiary bronchi in each lung. Each tertiary bronchus branches repeatedly. When the diameter of the passageway has narrowed to around 2 mm, cartilage disappear completely. This narrow passage represents a bronchiole.

Bronchioles

Varying the diameter of the bronchioles provides control over the amount of resistance to airflow and the distribution of air in the lungs. Sympathetic activation leads to a relaxation of smooth muscles in the walls of bronchioles, leading to dilation of the respiratory passageways. Constriction of these smooth muscles, can almost completely block the passageways.

After further branching, we reach the level of the terminal bronchioles supplies air to a lobule of the lung. A lobule is a segment of lung tissue that is bounded by connective tissue partitions and supplied by a single bronchiole within a lobule, a terminal brochiole divides to form several respiratory bronchioles. These passages, the finest branches of the bronchiol tree, deliver air to the respiratory surfaces of the lungs.

Alveolar Ducts and Alveoli

Respiratory bronchioles open into expansive chambers, called alveolar ducts. These passageways end at alveolar sacs, Common chamber connected to individual alveoli. Each lung contains approximately 150 million alveoli, their abundance gives the lungs an open spongy appearance.

The Respiratory Membrane

Gas exchange occurs across the respiratory membrane of the alveoli. The respiratory membrane consists of three components:

1. The squamous epithelial cells lining the alveolus.
2. The endothelial cells lining an adjacent capillary.
3. The fused basement membranes that lie between the alveolar and endothelial cells.

At the respiratory membrance, the total distance separating the alveolar air and the blood can be as little as 0.1 μm. Diffusion across the respiratory membrane proceeds very rapidly because (1) the distance is small, and (2) both oxygen and carbon dioxide are lipid-soluble. The membranes of the epithelial and endothelial cells thus do not pose a barrier to the movement of oxygen and carbon dioxide between the blood and alveolar air spaces.

Circulation to the Respiratory Membrane

The respiratory exchange surfaces receive blood from arteries to the pulmonary circuit. The pulmonary arteries enter the lungs and branch, following the bronchi to the lobules. Each lobule receives an arteriole and a venule, and a network of capillaries surrounds each alveolus directly beneath the epithelium. After passing through the pulmonary venules, venous blood enters the pulmonary veins that deliver it to the left atrium.

The Lungs

The left and right lungs occupy the left and right plural cavities. Each lung has distinct lobes separated by deep fissures. The right lung has three lobes (superior, middle and inferior) and the left lung has two lobes (superior and inferior).

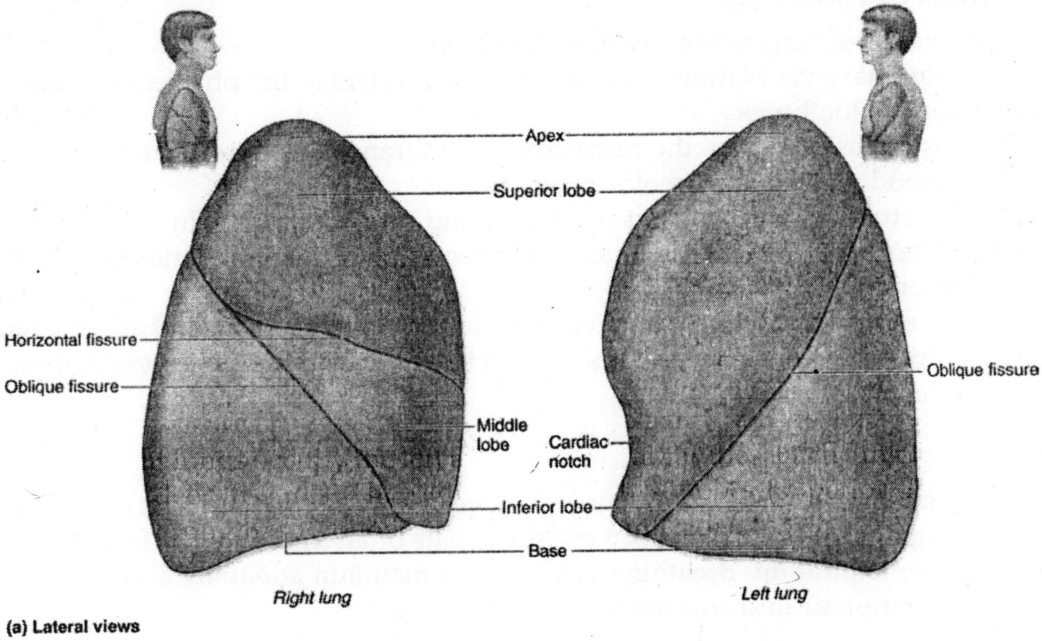

Fig. 2.3 : Gross Anatomy of the Lungs

The bluntly round apex of each lung extends into the base of the neck above the first rib, and the concave base rests on the superior surface of the diaphragm. The curving costal surface follows the inner contours of the rib cage. The mediastinum, which houses the heart great blood vessels, bronchi, oesophagus and other organs, in the thoracic cavity where lungs are present. Each cone-shaped lung is suspended in its own pleural cavity and connected to the mediastinum by vascular and bronchial attachments, collectively called its root. The anterior, lateral and posterior lung surfaces lie in close contact with ribs and term the continuously curving costal surface. On the medial surface of each lung is an indentation, the hilus. Blood vessels of the pulmonary and systemic circulations enter and leave the lungs by the hilus.

The smallest subdivision of the lung is the lobule. Each lobule is served by a large bronchiole and its branches.

The lung consists of fair spaces. The balance of lung tissue or its stroma, is mostly elastic connective tissue. As a result, the things are soft, spongy, elastic organs that together weigh just over 1 kg. The elasticity of healthy lungs helps to reduce the work of breathing.

The Pleural Cavities

The mediastinum divides the thorasic cavity into two pleural cavities. Each lung occupies a single pleural cavity lined by a serous membrane, or pleura. The parietal pleura covers the inner surface of the body wall and extends over the diaphragm and mediastinum. The visceral pleura covers the outer surface of the lungs, extending into the fissures between the lobes. A thin layer of fluid covering these surfaces provides lubrication that reduces friction and irritation of the pleura.

Respiratory Physiology

The process of respiration involves four steps :

1. Pulmonary ventilation or breathing which refers to the physical movement of air into and out of the lungs.
2. Gas diffusion across the respiratory membrane, which separates the alveolar air from the blood within the alveolar capillaries.
3. The storage and transport of oxygen and carbon dioxide. In this step, the blood stores and carries the respiratory gases between the alveolar capillaries and the capillary beds in other tissues.
4. The exchange of oxygen and carbon dioxide between the blood and the interstitial fluids. In this step, the blood delivers oxygen to body tissues and receives carbon dioxide for transport to the lungs.

Pulmonary Ventilation

Pulmonary ventilation is the physical movement of air into and out of the respiratory tract. A single breath or respiratory cycle, consists of an inhalation or inspiration and an exhalation or expiration. Breathing functions to maintain adequate alveolar ventilation, the movement of air into and out of the alveoli.

Pressure and Airflow to the Lungs

Air will flow from an area of higher pressure to an area of relatively low pressure, and this is the basis for pulmonary ventilation occurs when changes in the volume of the lungs create pressure gradients. These pressure differences cause air to move into or out of the respiratory tract. When the lungs expand, pressure falls inside the airways, and air moves into the respiratory tract. When lungs contract pressure increases and air moves out of the respiratory tract.

The volume of the lungs depends on the volume of the pleural cavities. The parietal and pleural membranes are separated by only a thin film of pleural fluid.

At the start of a breath, pressures inside and outside the lungs are identical and there is no movement of air. When the thoracic cavity enlarges, the pressure inside the lungs decreases. Air now enters the respiratory passageways because the pressure inside the lungs (Pi) is lower than atmospheric pressure (pressure outside or Po). During breathing, enlargement of the thorasic cavity involves the contractions of the diaphragm the muscular sheet that separates the thorasic and abdominopelvic cavities, aided by the external intercostal muscles.

The diaphragm forms the floor of the thorasic cavity. When relaxed, the diaphragm has the shape of dome and projects upward into thorasic cavity compressing the lungs. When the diaphragm contracts it flattends and increases the volume of the thorasic cavity expanding the lungs contraction of the diaphragm is controlled by the phrenic nerves, branches of cervical plexus.

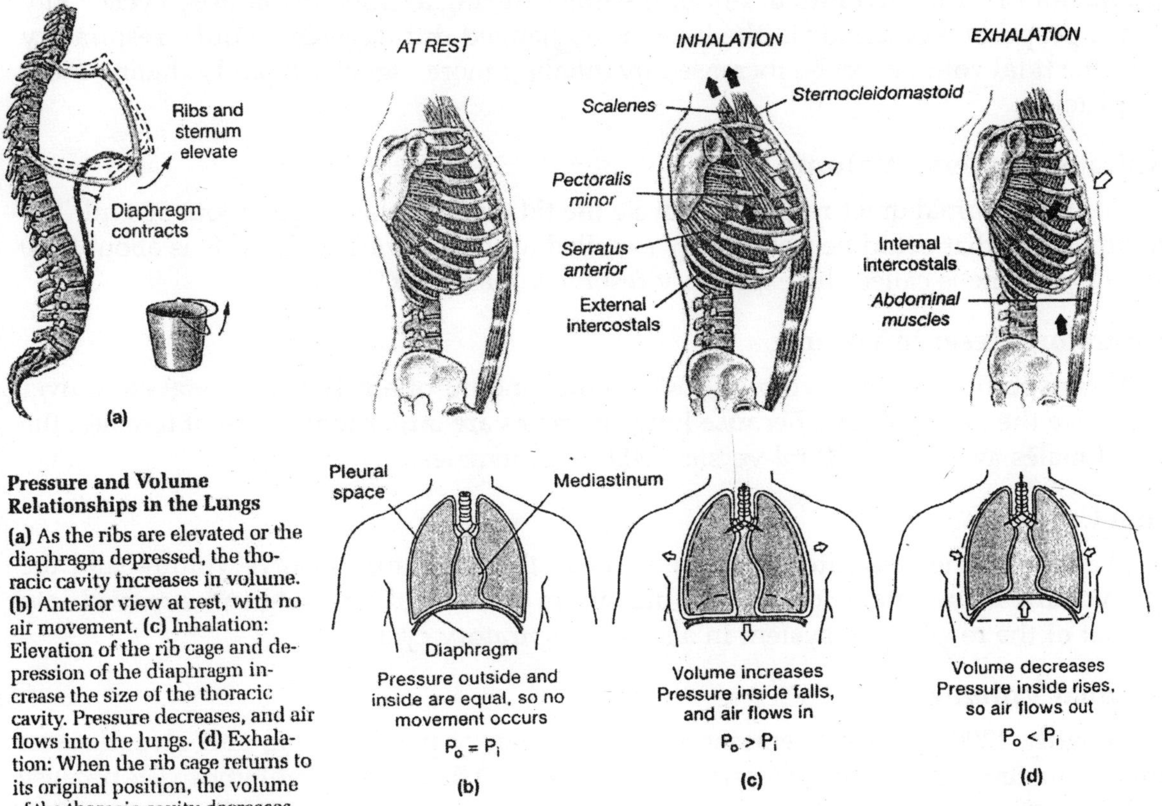

Pressure and Volume Relationships in the Lungs

(a) As the ribs are elevated or the diaphragm depressed, the thoracic cavity increases in volume. **(b)** Anterior view at rest, with no air movement. **(c)** Inhalation: Elevation of the rib cage and depression of the diaphragm increase the size of the thoracic cavity. Pressure decreases, and air flows into the lungs. **(d)** Exhalation: When the rib cage returns to its original position, the volume of the thoracic cavity decreases. Pressure rises, and air moves out of the lungs. *Accessory muscles* may assist such movements of the rib cage to increase the depth and rate of respiration.

Fig. 2.4 : Pressure and Volume Relationships in the Lungs

The external intercoastal elevate the rib cage. Because of the nature of the articulations between the ribs and the vertebrae this movement increases the volume of thorasic cavity. Contraction of the external intercostals is controlled by the inter costal nerves, branches of the thorasic spinal nerves.

Downward movement of the rib cage and upward movement of the diaphragm reverse the process and reduce the size of the lungs, pressure inside the lungs now exceeds atmospheric pressure, and air moves out of the lungs. During quiet breathing, expansion of the lungs stretches their elastic fibres. In addition, elevation of the rib cage, stretches opposing skeletal muscles and the elastic fibres in the body wall. When the inspiratory muscles relax, these elastic components recoil, returning the diaphragm and rib cage to their original positions. When breathing heavily, contractions of the internal intercostal muscles, and the abdominal muscles may assist in exhalation.

Respiratory Volumes and Rates

A respiratory cycle is a single cycle of inhalation and exhalation. The tidal volume is the amount of air moved into or out of the lungs during a single respiratory cycle. Only a small proportion of the air in the lungs is exchanged during a single quiet respiratory cycle, the tidal volume can be increased by inhaling more vigorously and exhaling more completely.

Expiratory Reserve Volume

During a normal quiet respiratory cycle the tidal volume averages about 500 ml. The amount of air that could be voluntarily expelled at the end of a tidal cycle is about 1000 ml. This volume is called the expiratory reserve volume (ERV).

Inspiratory Reserve Volume

The inspiratory reserve volume (IRV) is the amount of air that can be taken in over and above the tidal volume. Because lungs in males are larger than those of females, the IRV of males averages 3300 ml versus 1900 ml in females.

Vital Capacity

The sum of the inspiratory reserve volume, the expiratory reserve volume and the tidal volume is the vital capacity, the maximum amount of air that can be moved into and out of the respiratory system in a single respiratory cycle.

Residual Volume

Roughly 1200 ml of air remains in the respiratory passageways and alveoli, even after exhausting the expiratory reserve volume. Most of this residual volume exists because the lungs are held against the thoracic wall, preventing their elastic fibres from contracting further.

Minimal Volume

When the chest cavity is opened as in pneumothorax, the lungs collapse and the amount of air in the respiratory system is reduced to the minimal volume. Some air remains in the lungs even at minimal volume because the surfactant coating the alveolar surfaces prevents their collapse.

Not all of the inspired air reaches the alveolar exchange surfaces within the lungs. A typical tidal inspiration pulls around 500 ml of air into the respiratory system. The first 350 ml travels along the conducting passageways and enters the alveolar spaces. The last 150 ml never gets further, then the conducting passageways does not participate in gas exchange with the blood. The volume of air in the conducting passages is known as the dead space of the lungs.

Gas Exchange at the Respiratory Membrane

In pulmonary ventilation the alveoli are supplied with oxygen, and the accumulated carbon dioxide is removed. The actual process of gas exchange occurs between the blood and alveolar air across the respiratory membrane. This process depends on (1) the partial pressure of the gases involved, and (2) The diffusion of molecules from a gas into a liquid.

Oxygen Transport

Only 1.5 per cent of the oxygen content of arterial blood consists of oxygen molecules in solution. All the rest is bound to hemoglobin (Hb) molecules specifically to the iron atoms in the centre of heme units. Hemoglobin (Hb) is composed of four polypeptide chains, each bound to an iron-containing heme group. Since the iron atoms bind oxygen, each hemoglobin molecule can combine with four molecules of oxygen, and the process of oxygen loading is rapid and reversible.

The hemoglobin-oxygen combination called oxyhemoglobin (HbO_2). Hemoglobin that has released oxygen is called reduced hemoglobin or deoxyhemoglobin (HHb) as below :

$$HHb+O_2 \underset{\text{Tissues}}{\overset{\text{Lungs}}{\rightleftharpoons}} HbO2+H^+$$

The first O_2 molecule binds to iron, the hemoglobin molecule changes shape. As a result. hemoglobin more readily takes up two more oxygen molecules and uptake of the fourth oxygen molecule is more facilitated. When all four heme groups are bound to oxygen, a hemoglobin molecule is said to be fully saturated. When one, two or three oxygen molecules are bound, hemoglobin is partially saturated.

The rate at which hemoglobin reversibly binds or releases oxygen is regulated by several factors, PO_2, temperature, blood Ph, PCO_2 and the concentration of an organic chemical called BPG in the blood. These factors interact to ensure adequate deliveries of oxygen to tissue cells. The lower the oxygen content of a tissue the more oxygen wiil be released by hemoglobin molecules. At a normal tissue PO_2 of 40 mmHg, hemoglobin releases roughly 25 per cent of its stored oxygen. Active tissue consume oxygen at an accelerated rate and when the PO_2 declines it automatically increases the amount of oxygen released by hemoglobin molecules passing through local capillaries.

The amount of oxygen released by hemoglobin is also influenced by PH and temperature. When PH declines, the hemoglobin molecules release their bound oxygen molecules more readily, hemoglobin also releases more oxygen when the temperature rises.

BPG levels in blood decreases Hb's affinity for O_2 causes the oxygen hemoglobin dissociation curve to shift to the right BPG levels decrease as RBCs age.

Carbon Dioxide Transport

Carbon dioxide is transported in the blood from the tissue cells to the lungs in three forms.

Plasma Transport–Roughly 7 percent of the carbon dioxide, simply dissolved in plasma. The rest diffuses, into the red blood cells.

Hemoglobin Binding–Over 20 per cent of transported carbon dioxide is carried within RBCs as carbaminohemoglobin, bound to globin portions of hemoglobin molecules. At the pulmonary capillaries, the plasma PCo_2 declines and the bound carbon dioxide is released Deoxygenated hemoglobin combines more readily with carbon dioxide than does oxygenated hemoglobin.

Carbonic Acid Formation

The rest of carbon dioxide molecules roughly 70 per cent of the total are converted to carbonic acid through the activity of the enzyme carbonic anhydrase. When carbon dioxide diffuses into the RBCs, it combines with water, forming carbonic acid (H_2CO_3). H_2CO_3 is unstable and quickly dissociates into hydrogen ions and bicarbonate ions.

$$CO_2 + H_2O \rightleftharpoons H_2CO_3 \rightleftharpoons H^+ + HCO_3$$

Carbon dioxide Water Carbonic acid Hydrogen ion Biocarbonate ion

Although this reaction also occurs in plasma, it is thousand of times faster in erythrocytes because they contain carbonic anhydrase that reversibly catalyzes the conversion of carbon dioxide and water to carbonic acid. Hydrogen ions released during the reaction bind to hemoglobin thus oxygen release is entranced by carbon dioxide loading. Because of the buffering effect of hemoglobin, the liberated hydrogen ions cause little change in pH under resting condition.

Once generated bicarbonate ions diffuse quickly from the RBCs into the plasma, where they are carried to the lungs. To counterbalance the outrash of negative bicarbonate ions from the RBCs, chloride ions (Ci) move from the plasma into the erythrocytes. This ionic exchange process is called the chloride shift.

In the lungs when venous blood reaches the alveoli through the pulmonary capillaries its PCO_2 declines. Carbon dioxide first became free from its "bicarbonate housing". Bicarbonate ions re-enter the RBCs and bind with hydrogen ions to form carbonic acid which is then split by carbon anhydrase to release carbon dioxide and water.

Control of Respiration

Our breathing is very simple but its control is fairly complex. The control of breathing involve the activity of neurons in the medulla pens.

Medullary Respiratory Centres

The respiratory rhythmicity centre of the medulla oblongata sets the pace for respiration. It can be subdivided into a dorsal respiratory group (DRG) or inspiratory centre, and a ventral respiratory group (VRG) or expiratory centre.

The inspiratory centres functions in every respiratory cycle, whether quiet or forced. When its neurons fire, a burst of nerve impulses travels along the phrenic and intercostal nerves to excite the diaphragm and external intercostal muscles, respectively. As a result the thorax expands and air rushes into the lungs. The DRG then becomes dormant, and expiration occurs passively as the inspiratory muscles relax and the lungs recoil. This cycle repeats continuously and produces a respiratory rate of 12-15 breaths per minute with inspiratory phases lasting for about 2 seconds followed by expiratory phases lasting about 3 seconds.

Unlike the DRG which contains neurons mostly involved in initiating inspiration, the URG contains mix neurons involved in inspiration and expiration.

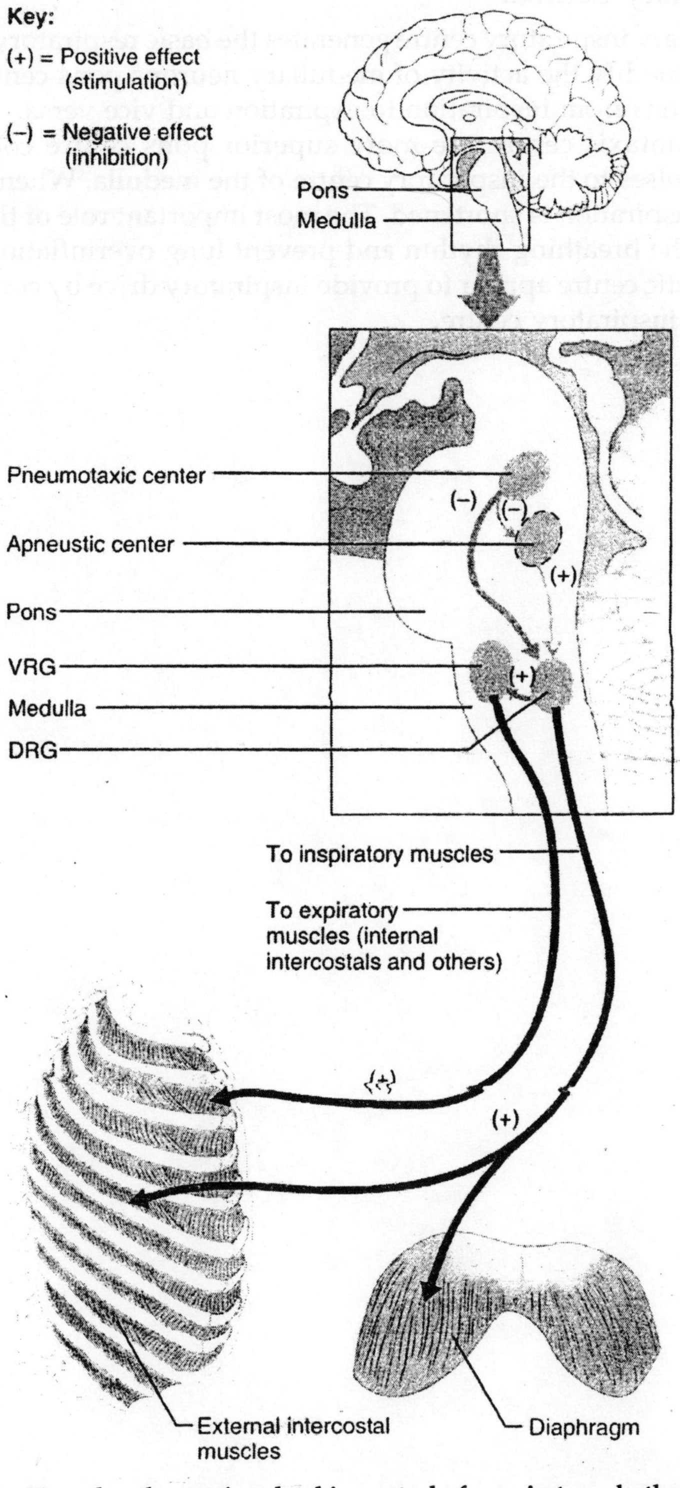

Fig. 2.5 : Neural pathways involved in control of respiratory rhythm

Pons Respiratory Centres

The medullary inspiratory centre generates the basic respiratory rhythm, pons centres influence and modify the activity of medullary neurons pons centres appear to smooth out the transitions from inspiration to expiration and vice versa.

The pneumotaxic centre the more superior pons centre continuously transmits inhibitory impulses to the inspiratory centre of the medulla. When its signals are strong, the period of inspiration is shortened. The most important role of the pneumotaxic centre is to finetune the breathing rhythm and prevent lung overinflation.

The apneustic centre appear to provide inspiratory drive by continuously stimulating the medullary inspiratory centre.

③

Blood Circulation

Introduction

Blood is the river of the life that surges within us, transporting nearly everything that must be carried from one place to another within the body. Blood is the only fluid tissue in the body. Although blood appears to be a thick, homogeneous liquid, the microscope reveals that it has both cellular and liquid components. Blood is a specialized type of connective tissue in which living blood cells, the formed elements are suspended in the non-living fluid matrix called plasma. The collagen and elastic fibres of other connective tissues are absent from blood but dissolved fibrous proteins become visible as fibrin strands when blood clotting occurs.

Blood is sticky, opaque fluid with a characteristic metallic taste-depending on the amount of oxygen it is carrying, the colour of blood varies from scarlet (oxygen-rich) to a dark red (oxygen-poor). Blood is heavier than water and about five times more viscous, largely because of its formed elements. Blood is slightly alkaline with a pH between 7.35 and 7.45. Its temperature (38°C or 100.4°F) is always slightly higher than body temperature.

Blood accounts for approximately 8 per cent of body weight. Its average volume in healthy adult males is 5-6 L. Somewhat greater than in healthy females 4-5 L.

Functions

Blood performs a number of functions all concerned in one way or another with substance distribution, regulating blood levels of particular substances or body protection. These functions overlap and interact to maintain the constancy of our internal environment.

Distribution

The distribution and functions of blood include:

- Delivering oxygen from the lungs and nutrients from the digestive tract to all body cells.
- Transporting metabolic waste products from cells to elimination sites (to the lungs

for elimination of carbon dioxide and to the kidneys for disposal of nitrogenous wastes in urine).

- Transporting hormones from the endocrine organs to their target organs.

Regulation

The regulatory functions of blood include:

- Maintaining appropriate body temperature by absorbing and distributing heat throughout the body and to the skin surface to encourage heat loss.
- Maintaining normal PH in body tissues. Many blood proteins and other blood, borne solutes act as buffers to prevent excessive or abrupt changes in Blood PH which could perform normal cellular activities. Additionally, blood acts as the reservoir for the body's "alkaline reserve" of bicarbonate atoms.
- Maintaining adequate fluid volume in the circulatory system. Salts (Sodium chlroride and others) and blood proteins act to prevent excessive fluid loss from the blood stream into the tissue spaces. As a result the fluid volume in the blood vessels remains ample to support efficient blood circulation to all parts of the body.

Protection

The protective functions of blood include preventing blood loss. When a blood vessel is damaged, platelets and plasma proteins initiates clot formation halting blood loss, Preventing infection. Drifting along in blood are antibodies complement proteins and white blood cells all of which help to defend the body against foreign invaders such as bacteria and viruses.

Blood Plasma

Blood Plasma is a straw coloured sticky fluid, although it is mostly water(about 90 percent), plasma contains over 100 different dissolved solutes. These includes nutrients, gases, harmones, various wastes and products of cell activity ions and proteins. There are about 7 gram protein in each 100ml of plasma. The large size and globular shapes of most blood proteins prevent them from crossing capillary walls and they remain trapped within the circulatory system. There are three primary classes of plasma proteins albumins globulins and fibrinogen.

Albumen constitute roughly 60 per cent of the plasma proteins. They are major contributors to the osmotic pressure of the plasma. Globulins accounting for 35 percent of the protein population include immunoglobulins and transport proteins. Immunoglobulin also called antibodies attack foreign proteins and pathogens.

Both albumins and globulins can attached to lipid such as triglycerides, fatty acids or cholesterol. These lipids are not water soluble in themselves but the protein-lipid combination readily dissolved in plasma if in this way the circulatory system transports insoluble lipid to peripheral tissues. Globulins involved in lipid transport are called lipoproteins.

The third type of protein, fibrinogen, functions in the clotting reaction under certain conditions, fibrinogen molecules interact to form large insoluble strands of fibrin, the basic framework for a blood clot.

The liver synthesizes and releases more than 90 percent of the plasma proteins including all of the albumin, fibrinogen and prothrombin and most of the globulins. Liver is the primary source of plasma proteins, liver disorder can alter the composition and functional properties of the blood. For example, some forms of liver disease can lead to uncontrolled bleeding caused by inadequate synthesis of fibrinogen, prothrcmbin and other plasma proteins involved in the clotting response.

Formed Elements

Formed elements are produced through the process of hemopoiesis or hematopoiesis. Blood cells appear in the circulation during the third week of embryonic development. These cells divide repeatedly, increasing in number. The vessels of the embryonic yolk sac are the primary site of blood formation for the first 8 weeks of development. As other organ systems appear, Some of the embryonic blood cells move out of the circulation and into the liver, spleen, thymus and bone marrow. These embryonic cells differentiate into stem cells. These stem cells called hemolytoblasts produce all of the blood cells.

These blood cells are erythrocytes, leucocytes and platelets. Erythrocytes have no nuclei or organ cells, platelets are just cell fragments. Only leucocytes are complete cells.

Erythrocytes

Erythrocytes or red blood cells (RBCs) are small cells about 7.5 μm in diameter. Shaped like biconcave discs, their thin centres appear lighter in colour than their edges. They are little "bags" of hemoglobin (Hb), the RBC protein that functions in gas transport. It picks up oxygen in the capillary beds of the lungs and releases it to tissue cells across other

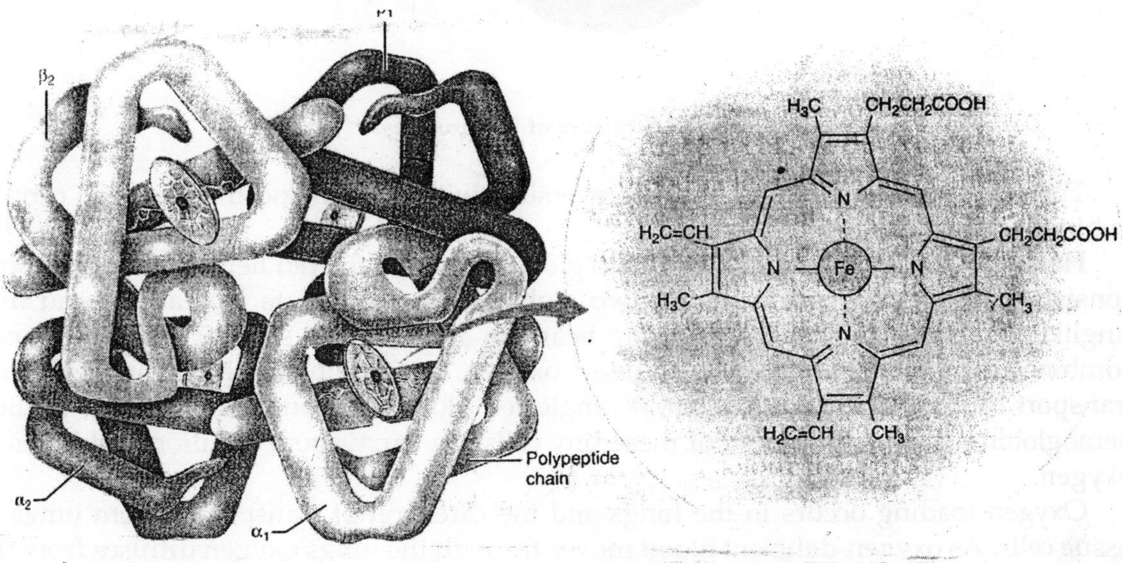

(a) Hemoglobin (b) Iron-containing heme group

Fig. 3.1 Structure of Hemoglobin

capillaries throughout the body. It also transports about 20 per cent of the carbon dioxide released by tissue cells in the opposite direction back to the lungs. Each erythrocyte contributes to its gas transport function because its small size and biconcave shape provides a huge surface area relative to volume. This biconcave disc shape is ideally suited for gas exchange. Secondly discounting its water content an erythrocyte is over 97 per cent hemoglobin, the molecule that binds to and transports respiratory gases.

Erythrocytes lack mitochondria and generate ATP by anaerobic mechanisms, they do not consume any of the oxygen they are transporting, making them very efficient oxygen transporters.

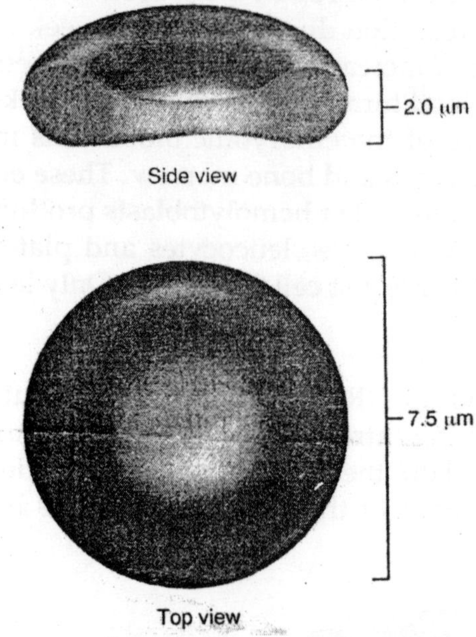

Fig.3.2 Structure of Erythrocytes.

Their hemoglobin binds easily and reversibly with oxygen and most oxygen carried in blood is bound to hemoglobin.

Hemoglobin is made up of the protein globin bound to the red heme pigment. Globin consists of four polypeptide chains–two alpha (α) and two beta (β) each bound of a ringlike heme group. Each heme group bears an atom of iron set. Each iron atom can combine reversibly with one molecule of oxygen, hence a hemoglobin molecule can transport four molecules of oxygen. A single red blood cell contains about 250 million hemoglobin molecules. So each of these tiny cells can carry about 1 billion molecules of oxygen.

Oxygen loading occurs in the lungs and the direction of transport is from lungs to tissue cells. As oxygen-deficient blood moves through the lungs oxygen diffuses from the air sacs of the lungs into the blood and then into the erythrocytes, where it binds to hemoglobin. When oxygen binds to iron, the hemoglobin now called oxyhemoglobin and becomes bright red. In the tissues, the process is reversed and oxygen detached from iron hemoglobin resumes its former shape and the resulting deoxyhemoglobin are reduced to hemoglobin, and becomes dark red.

About 20 per cent of the carbon dioxide transported in the blood combines with hemoglobin but it binds to amino acids of globin rather than with the heme group. This formation of carbaminohemoglobin occurs more readily when hemoglobin is in the reduced state.

Blood cell formation is referred to as hematopoiesis or hemopoiesis. This process occurs in the red bone marrow. The direct stimulus for erythrocyte formation is provided by erythropoietin. Normally small amount of erythropoietin circulates in the blood at all times and sustains red blood cell production at a basal rate. Although liver produce some, the kidneys play the major role in erythropoietin production. When certain kidney cells become hypoxia, they acclerate the release of erythropoietin.

Erythropoietin formation can result from:

1. Reduced numbers of red blood cells due to hemorrhage or excess RBC destruction.
2. Reduced availability of oxygen, occur at high altitudes or during pneumonia.
3. Increased tissue demands for oxygen.

Too many erythrocytes or excessive oxygen in the blood stream depresses erythropoietin production. Bloodborn erythropoietin stimulates red marrow cells that are already committed to becoming erythrocytes, causing them to mature more rapidly. Hypoxia does not activate the bone marrow directly. Instead it stimulates kidneys, which in turn provide the hormonal stimulus that activates their bone marrow.

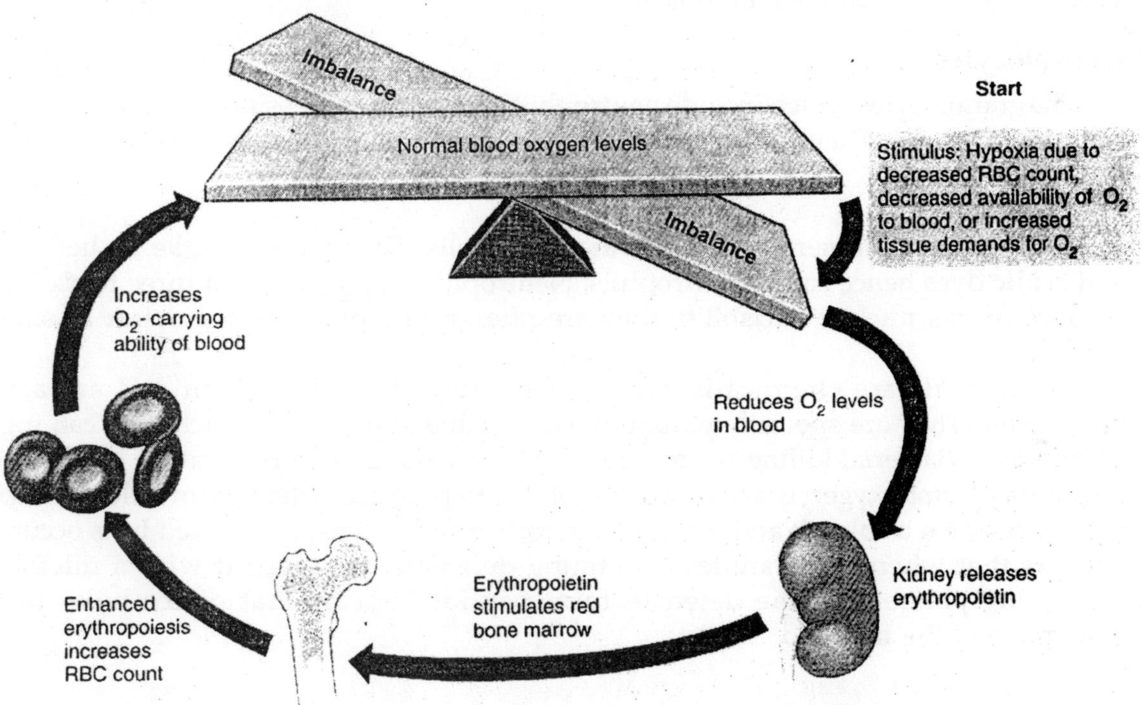

Fig.3.3 :Erythropoietin Mechanism for regulating the rate of Erythropoiesis.

The raw materials required for erythropoiesis include the usual nutrients and structural materials, proteins, lipids and carbohydrates. Iron is essential for hemoglobin synthesis, which is available from the diet and absorbed into bloodstream is controlled by intestinal cells.

An erythrocyte is exposed to severe physical stress. A single roundtrip of the circulatory system usually takes less than 30 seconds. A red blood cell has a relatively short life span of about 120 days. The continual elimination of red blood cells is usually unnoticed because new erythrocytes are entering the circulation at a comparable rate. About 1 per cent of the circulating erythrocytes are replaced each day.

Leukocytes

Leukocytes (leuko-white) or while blood cells (WBCs) are the only formed elements that are complete cells with nuclei and usual organelles. Leukocytes accounting for less than 1 per cent of total blood volume than red blood cells. On average, there are 4000-11,000 WBCs per cubic millimeter of blood.

Leukocytes are defensive against diseases. They protect body from damage by bacteria, viruses, parasites, toxins and turnover cells. These cells are able to slip out of the capillary blood vessels–a process called diapodosis. They gather in large numbers at areas of tissue damage and infection to destroy foreign substances or dead cells.

Leukocytes are grouped into two categories on the basis of structural and chemical characteristics. Granulocytes contain specialized membrane bound cytoplasmic granules, agranulocytes lack obvious granules.

Granulocytes

The granulocytes which include neutrophils, basophils and eosinophils are all roughly spherical in shape. They have lobed nuclei and membrane bound cytoplasmic granules.

Neutrophils

They are most numerous of the white blood cells. Their granules take up both basic and acidic dyes hence called neutrophils. Neutrophil nuclei consist of three to six lobes. Because of this nuclear variability they are often called polymorphonuclear as simply polyps.

Neutrophils are chemically attracted to sites of inflammation and are active phagocytes. They are specially partial to bacteria and some fungi which they can ingest and destroy. Bacterial killing is promoted by a process called a respiratory burst. In the respiratory burst oxygen is actively metabolized to produce potent germ killer oxidizing substances such as bleach and hydrogen peroxide and defensin mediated lysis occurs. It appears that when the granules containing defensins are merged with a microbeg-containing phagosome the defensin form peptide "Spears that pierce holes in the membrane of the ingested "foe".

Summary of Formed Elements of the Blood

Illustration	*Description**	*Number of cells/mm3 (μl) of blood*	*Duration of development (D) and life span (LS)*	*Function*
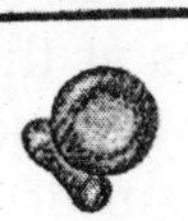	Biconcave, anucleate disc; salmon-colored; diameter 7–8 μm	4–6 million	D: 5–7 days LS: 100–120 days	Transport oxygen and carbon dioxide
	Spherical, nucleated cells	4,800–10,800		
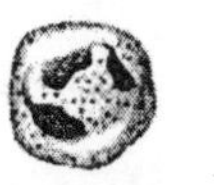	Nucleus multilobed; inconspicuous cytoplasmic granules; diameter 10–14 μm	3000–7000	D: 6–9 days LS: 6 hours to a few days	Phagocytize bacteria
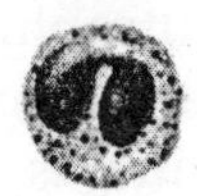	Nucleus bilobed; red cytoplasmic granules; diameter 10–14 μm	100–400	D: 6–9 days LS: 8–12 days	Kill parasitic worms; destroy antigen-antibody complexes; inactivate some inflammatory chemicals of allergy
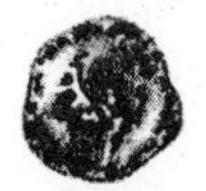	Nucleus lobed; large blue-purple cytoplasmic granules; diameter 10–12 μm	20–50	D: 3–7 days LS: ? (a few hours to a few days)	Release histamine and other mediators of inflammation; contain heparin, an anticoagulant
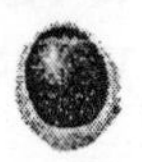	Nucleus spherical or indented; pale blue cytoplasm; diameter 5–17 μm	1500–3000	D: days to weeks LS: hours to years	Mount immune response by direct cell attack or via antibodies
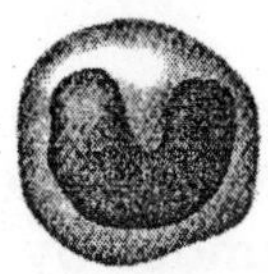	Nucleus U or kidney shaped; gray-blue cytoplasm; diameter 14–24 μm	100–700	D: 2–3 days LS: months	Phagocytosis; develop into macrophages in tissues
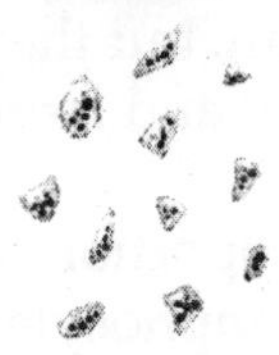	Discoid cytoplasmic fragments containing granules; stain deep purple; diameter 2–4 μm	250,000–500,000	D: 4–5 days LS: 5–10 days	Seal small tears in blood vessels; instrumental in blood clotting

Table 3.1 : Summary of formed elements of the Blood

Eosinophils

Eosinophils account for 1.4 per cent of all leukocytes and are approximately the size of neutrophils. Their deep red nucleus usually resembles an old-fashioned telephone receiver that is, it has two lobes connected by a broad band of nuclear material. Large coarse granules that stain from brick red to crimson with acid (eosin) dyes pack the cytoplasm. These granites are lysosome like and filled with a unique variety of digestive enzymes. They lack enzymes that specifically digest bacteria.

Eosinophils perform several functions but perhaps their most important role is to lead the counterattack against parasitic worms. Such as flatworms (tapeworms and flukes) that are too large to be phagocytized. These worms are ingested in food specially raw fish or invade the body via the skin and then typically burrow into the intestinal or respiratory mucosae. Eosinophils tend to reside in the loose connective tissues at the same body sites, and when a parasitic warm "prey" is encountered they gather around and release the enzymes from their cytoplasmic granules onto the parasite's surface, thus digesting it away. Eosinophils also losses the severity of allergies by phagocytizing immune (antigen-antibody) complexes involved in allergy attacks and inactivating certain inflammatory chemicals released during allergic reductions.

Basophils

Basophils are the rarest white blood cells averaging only 0.5 per cent of the leukocytes population (1 in 200). Basophils are the same size as or slightly smaller than neutrophils. Their cytoplasm contains large, coarse histamine containing granules that have an affinity for the basic dyes (basophils="base loving") and stain purplish-black. Histamine is an inflammatory chemical that acts as a vasodilation and attracts other white blood cells to the inflamed site. The deep purple nucleus is generally U or S-shaped with two or three constrictions.

Agranulocytes

The agranulocytes include lymphocytes and monocytes, WBCs that lack visible cytoplasmic granules. Although they are similar stucturally, they are functionally distinct and unrelated cell types. Their nuclei are typically spherical or kidney-shaped.

Lymphocytes

Lymphocytes are the second most numerous leukocytes in the blood, when stained a typical lymphocyte has a large, dark purple nucleus that occupies most of the cell volume. The nucleus is usually spherical but may be slightly indented, and it is surrounded by a thin rim of pale-blue cytoplasm. Lymphocyte diameter ranges from 5 to 17 μm, but they are often classified according to size as small (5 to 8 μm), medium (10 to 12 μm) and large (14 to 17 μm).

Although large numbers of lymphocytes exist in the body, only a small proportion of them (mostly the small lymphocytes) is found in the blood stream. In fact, lymphocytes are so-called because most are firmly enmeshed in lymphoid tissues (lymphnodes, spleen, etc.) where they play a crucial role in immunity. T lymphocytes (T cells) function in the immune response by acting directly against virus infected cells and tumour cells. B lymphocytes (B cells) give rise to plasma cells which produce antibodies (immunoglobulins) that are released to the blood.

Monocytes

Monocytes, which account for 4-8 per cent of WBCs, have an average diameter of 18 μm and are the largest leukocytes. They have abundant pale blue cytoplasm and a darkly staining purple nucleus, which is distinctively U or kidney-shaped. Once in the tissues, monocytes differentiate into highly mobile macrophages with prodigious appetites. In chronic infections such as tuberculosis, the macrophage increase in number and are actively phagocytic and they are crucial in the body's defense against viruses and certain intracellular bacterial parasites.

Production and Life Span of Leukocytes

Like erythropoiesis, leukopoiesis, or the production of white blood cells, is hormonally stimulated. These hormones are glycoproteins, generally referred to as cytokines.

Stem cells responsible for the production of white blood cells originate in the bone marrow. Neutrophils, eosinophils, and basophils complete their development in myeloid tissue, monocytes begin their differentiation in the bone narrow, enter the circulation and complete their development when they become free macrophages in peripheral tissues.

Production of lymphocytes originate also in the bone marrow, but many of these subsequently migrate to peripheral lymphoid tissues including the thymus, spleen and lymphnodes. As a result, lymphocytes are produced in these organs as well as in the bone marrow.

Factors that regulate lymphocyte maturation are as yet incompletely understood prior to maternity, the "thymosins" produced by the thymus gland promote the differentiation maintenance of different T cell populations.

Several hormones called colony-stimulating factors (CSFs) are involved in the regulation of other white blood cell populations.

Platelets

Platelets are not cells, they are cytoplasmic fragments of extraordinarily large (up to 60 μm in diameter) cells called megakaryocytes. In blood smears, each platelet exhibits a blue staining outer margin and an inner area containing granules that stain purple. The granules contain chemicals that act in the clotting process, including serotonin, Ca^{2+} a variety of enzymes, ADP and platelet-derived growth factor (PDGF).

Although platelets are sometimes called thrombocytes (thromb=clot). They are essential for the clotting process that occurs in plasma when blood vessels are ruptured or their lining is injured. By sticking to the damaged site, platelets form a temporary plug that helps seal the break. Because platelets are anucleate, they age quickly and degenerate in about ten days if they are not involved in clotting.

Platelet formation is regulated by a hormone called thrombopoietin. Their ancestral cells, the megakaryocytes, are progeny of the hemocytoblast and the myloid stem cell, but their formation is quite unusual. Repeated mitosis of the megakaryoblast occur, but cytokinesis does not. The final result is the megakaryocyte, a cell with a huge multilobed nucleus and a large cytoplasmic mass. When formed the megakaryocyte presses up against a sinusoid and sends cytoplasmic extensions through the sinusoid wall into the blood stream. These extensions then rupture releasing the platelet fragments like stamps being torn from a sheet of postage stamp, to seed the blood with platelets. The plasma membranes associated with each fragment quickly seal around the cytoplasm to form the grainy roughly disc-shaped platelets each with a diameter of 2 to 4 μm. Each cubic millimeter of blood contains between 25,000 and 500,000 of the tiny platelets.

Platelet are continually replaced and an individual platelet circulates for 10-12 days before being removed by phagocytes 350,000/μl represents the average concentration. An abnormally low platelets count (80,000/μl or less) is known as thrombocytopenia and usually indicates excessive platelet destruction or inadequate platelet production. Symptoms include bleeding along the digestive tract within the skin, and occasionally inside the CNS.

Hemostasis

The process of hemostasis (haiema, blood+stasis, halt) prevents the loss of blood through the walls of damaged vessels. In doing so, it not only restricts blood loss but also establishes a framework for tissue repair. The major steps in hemostasis include the vascular, platelet, and coagulation.

Step 1: The vascular phase : Cutting the wall of a blood vessel triggers a contraction in the smooth muscle fibres in the vessel wall that decreases the vessel's diameter. This contraction produces a local vascular spasm, which can slow or even stop the loss of blood through the wall of a small vessel. This period of local vasoconstriction called the vascular phase of hemostasis lasts about 30 minutes.

Step 2:The Platelet Phase: During the vascular phase, the membranes of endothelial cells at the injury site become "sticky" and in small capillaries endothelial cells may stick together and block the opening completely. In larger vessels platelets begin to attach to exposed endothelial surfaces. This attachment marks the start of the platelet phase of hemostasis. As more platelets arrive they form a mass that may plug the break in the vascular lining.

Step 3: The coagulation Phase : The vascular and platelet phases begin within a few seconds after the injury. The coagulation phase does not start until 30 seconds to several minutes later. Blood clotting or coagulation involves a complex sequence of steps leading to the conversion of circulating fibrinogen into the insoluble protein fibrin. As the fibrin network grows blood cells and additional platelets are trapped within the fibrous forming a blood clot that effectively seals off the damaged portion of the vessel.

Coagulation

Coagulation or blood clotting is a process in which blood is transformed from a liquid to a gel is a multi-step process that leads to its critically important last three steps:

1. A complex substance called prothrombin activator is formed.
2. Prothrombin activator converts a plasma protein called prothrombin into thrombin and enzyme.
3. Thrombin catalyzes the joining of fibrinogen molecules present in plasma to a fibrin mesh which traps blood cells and effectively seals the hole until the blood vessel can be permanently repaired.

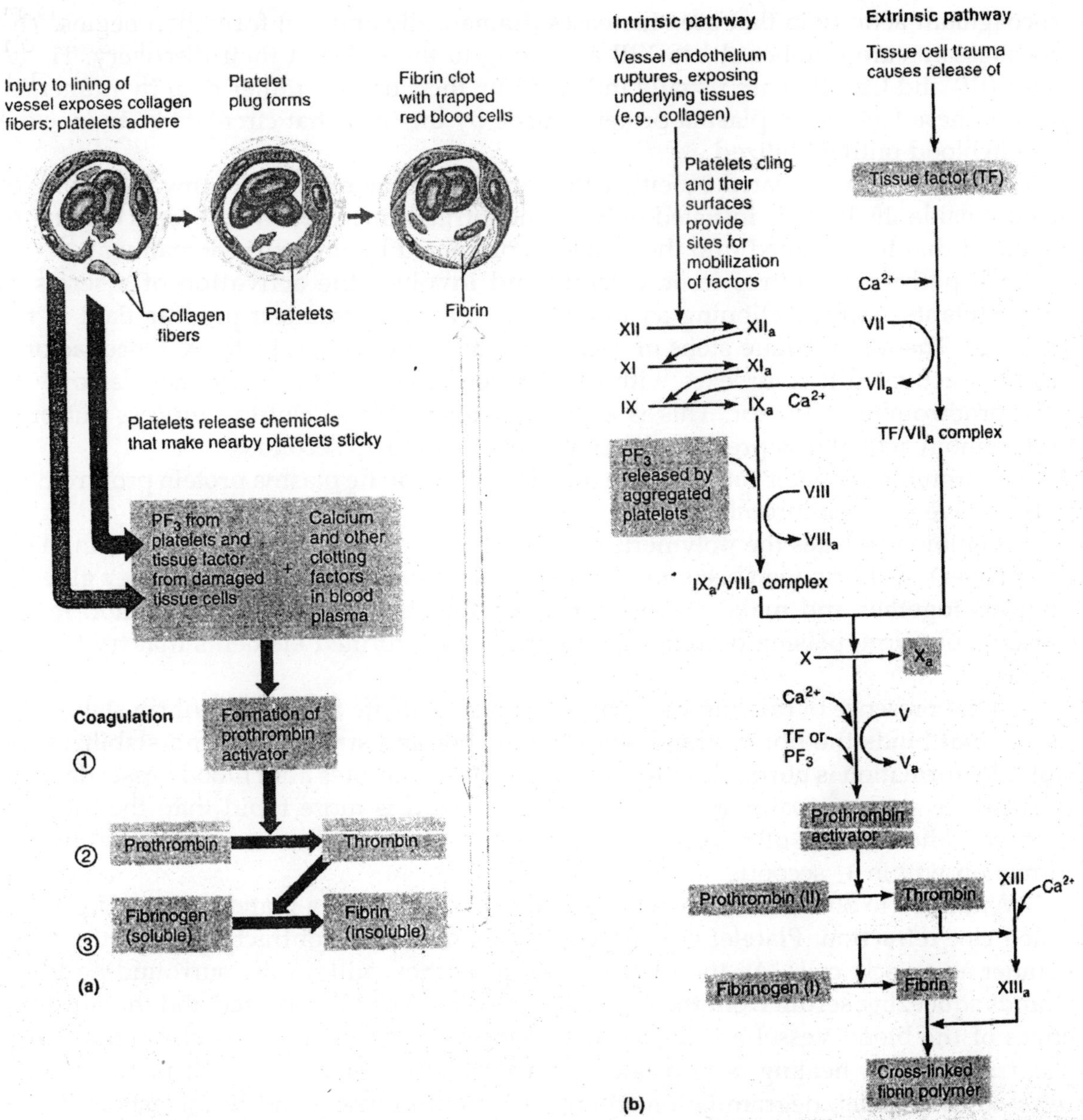

Fig.3.4 : Events of Platelet Plug Formation and Blood Clotting.

The complete coagulation process is much more complicated, however, over 30 different substances are involved. Factors that enhance clot formation are called clotting factors or procoagulants. Although vitamin K is not directly involved in coagulation, this fat soluble vitamin is required for the synthesis of four of the procoagulants made by the liver. Factors that inhibit clotting are called anti-coagulants. Whether or not blood clots depends on a delicate balance between these two groups of factors. Normally anticoagulants dominate and clotting is prevented, but when a vessel is ruptured, procoagulant activity in that area increases dramatically and clot formation begins. The procoaguiants are numbered I to XIII according to the order of their discovery. Tissue factor (III) and Ca+ (IV) are usually indicated by their names, rather than by numerals. Most of these factors are plasma proteins made by the liver that circulate in an inactive form in blood until mobilized.

Clotting may be initiated by either the intrinsic or the extrinsic pathway clotting of blood outside the body is initiated only by the intrinsic mechanism, whereas clotting of the blood that has escaped into the tissues is promoted by the extrinsic pathways.

Each pathway requires ionic calcium and involves the activation of a series of procoagulants, each functioning as an enzyme to activate the next procoagulant in the sequence. The intermediate steps of each pathway is a common factor X. Once factor X has been activated it complexes with calcium ions tissue factor or PF^3 and factor V to form prothrombin activator. This is a slowest step in blood clotting process but once prothrombin activator is present, the clot forms in 10 to 15 seconds.

Prothrombin activator catalyzes the transformation of the plasma protein prothrombin to the active enzyme thrombin.

Thrombin catalyzes the polymerization of fibrinogen (another plasma protein made by the liver). As fibrinogen become a long hair like insoluble fibrin strands, they glue the platelets together and make a web that forms the structural basis of the clot. In the presence of fibrin, plasma becomes get like and traps formed elements that try to pass through it.

In the presence of calcium ions, thrombin also activate factor XIII (fibrin stabilizing factor) that binds the fibrin strands tightly together and strengthens and stabilizes the clot. Clot formation is normally complete within 3 to 5 minutes after blood vessel damage because the extrinsic pathway involves fewer steps it is more rapid than the intrinsic pathway and in case of severe trauma the extrinsic mechanism can provide clot formation within 1 seconds.

Within 30 to 50 minutes, the clot is stabilizes further by a platelet induced process called clot retraction. Platelet contain contractile and they contract in much the same manner as muscle cells. As the platelets contracts they pull on the surrounding fibrin strands squeezing serum from the mass. As a result the clot compacted and the ruptured edges of the blood vessel are drawn more closely together, even as clot retraction is occurring vessels healing is also taking place platelet derived growth factor (PDGF) released by platelet, degranulation stimulates smooth muscle and fibroblasts to divide and rebuild the wall as fibroblast form a connective tissue patch in the injured area, endothelial cells multiply to restore the endothelial lining.

A clot is not permanent solution to blood vessel injury and a process called fibrinolysis removes unneeded clots when healing has occurred without fibrinolysis, blood vessel would gradually become completely blocked.

The fibrin digesting enzyme called plasmin produced when the blood protein plasminogen is activated. The presence of clot causes endothelial cells to secret tissue plasminogen activator. As a result plasmin that strays into the plasma is quickly destroyed by circulating enzymes. Fibrinolysis begins within two days and continues slowly over several days until the clot is finally dissolved.

The Heart

The heart is a transport system pump, the hollow blood vessels are the delivery routes. The heart continually propels oxygen, nutrients, wastes and many other substances into the blood vessels that move to and past the body cells.

The weight of hollow cone-shaped heart is between 250 and 350 grams. It enclosed within the medial cavity of the thorax. As it rests on the superior surface of the diaphragm, the heart lies anterior to the vertebra column and posterior to the sternum. The lungs flank the heart laterally. Its broad base or posterior surface, is about 9 cm wide and directed towards the right shoulder. Its apex points inferiorly toward the left hip.

The heart is enclosed in a double walled sac called the pericardium. This dense connective tissue layer protects the heart anchors it to surrounding structures. Such as diaphragm and the great vessels that issue from the heart and prevents overfilling of the heart with blood.

Deep to the fibrous pericardium is the serious pericardium, a thin serious membrane composed of two layers. Its parietal layer lines the internal surface of the fibrous pericardium. At the superior margin of the heart, the parietal layer attaches to the large arteries existing from the heart and then turns inferiorly and continues over the external heart surface as the visceral layer, also called the pericardium (upon the heart). This epicardium is an integral part of the heart wall.

Between the two layers of serious pericardium is the slitlike pericardial cavity, which contains serous fluid. The serous membranes, lubricated by the fluid, glide smoothly against one another during heart activity, allowing the mobile heart to work in a friction free movement.

Layers of the Heart wall

The heart wall is composed of three layers a superficial epicardium, a middle myocardium, and a deep endocardium. All these three layers are richly supplied with blood vessels.

The epicardium or visceral layer of the serous pericardium is often infiltrated with fat, especially in older people.

The myocardium (muscle heart) composed of mainly cardiac muscle forms the bulk of heart. It is the layer that actually contracts within this layer, the branching cardiac muscle cells are tethered to each other by crisscrossing connective tissue fibres and arranged in spiral or circular bundles. These interlacing bundles effectively link all parts of the heart together.

The endocardium ("inside the heart") is a white sheet of endothelium resting on a thin connective tissue layer located on the inner myocardial surface, it lines the heart chambers and covers the connective tissue skeleton of the valves. The endocardium is continuous with the endothelial linings of the blood leaving and entering the heart.

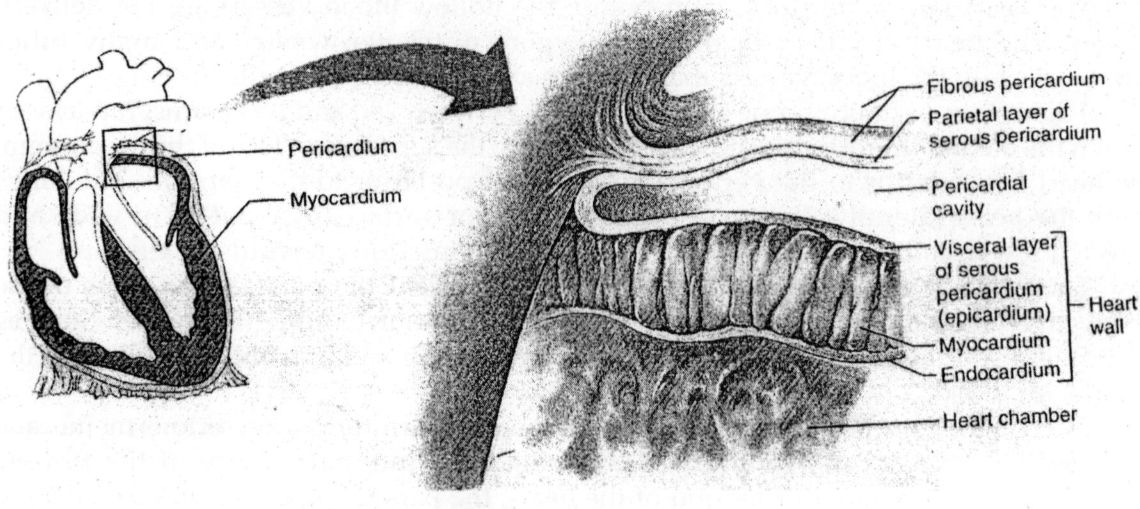

Fig. 3.4 The Pericardial layers and layers of the heart wall

Chambers and associated great vessels

The heart has four chambers, two superior atria and two inferior ventricles. The internal partition that divides the heart longitudinally is called the interatrial septum, when it separates the atria and the interventricular septum when it separates the ventricles. The right ventricle forms most of the anterior surface of the heart. The left ventricle dominates the inferoposterior aspect of the heart and forms the heart apex.

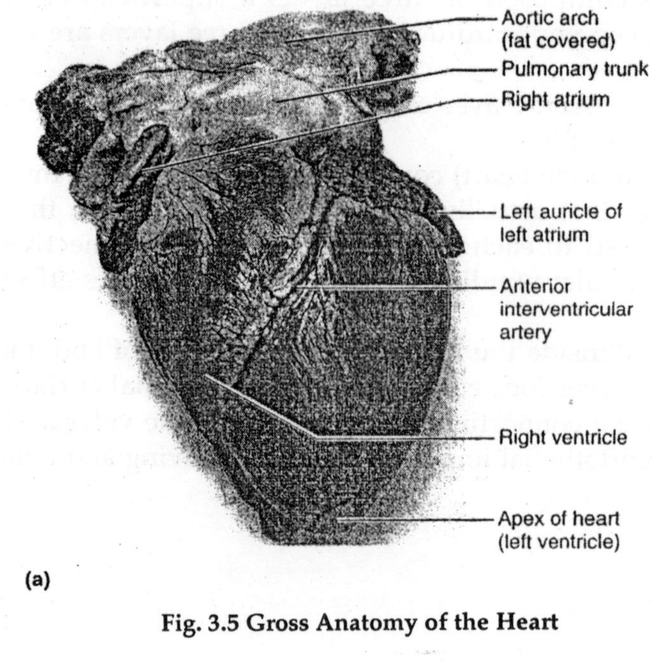

Fig. 3.5 Gross Anatomy of the Heart

Two grooves visible on the heart surface indicate the boundaries of its four chamber and carry the blood vessels that supply the myocardium. The atrioventricular groove or coronary sulcus, encircles the junction of the atria and ventricles.

Atria : The receiving chambers

A wrinkled, protruding appendages called auricles which increase the atrial volume. The right and left atria are remarkably free of distinguishing surface features. Internally the atrium has two basic parts, a smooth walled posterior part and an anterior partition in which the walls are ridged by bundle of muscle tissue. These two atrial regions are separated by a C-shaped ridge called the crista terminals.

Functionally, the atria are receiving chambers for blood returning to the heart from the circulation. Because they need contract only minimally to push blood "next door" into the ventricles, the atria are relatively small, thin walled chambers. As a rule, they contribute little to the propulsive pumping activity of the heart.

Blood enters the right atrium via three veins : (1) The superior vena cava returns blood from body regions superior to the diaphragm, (2) The inferior vena cava returns blood from body areas below the diaphragm, and (3) the coronary sinus collects blood draining from the myocardium itself. Four pulmonary veins enter the left atrium which makes upmost of the heart's base. The pulmonary veins transport blood from the lungs back to the heart.

Ventricles : The discharging chambers

Together the ventricles make up most of the mass of the heart. The right ventricle forms most of the heart's anterior surface while the left ventricle dominates its postero-inferior surface.

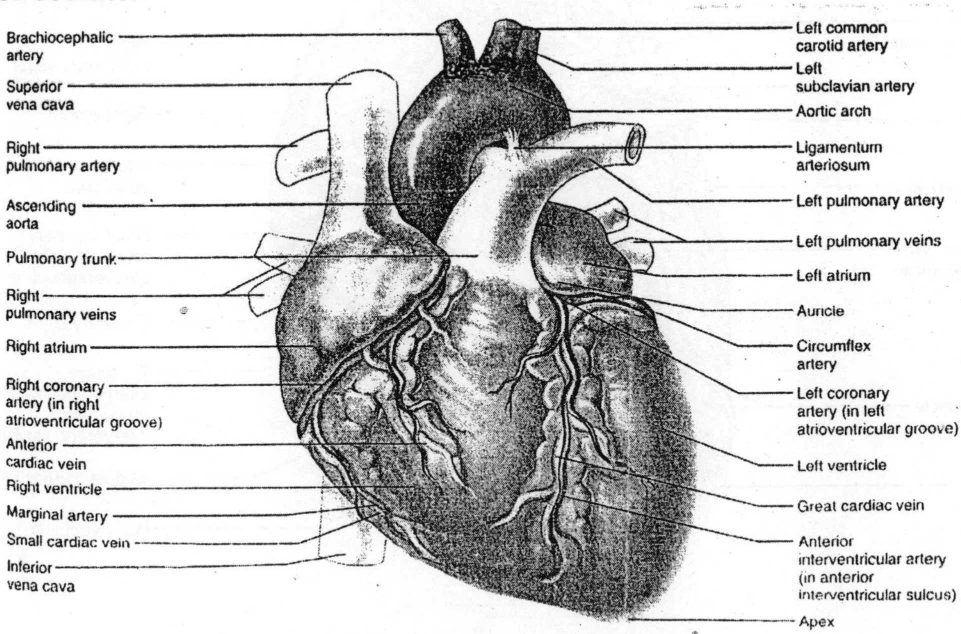

Fig. 3.6 Gross Anatomy of the Heart.

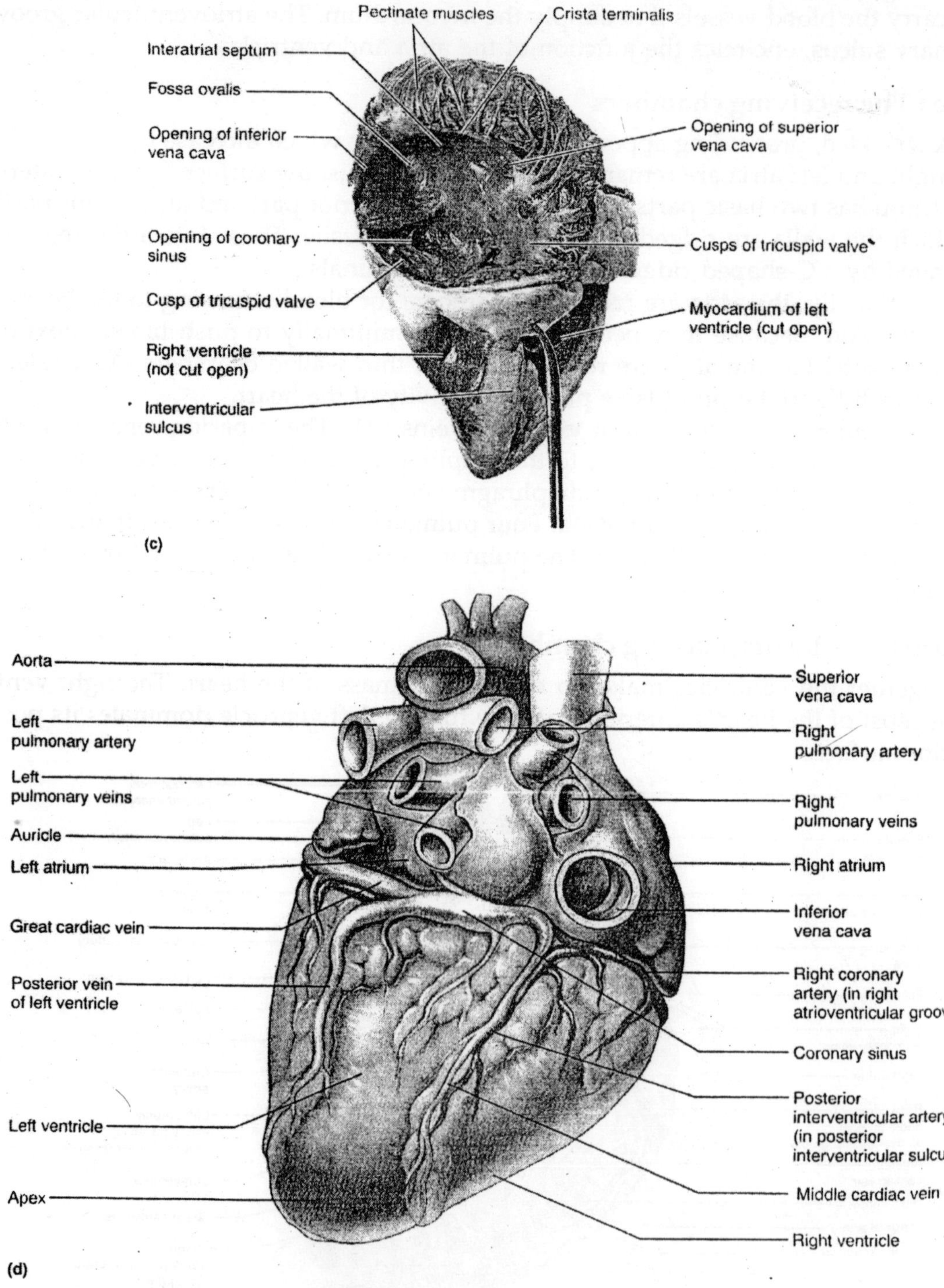

Fig. 3.7 Gross Anatomy of the Heart.

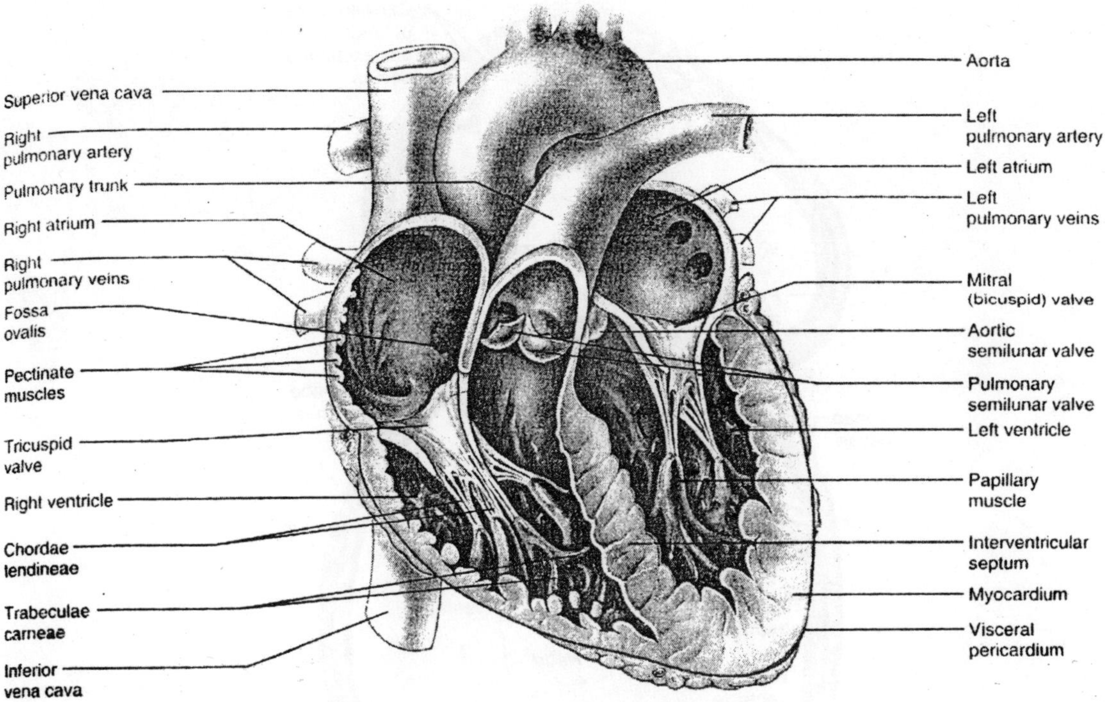

Fig. 3.8 Anatomy of the Heart.

The ventricles are the discharging chamber or actual pumps of the heart. When the ventricles contract, blood is propelled out of the heart into the circulation. The right ventricle pumps blood into the pulmonary trunk, which routes the blood to the lungs where gas exchange occurs. The left ventricle ejects blood into the aorta, the largest artery in the systemic circulation.

Pathway of blood through the Heart

The blood vessel that carry the functional blood supply to and from all body tissues constitute the systemic circuit.

The right side of the heart is the pulmonary circuit pump. Blood returning from the body which is oxygen poor and carbon dioxide rich, enters the right atrium and passes into the right ventricle, which pumps it to the lungs via the pulmonary trunk. In the lungs, the blood unlc ads carbon dioxide and picks up oxygen. The freshly oxygenated blood is carried by the pulmonary veins back to the left side of the heart veins are vessels that carry blood that is relatively oxygen-poor to the heart and arteries as transporters of oxygen-rich blood from the heart to the rest of the body. Exactly the opposite condition exists in the pulmonary circuit.

The left side of the heart is the systemic circuit pump. Freshly oxygenated blood leaving the lungs is returned to the left atrium and passes into the left ventricle which pumps it into the aorta. From there the blood is transported by small systemic arteries to the body tissues. Where gases and nutrients are exchanged across the capillary walls.

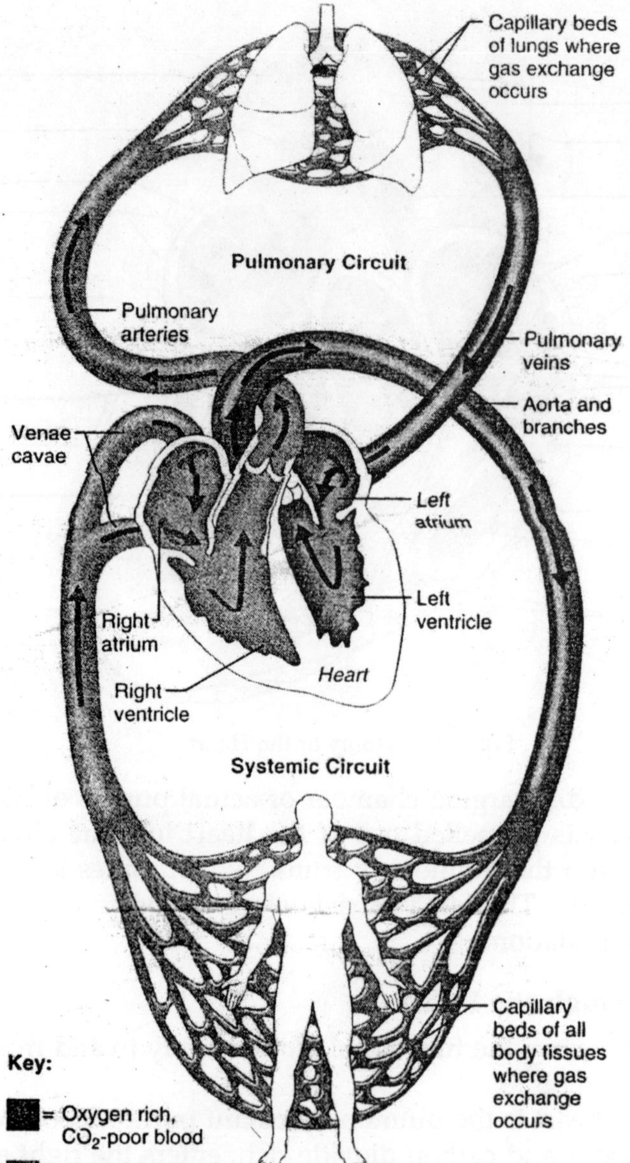

Fig. 3.8 The Systemic and Pulmonary Circuits.

Then the blood once again loaded with carbon dioxide and oxygen depleted returns through the systemic veins to the right side of the heart, where it enters the right atrium through the superior and inferior venae cavae. This whole cycle repeats itself continuously.

Although equal volumes of blood are being pumped to the pulmonary and systemic circuits at any moment, the two ventricles have very unequal workloads. The pulmonary circuit, served by the right ventricle is a short, low pressure circulation, whereas the systemic circuit, associated with the left ventricle takes a long pathway through the entire body and encounters about five times as much friction or resistance to blood flow. This functional difference is revented in the comparative anatomy of the two articles. The walls of the left ventricle are three times on thick as those of the right ventricle and its cavity is nearly circular. The right ventricular cavity is flattened into a crescent shape that partially encloses the left ventricle. The left ventricle can generate much more pressure than the right and is a far more powerful pump.

Coronary circulation

The coronary circulation, the functional blood supply of the heart, is the shortest circulation in the body. The arterial supply of the coronary circulation is provided by the right and left coronary arteries, both of which arise from the base of the aorta and encircle the heart in the atrioventricular groove. The left coronary artery runs toward the left side of the heart and then divides into its major branches, the anterior interventricular artery, which follows the anterior interventricular sulcus and supplies blood to the interven-tricular spectrum and anterior walls of both ventricles, and the circumflex artery which supplies the left atrium and the posterior walls of the left ventricle.

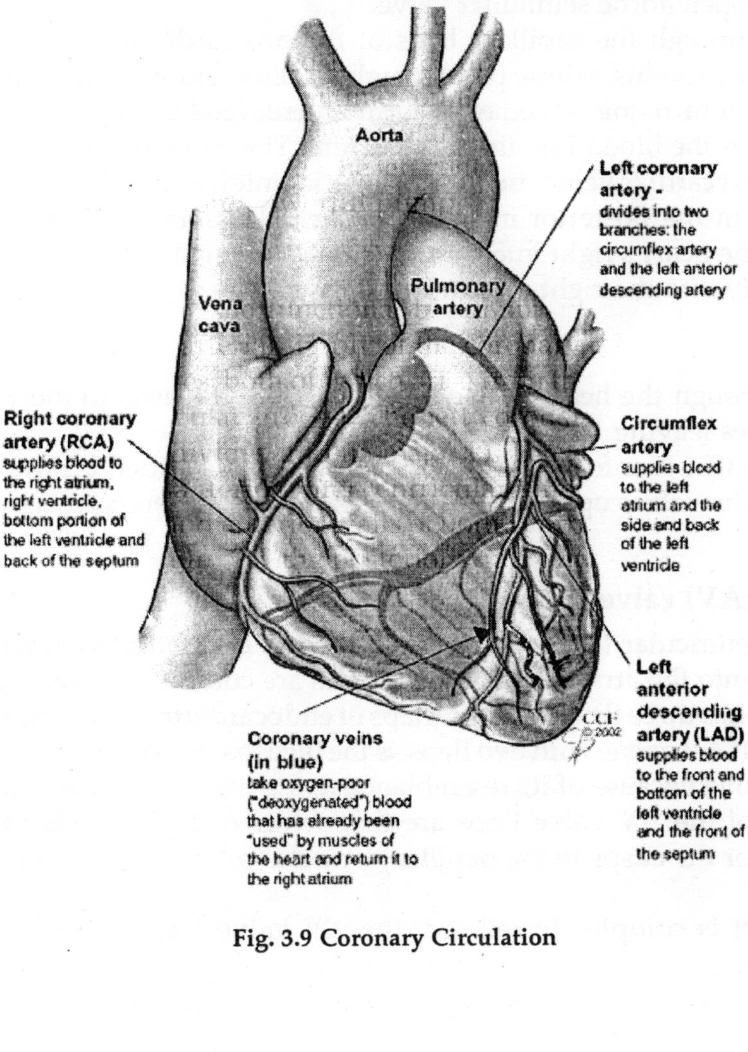

Fig. 3.9 Coronary Circulation

The right coronary artery courses to the right side of the heart, where it also divides into two branches. The marginal artery serves the myocardium of lateral part of the right side of the heart. The more important posterior inerventricular artery runs to the heart apex and supplies the posterior ventricular walls. Near the apex of the heart, it merges with the anterior interventricular artery overall the branches of the right coronary artery supply the right atrium and nearly all of the right ventricle.

The arterial supply of the heart varies considerably. For example, in 15 percent of people the left coronary artery gives rise to both interventricular arteries in about 4 per cent, a single coronary artery supplies the whole heart. Additionally, there are many anastomoses among the coronary arterial branches. These fusing networks provide additional routes for blood delivery to the heart muscle.

The coronary arteries provide a pulsating blood flow to the myocardium. These vessels and their main branches lie in the epicardium and send branches deep to nourish the myocardium. They actively deliver blood when the heart is relaxed, but they are fairly ineffective when the ventricles are contracting because (1) they are compressed by the contracting myocardium and (2) the entrance to the coronary arteries are partly blocked by the flaps of the open aortic semilunar valve.

After passing through the capillary beds of the myocardium, the venous blood is collected by the cardiac veins, whose paths roughly follow those of the coronary arteries. The cardiac veins, in turn, join together to form an enlarged vessel called the coronary sinus, which empties the blood into the right atrium. The coronary sinus has three large tributaries—the great cardiac vein found in the anterior interventricular sulcus, the middle cardiac vein lying in the posterior interventricular sulcus, and the small cordial vein which runs along the heart's right inferior margin. Additionally, several anterior cardiac veins empty directly into the right atrium anteriorly.

Heart Valves

Blood flows through the heart in one direction, from the atria to the ventricles and out the great arteries leaving the superior aspect of the heart.

This one-way traffic is enforced by four heart valves, the paired atrioventricular and semilunar valves. The valves open and close in response to differences in blood pressure on their two sides.

Atrioventricular (AV) valves

The two atrioventricular (AV) valves are located at each atrial-ventricular junction, prevent back flow into the atria when the ventricles are contracting. The right AV valve the tricuspid valve, has three flexible cusps (flaps of endocardium reinforced by connective tissue cores). The left AV valve, with two flaps, is the bicuspid valve, but is more commonly called the mitral valve because of its resemblance to the two-sided bishop's miter or hat. Attached to each of the AV valve flaps are tiny white collagen cords called chordae tendinae that anchor the cusps to the papillary muscles protruding from the ventricular walls.

When the heart is completely relaxed, the AV valve flaps hang simply into the

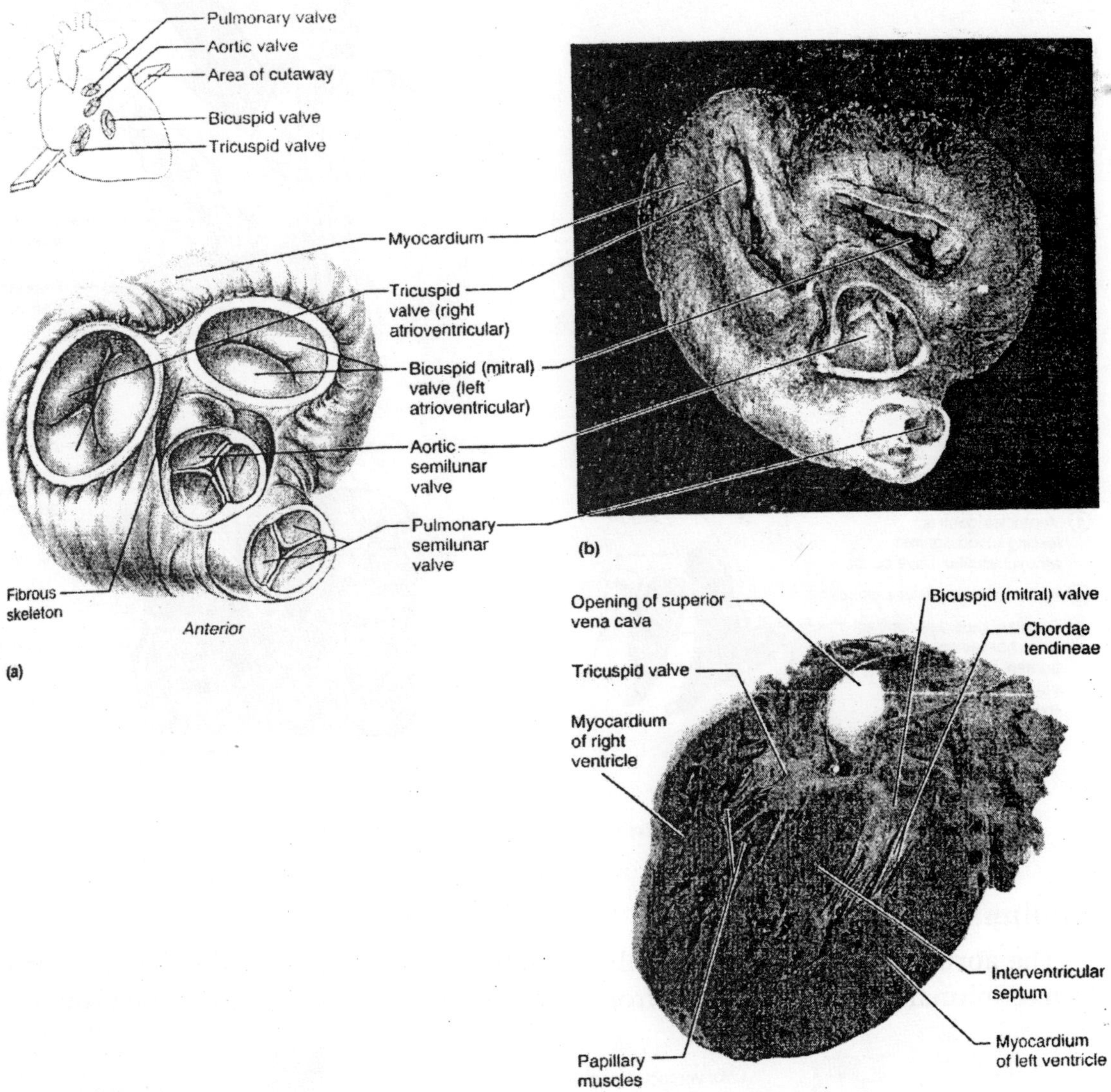

Fig. 3.10 Heart Valves

ventricular chambers below, blood flows into the atria and then through the AV valves into the ventricles. When the ventricles begin to contract, compressing the blood in their chambers, the intraventricular pressure rises, forcing the blood superiorly against the valve flaps. As a result, the valve flap edges meet closing the valve. The chordae tendineae and the papillary muscles serve as guagewires to anchor the valve flaps in their closed position.

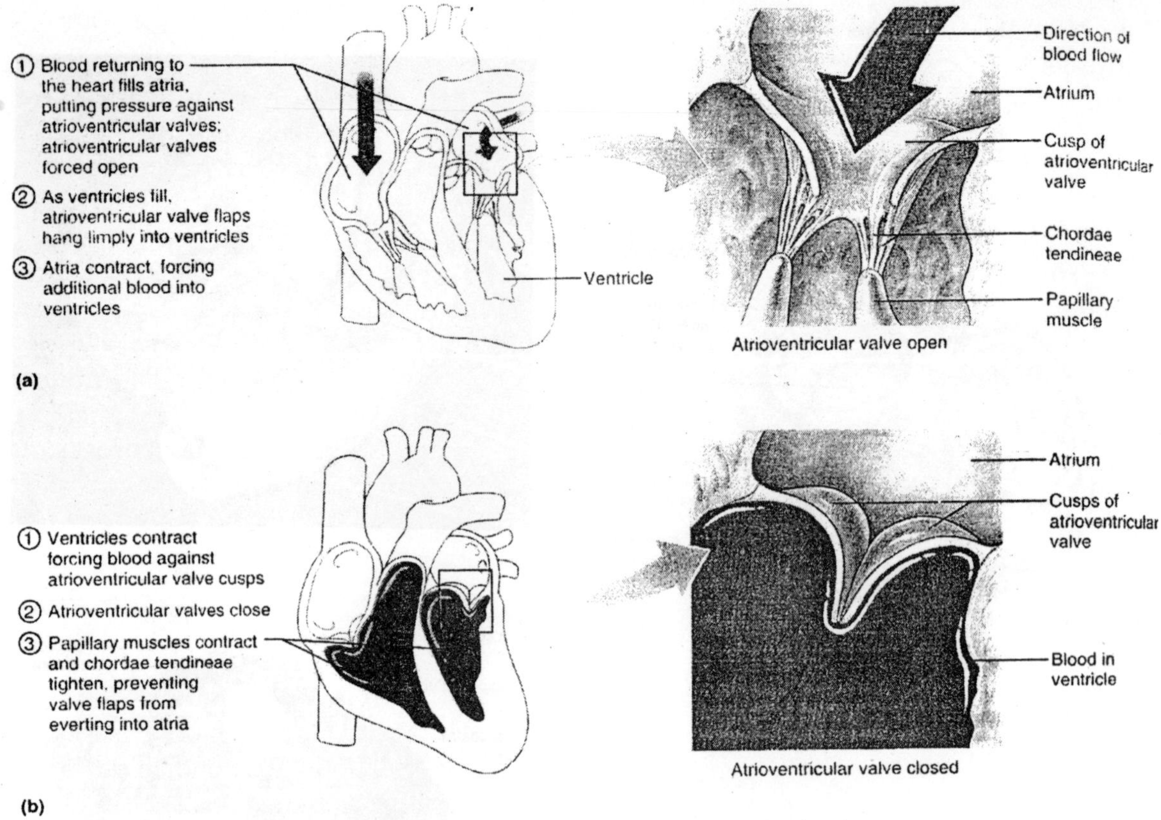

Fig 3.11 : Atrioventricular valves of the Heart

Semilunar (SL) Valves

The aortic and pulmonary semilunar valves guard the bases of the large arteries. Each semilunar valve is fashioned from three pocket like cusps, each shaped roughly like

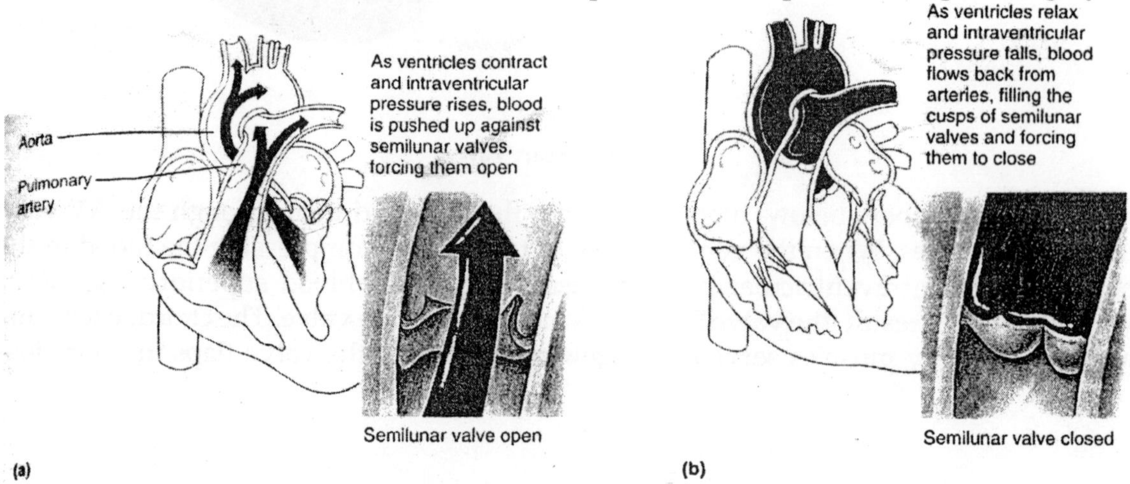

Fig. 3.12 Semilunar Valves

a crescent moon (semilunar = half moon) when the ventricles are contracting and interventricular pressure rises above the blood pressure in the aorta and pulmonary trunk, the semilunar valves are forced open and their cusps flatten against the arterial walls on the blood rushes past them. When the ventricles relax, and the blood flows backward towards the heart, it fills the cusps and closes the valves.

The Heart Beat

The heart's remarkably steady performance is a direct result of the unusual structural characteristics of its cardiac muscle tissues. Two types of cardiac muscle cells are involved in a normal heart beat. Contractile cells produce the powerful contractions that propel blood while specialized muscle cells of the conducting system control and coordinate the activities of the contractile cells.

In a cardiac muscle cells the complete depolarization-repolarization process lasts 250-300 m sec. Some 30 times larger than the duration of an action potential in a skeletal muscle sarcolemma. Cardiac muscle tissue contracts on its own in the absence of neural or hormonal stimulation. This properly called automaticity or autorhythmicity.

Autorhythmic cardiac cells are localized in SA node, AV node, bundle of his, right and left bundle branches and ventricular walls as purkinje fibres. Impulses pass across the heart in the same order.

The SA node typically generates impulses about 75 times every minute. Because no other region of the conduction system or myocardium has faster depolarization rate. The SA seecs pace hence it is called pacemaker. From SA node the depolarization wave spread throughout the atria. At the AV node, the impulse is delayed, allowing the atria to respond and complete their contraction before the ventricles contract.

From AV node, the impulse sweeps to the bundle of his. This bundle of conducting cells travels along the interventricular septum before dividing into left and right bundle branches. At this point special purkinje fibres convey the impulses to the contractile cells of the ventricular myocardium, ventricular contraction follows the ventricular depolarization wave.

The Electrocardiogram

The electrical events occurring in the heart are powerful enough that they can be detected by electrodes on the body surface. A recording of these electrical activities constitutes an electro cardiogram also called ECG or EKG. Each time the heart beats, a wave of depolarization radiates through the atria, reaches the AV node travels down the interventricular septum to apex turns and spreads through the ventricular myocardium towards the base.

In an electrocardiogram the small p wave accompanies the depolarization of the atria. The atria begin contracting around 100 m sec. after the start of the p wave.

The QRS complex appears as the ventricles depolarize. This is a strong electrical signal, because the mass of the ventricular muscle is much larger than that of the atria. The ventricles begin contracting shortly after the peak of the R wave. The smaller T wave indicates ventricular repolarization.

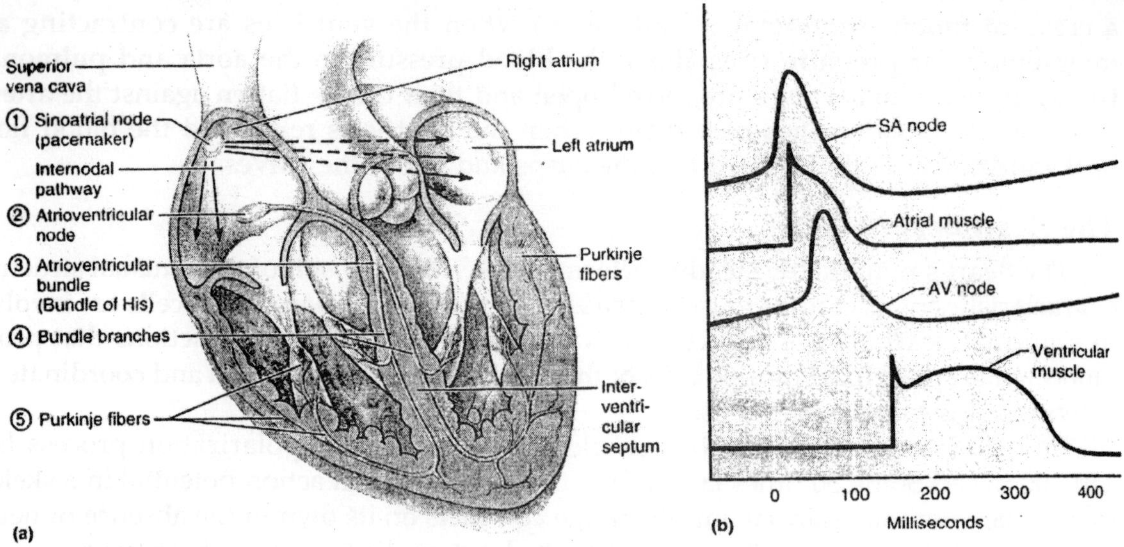

Fig. 3.13: The Intrinsic Conduction system of the Heart and succession of the action potential through selected areas of the Heart during one Heart Beat

The Cardiac Cycle

The heart alternately contracts forcing blood out of its chambers, then relaxes allowing its chamber to refill with blood. The term systole and diastole refer to these contraction

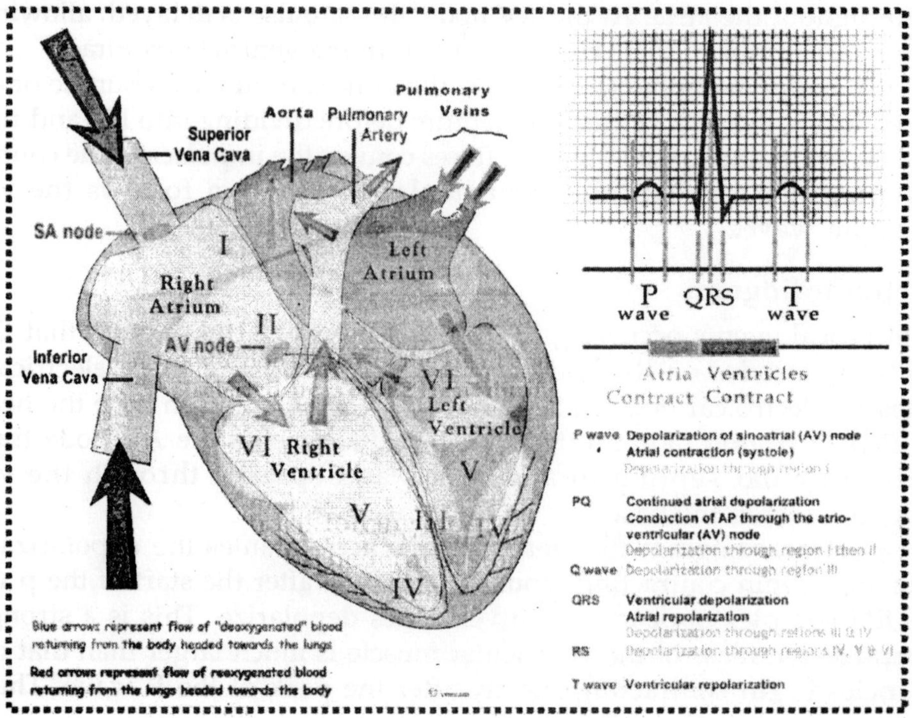

Fig. 3.14 : The Cardiac Cycle

and relaxation periods of heart activity. The cardiac cycle includes all events associated with the flow of blood through the heart during one complete heartbeat that is atrial systole and diastole followed by ventricular systole and diastole.

The cardiac cycle begins with atrial systole. At the start of atrial systole, the ventricles are already filled to around 70 per cent of capacity and atrial systole essentially tops them off by providing the additional 30 per cent. As atrial systole ends, ventricular systole begins. The blood pushes open the semilunar valves and flows into the aortic and pulmonary trunks. This blood flow continues for the duration of ventricular systole.

When ventricular diastole begins, ventricular pressure decline rapidly, the semilunar valves close ventricular pressures continue to drop and AV valves open, blood flows from atria into the ventricles. Both the ventricles, and atria are now in diastole, blood now flows from the major veins through the relaxed atria and into the ventricles. By the time atrial systole marks the start of another cardiac cycle.

Heart Sounds

With a stethoscope a sound "lubb-dupp" hear at each heartbeat. These sounds accompany the action of the heart valves. The first heart sound "lubb" lasts a little longer than the second. It marks the start of ventricular systole, and the sound is produced as the AV valves close and the semilunar open. The second heart sound "dupp" occurs at the beginning of ventricular diastole, when the semilunar valves close.

Third and fourth heart sounds may be audible as well but they are usually very faint and are seldom detectable in healthy adults. These sounds are associated with artrial contraction and blood flowing into the ventricles, rather than valve action.

Cardiac Output

Cardiac output (CO) is the amount of blood pumped out by each ventricle in 1 minute. It is the product of heart rate (HR) and stroke volume (SV). Stroke volume is the volume of blood pumped out by a ventricle with each beat.

Using the normal resting valves for heart rate (75 beats/min) and stroke volume (70 ml/beat) the average cardiac output can easily be computed. CO (m1/min) \ HR (76 beats/min) × SV (70 ml/beat).

Thus CO=5250 ml/min (5.25 l/min.).

The normal adult blood volume is about 5 liter. Thus the entire blood supply passes through each side of the heart once each minute. Thus Co increases when the stroke volume increases or the heart beats faster or both, and decreases when either or both of these factors decrease.

Blood Vessels

The walls of all blood vessels except the very smallest are composed of three distinct layers or tunics. These tunics surround a central blood containing space, the vessel lumen.

The innermost tunic is the tunica interna or tunica intima. This tunica contains the endothelium the simple squamous epithelium that lines the lumen of all vessels. The endothelium is a continuation of the endocardial lining of the heart.

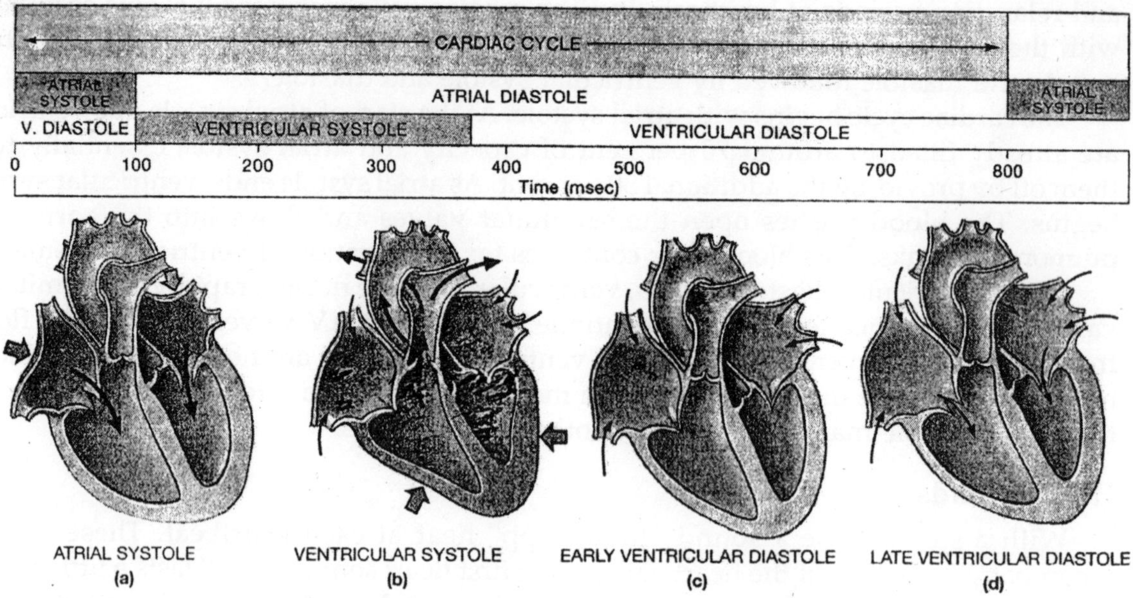

Fig 3.15 Generalized Structure of Arteries, Veins, and Capillaries.

The middle tunic, tunica media is circularly arranged smooth muscle cells and sheaths of elastin. Generally, the tunica media is the bulkiest layer in arteries, which bear the chief responsibility for maintaining blood pressure and continuous blood circulation.

The outermost layer of blood vessel wall is the tunica externa or tunica adventitia. This tunic is composed of loosely arranged collagen fibres that protect the blood vessel and anchor it to surrounding structures. In larger vessels a system of tiny blood vessels the vasa vasorum (vessels of the vessels).

The three vessel types vary in length, diameter and the relative thickness and tissues makeup of their walls.

Arterial System

Arteries are vessels that transport blood away from the heart. Although systemic arteries always carry oxygenated blood and systemic veins always carry oxygen-poor blood, this is not true for the vessels of the pulmonary circulation.

In terms of relative size and function arteries can be divided into three groups, elastic arteries, muscular arteries and arterioles.

Elastic (Conducting) Arteries

Elastic arteries are the thick-walled arteries near the heart are the major branches. These arteries are the largest in diameter, ranging from 2.5 cm to 1 cm and the most elastic. Their large lumen allows them to serve is low resistance pathways that conduct blood from the heart to medium-sized arteries. For this reason they are sometimes referred to as conducting arteries. Elastic arteries contain more elastin. They also contain smooth muscle.

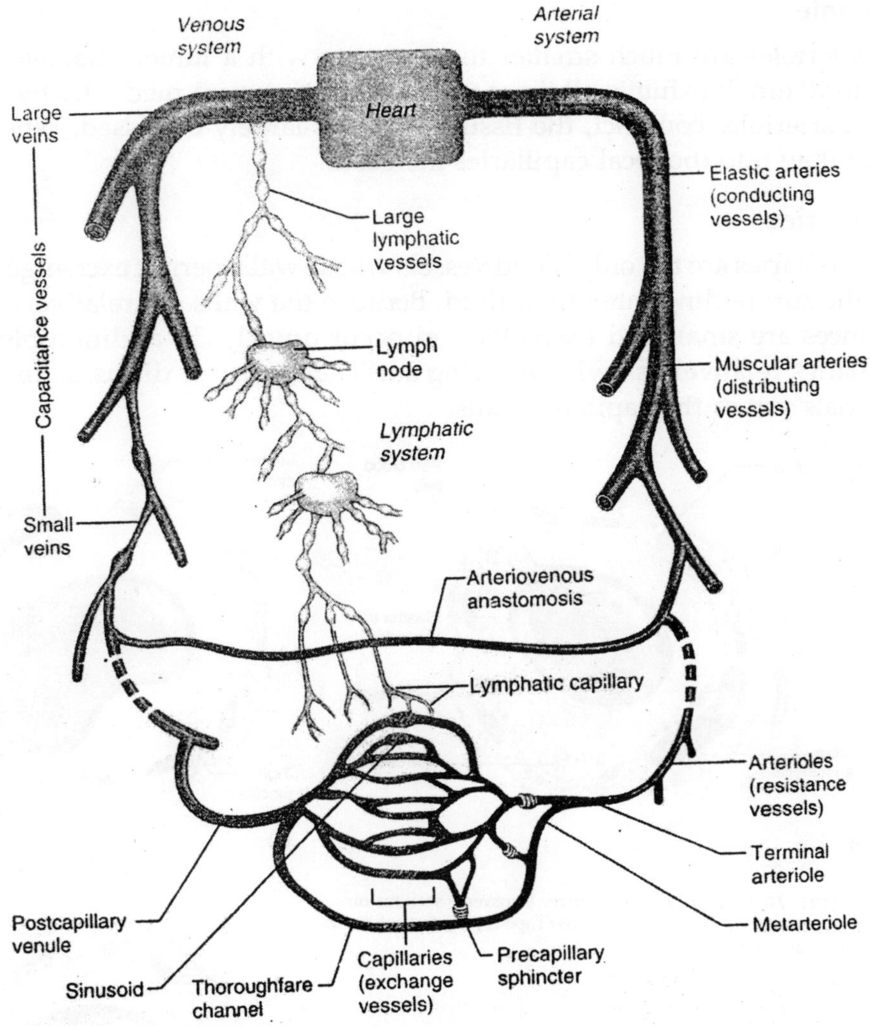

Fig. 3.16 : Relationship of vessels of the blood vascular system to each other and vessels of the lymphatic system.

The elastic arteries expand and recoil passively to accommodate changes in blood volume consequently, blood flows fairly continuously rather than starting and stopping with the pulsating rhythm of the heartbeat.

Muscular (distributing) Arteries

Distally the elastic arteries give way to the muscular or distributing arteries. The muscular arteries deliver blood to specific body organs. Their internal diameter ranges from 1 m to about 0.3 mm. They have thickest media, contains more smooth muscle and less elastic tissue. They are more active in vasoconstriction and are less distensible.

Arterioles

Arterioles are much smaller than arteries with a lumen diameter ranging from 0.3 mm to 10 μm. It exhibits all three tunics but their tunica media is chiefly smooth muscle. When arterioles constrict, the tissue served as largely bypassed. When arterioles dilate, blood flow into the local capillaries increases.

Capillaries

Capillaries are the only blood vessels whose walls permit exchange between the blood and the surounding interstitial fluid. Because the walls are relatively thin, the diffusion distances are small and exchange can occur quickly. In addition blood flows through capillaries relatively slowly, allowing sufficient time for diffusion or active transport of materials across the capillary walls.

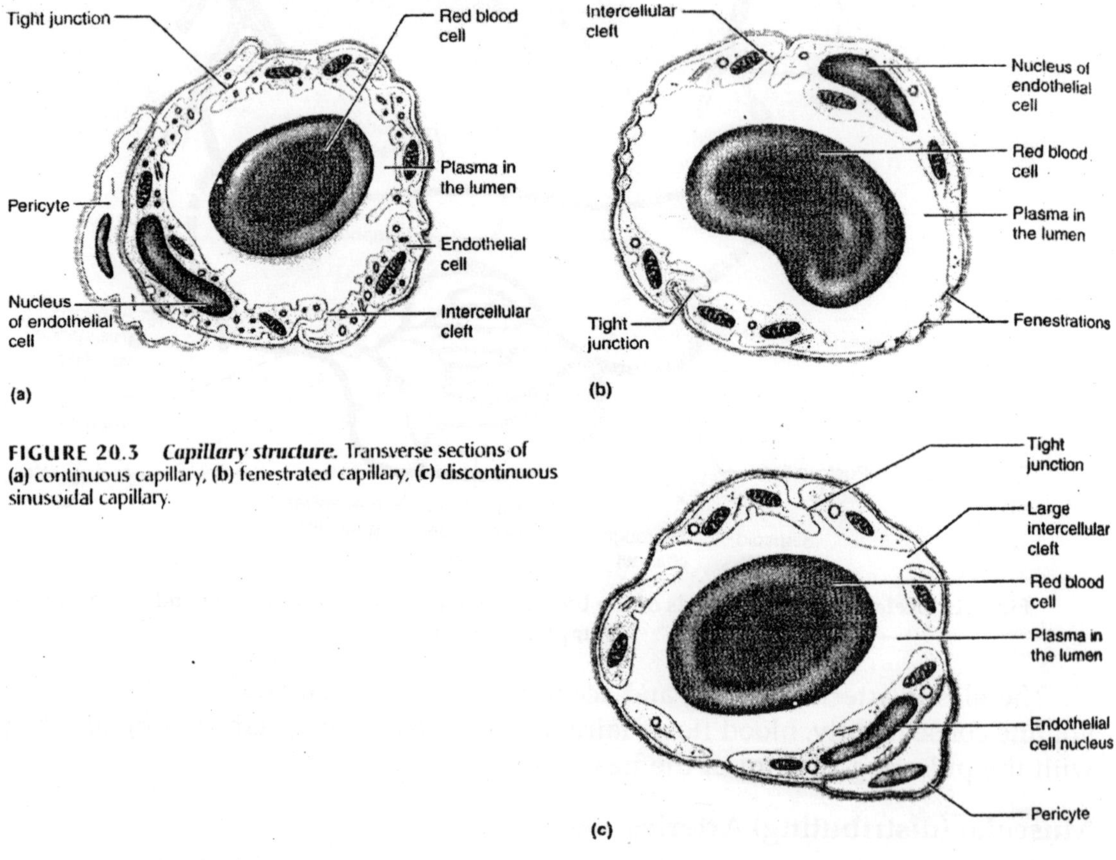

Fig. 3.17 : Capillary Structure.

Types of Capillaries

Structurally there are three types of capillaries, continuous, fenestrated and sinusoidal. In continuous capillaries endothelial cells provide an uninterrupted lining, adjacent cells are joined laterally by tight junctions.

Fenestrated capillaries are similar to the continuous variety except their endothelial cells with oval pores or fenestrations. Fenestrated capillaries are found where active capillary absorption or filtrate formation occurs. For example, in the small intestine receive the digested food nutrients and those in endocrine organs allow hormones rapid entry into the blood. It also occurs in the kidneys where rapid filtration of blood plasma is essential.

Sinusoids or sinusoidal capillaries are found only in certain organs (liver, bone marrow, lymphoid tissues and some endocrine organs). Sinusoids have large irregularly shaped lumen and are usually fenestrated. These structural adaptations allow large molecules (such as proteins) and even blood cells to pass between the blood and surrounding tissues.

Capillary Beds

Capillaries do not function independently. They form networks called capillary bed. The flow of blood from an arteriole to a venule, that is through a capillary bed is called microcirculation.

Venous System

Blood is carried from the capillary beds toward the heart by veins. The venous vessels increase in diameter and their walls gradually thicken as they progress from venules to the larger and larger veins.

Venules ranging from 8 to 100 μm in diameter, are formed when capillaries unite. The smallest venules consist entirely of endothelium. They are extremely porous.

Venules join to form veins. Veins have three tunics. The tunica externa is heaviest with thick bundle of collagen and elastic fibres. It is several times thick than tunica media. Veins are called blood reservoirs. Blood pressure within veins is low. Low pressure help return blood to the heart at the same rate it was pumped into the circulation. Venous valves are formed from folds of the tunica interna and they resemble the semilunar valves of the heart in both structure and function. Venous valves are most abundant in the veins of the limbs, where the upward flow of blood is opposed by gravity. They are absent in veins of the ventral body cavity.

Physiology of Circulation

The components of the cardiovascular system (the blood heart and blood vessels) are functionally integrated to maintain an adequate blood flow through peripheral tissues and organs under normal circumstances, blood flow is equal to cardiac output when cardiac output goes up, so does capillaryblood flow, when cardiac output declines, blood flow is reduced. Two factors, presume and resistance affect the flow rates of blood through the capillaries.

Pressure : Liquids, including blood, will flow from an area of higher pressure toward an area of relatively lower pressure. The flow rate is directly proportional to the pressure difference the greater the difference in pressure, the faster the flow. In the systemic circuit, the overall pressure difference is measured between the base of the ascending aorta (as blood leaves the left ventricle) and the entrance to the right atrium (as it returns).

This pressure difference called the circulatory pressure averages around 100 mm Hg. This relatively high circulatory pressure is needed primarily to force blood through the arterioles and into the capillaries.

Arterial Blood Pressure

Blood pressure in large and small arteries rises and falls, rising during ventricular systole and falling during ventricular diastole. Systolic pressure is the peak blood pressure measured during ventricular systole, and diastolic pressure is the minimum blood pressure at the end of ventricular diastole. The difference between the systolic and diastolic pressures is the pulse pressure. The pulse pressure becomes smaller on the distance from the heart increases.

As the left ventricle contracts and expels blood into the aorta, it imports kinetic energy to the blood, which in turn stretches the elastic aorta as aortic pressure reaches its peak. Indeed, if the aorta were opened during this period, blood would spurt upward 5 or 6 feet. This pressure peak, called the systolic pressure, averages about 120 mm Hg in healthy adults. Blood moves forward into the arterial bed because the pressure in the aorta is higher than the pressure in the more distal vessels. During diastole, the aortic semilunar valve closes, preventing blood flow back into the heart, and the walls of the aorta recoil, maintaining adequate pressure on the reducing blood volume to keep the blood flowing forward into the smaller vessels. During this time, aortic pressure drops to its lowest level (approximately 70 to 80 mm Hg in healthy adults) called diastolic pressure.

Capillary Blood Pressure

As blood reaches the capillaries, blood pressure has dropped to approximately 40 mm Hg and by the end of the capillary beds is further reduced to 20 mm Hg or less such low capillary pressures are desirable because (1) high pressures would rupture them and (2) most capillaries are extremely permeable and thus even the low capillary pressure forces solute containing fluids (filtrate) out of the blood-stream into the interstitial space. These fluid flows help to distribute nutrients, gases and hormones between blood and tissue cells and continuously refresh the interstitial fluid.

Venous Blood Pressure

Unlike arterial pressure which passages with each contraction of the left ventricles venous blood pressure is steady and changes very little during the cardiac cycle. The entire pressure gradient in the veins from venules to the termini of the venae cavae only 20 mm Hg opposed to an average pressure gradient of 60 mm Hg from the aorta to the ends of the arterioles.

Two factors help to propel venous blood toward the heart:

1. Muscular compression : The contractions of skeletal muscles near a vein compress it, helping to push blood toward the heart. The valves in medium-sized veins ensure that blood flow occur in one direction only.

2. The respiratory pump : During inspiration, decreased pressure in the thoracic cavity draws air into lungs. This drop in pressure also pulls blood into the venae cavae and atria increasing venous return. On exhalation the increased pressure that forces air out of the lungs compresses the venae cavae pushing blood into the right atrium.

Cardiovascular Regulation

Homeostatic mechanisms regulate cardiovascular activity to ensure that tissue blood flows also called tissue perfusion, meets the demand for O_2 and nutrients. The factors that influence tissue blood flow are cardiac output, peripheral resistance and blood pressure. Other factors involved in the regulation of cardiovascular function include.

1. Local Factors : Local factors change the pattern of blood flow within capillary beds in response to chemical changes in the interstitial fluids. For example, at any given moment some of the precapillary sphincters are open and others are closed. As long as the proportion remains constant the total blood flow through the tissues will remain constant.

2. Neural mechanisms : Neural control mechanisms respond to changes in arterial pressure or blood gas level at specific sites. When those changes occur, the cardiovascular centres (cardiac and vasomotor) of the autonomic nervous system adjust. Cardiac output and peripheral resistance to maintain adequate blood flow.

The cardioacceleratory centre increases cardiac output through sympathetic innervation and a cardioinhibitory centre reduces cardiac output through parasymapathetic innervation.

The vasomotor center of the medulla oblongata primary controls the diameters of the arterioles. Inhibition of the vesomotor centre leads to vasodilation, a dilation of arterioles that reduces peripheral resistance. Stimulation of the vesomotor centre causes vasoconstriction and with very strong stimulation both of which increase peripheral resistance.

The cardiovascular centres detect changes in tissue demand by monitoring arterial blood especially blood pressure, pH and dissolved gas concentrations. The baroreceptors reflexes respond to changes in blood pressure and the chemoreceptor reflexes respond to changes in chemical composition.

Baroreceptor Reflexes

Baroreceptor reflexes are autonomic reflexes that adjust cardiac output and peripheral resistance to maintain normal arterial pressures, when blood pressure climbs, the increased output from the baroreceptors travels to the medulla oblongata where it inhibits the cardioacceleratory centre stimulates the cardioinhibitory center and inhibits the vesomotor centres.

Under the command of the cardioinhibitory centre, the vagus nerve release actyloboline, which reduces the rate and strength of the cardiac contractions lowering cardiac output. The inhibition of the vasomotor centre leads to the dilation of peripheral arterioles throughout the body. This combination of reduced cardiac output and decreased peripheral resistance then reduces the blood pressure.

This pattern is reversed if blood pressure becomes abnormally low. In that case, a corresponding reduction in baroreceptor output stimulates the cardioaccelaratory centre, inhibits the cardioinhibitory centre and stimulates the vasomotor centre. The cardioacceleratory centre stimulates sympathetic neurons innervating the SA node, AV node, and general myocardium. This stimulation increases heart rate and stroke volume, leading to an immediate increases in cardiac output vasomotor activity also carried by sympathetic motor neurons, produces a rapid vasoconstriction increasing peripheral resistance. These adjustments, increased cardiac output and increased peripheral resistance, work together to elevate blood pressure.

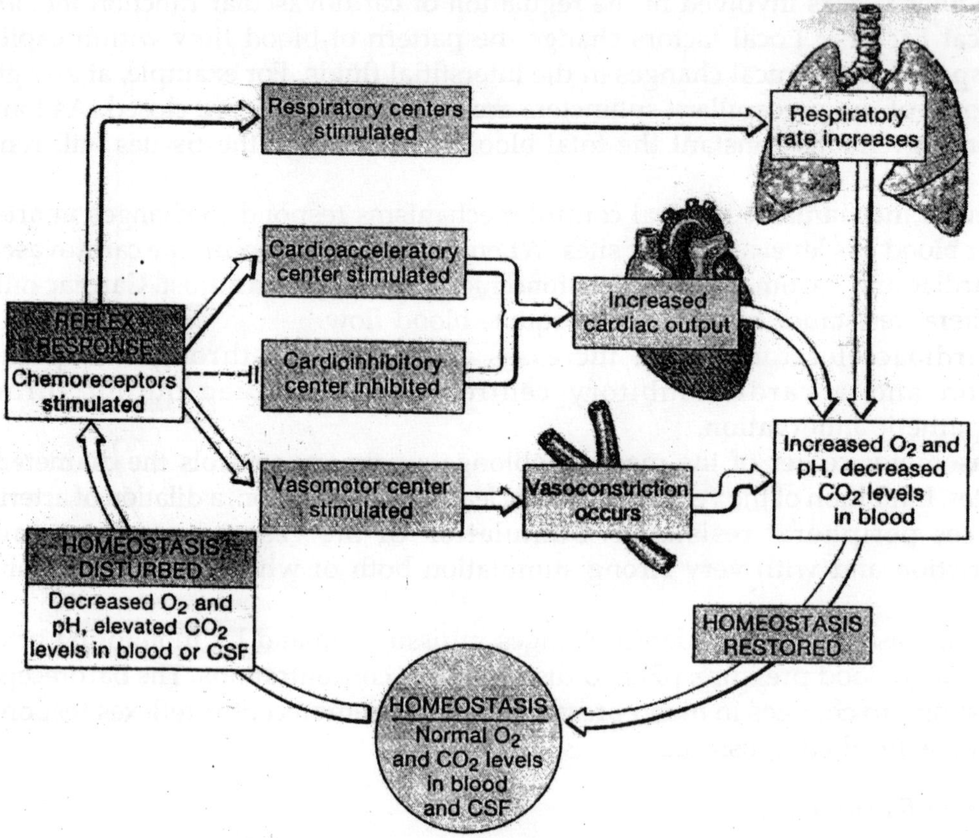

Fig. 3.18 The Chemoreceptor Reflexes

Chemoreceptor Reflexes

The chemoreceptor reflexes found the carotid bodies located in the neck near the carotid sinus and the aortic bodies situated near the arch of the aorta.

Activation of chemoreceptors occurs through a drop in PH, a rise in CO_2 levels or fall in plasma O_2. Any of these changes leads to a stimulation of the cardioacceleratory and vasomotor centres. This elevates arterial pressure and increases blood flow through peripheral tissues. Chemoreceptor output also affects the respiratory centres in the medulla oblongata. As a result, a rise in blood flow of blood pressure is associated with an elevated respiratory rate.

Hormones and Cardiovascular regulation

The endocrine system provides both short-term and long-term regulation of cardiovascular performance. Epinephrine (E) and norepinephrine (NE) from the adrenal medulla stimulate cardiac output and peripheral vasoconstriction. Other regulatory hormones include antidiuretic hormone (ADH), angiotensin II, erythropoietin (EPO) and atrial natriuteric peptide (ANP).

Angiotensin II: Angiotensin II appears in the blood following the release of renin by specialized kidney cells stimulated by a fall in blood pressure. Renin starts a chain reaction that ultimately converts an inactive protein, angiotensinogen, to the hormone angiotensin II. Angiotensin II causes an extremely powerful vesoconstriction that elevates blood pressure almost at once. It also stimulates the secretion of ADH by the pituitary and aldosterone by the adrenal cortex, and the two complement one another ADH stimulates water conservation at the kidneys and aldosterone stimulates the reabsorption of sodium ions and water from the urine. In addition angiotensin II stimulates thirst and the presence of ADH and aldosterone ensures that the additional water consumed will be retained delevating the plasma volume.

ADH also responds to an increase in the osmotic concentration of the plasma. The immediate result is a peripheral vasoconstriction that elevates blood pressure.

Erythropoietin (EPO) is released by the kidneys if the blood pressure declines or if oxygen contest of the blood becomes abnormally low. This hormone stimulates red blood cell production, elevating the blood volume and improving the oxygen carrying capacity of the blood.

Atrial Natriuteric Peptide (ANP)—ANP release is stimulated by increased blood pressure. This hormone is produced by specialized cardiac muscle cells in the artrial walls when they are stretched by excessive venous return. ANP reduces blood volume and blood pressure by (1) promoting the loss of sodium ions and water at the kidneys, (2) increasing water losses at the kidneys by blocking the release of ADH and aldosterone, (3) reducing thirst, (4) blocking the release of E and NE, and (5) stimulating peripheral vasodilation. As blood volume and blood pressure decline, the stress on the atrial walls is removed, and ANP production ceases.

Exercise and the Cardiovascular System

At rest the cardiac output averages around 5.6 liters per minute. During exercise, both cardiac output and the pattern of blood distribution change markedly. As exercise begins, a number of interrelated changes occur.

Extensive vasodilation occurs as the rate of skeletal muscle oxygen consumption increases peripheral resistance drops, blood flow through the capillaries increases, and blood enters the venous system at an accelerated rate.

The venous return increased as skeletal muscle constrictions squeeze blood along the peripheral veins and an increased breathing rate, pulls blood into the venae cavae.

Cardiac output rises as a result of the increased venous return. This increase occurs in direct response to ventricular stretching and in a reflexive response to atrial stretching. The increased output keeps pace with the elevated demand and atrial pressures are

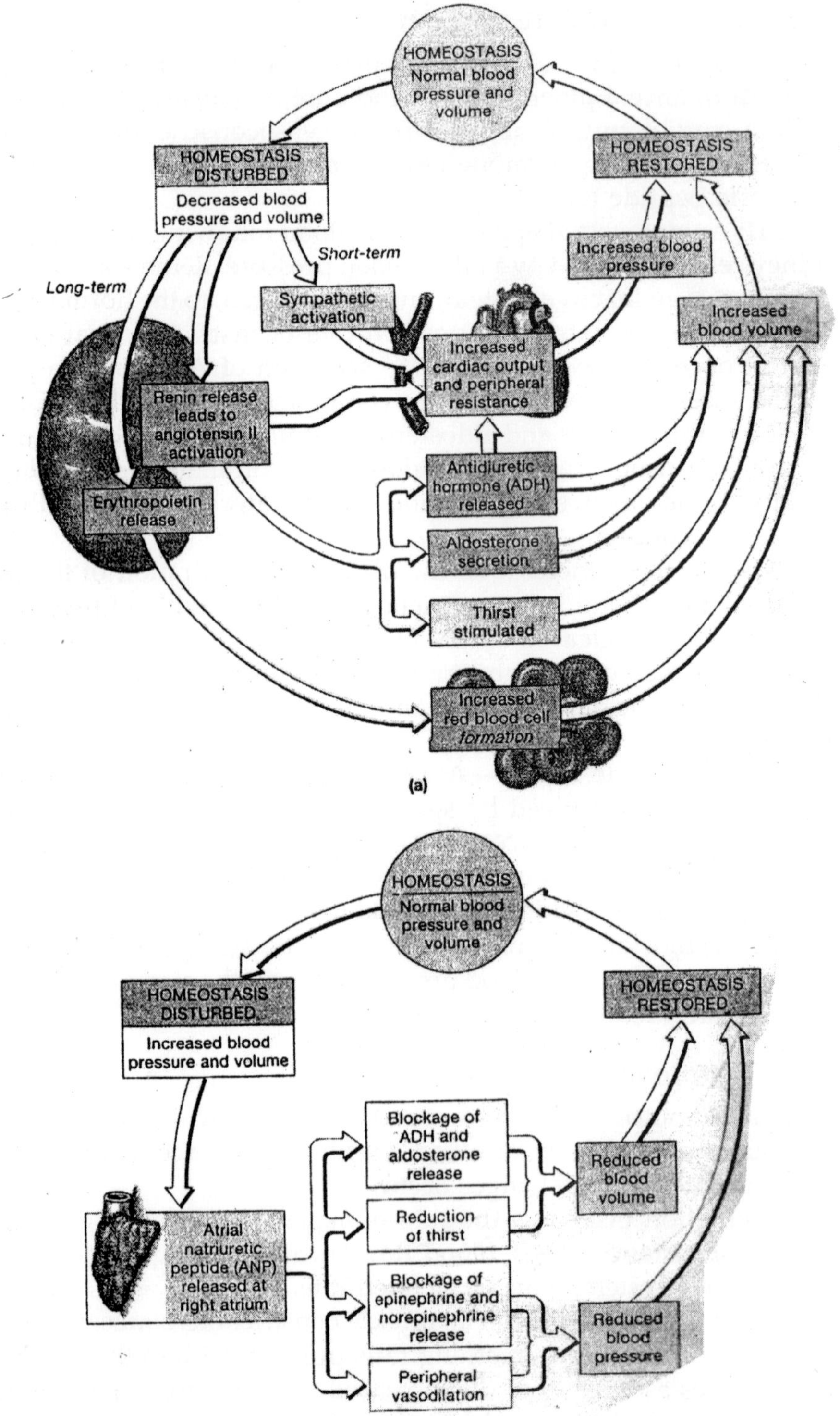

Fig. 3.19 Regulation of Blood Pressure and Blood Volume

maintained despite the drop in peripheral resistance.

This regulation by venous feedback gradually increases cardiac output to about double resting levels. Over this range typical of light exercises, the pattern of blood distribution remains relatively unchanged. At higher levels of exertion other physiological adjustments occur as the sympathetic nervous system stimulates the cardiac and vasomotor centres. Cardiac output increases and major changes in the peripheral distribution of blood increase the flow to active skeletal muscles. When one is exercising at maximal levels, the blood essentially races between the skeletal muscles, the lungs and the heart. Only the blood supply to the brain is unaffected.

④

Excretory System

The kidneys maintain constancy of fluids in our internal environment. Besides water and salt balances. Kidneys also regulate the concentrations of other ions and molecules and removes metabolic wastes from the body. The only true excretory products that are removed from the body during elimination are bile pigments, and the salts of certain minerals. Everyday the kidneys filter nearly 200 liters of fluid from the bloodstream, allowing toxins, metabolic wastes, and excess ions to leave the body in urine while returning needed substances to the blood. Although the lungs and skin also participate in excretion, the kidneys are the major excretory organs.

As the kidneys perform these excretory functions, they simultaneously regulate the volume and chemical make up of the blood, maintaining the proper balance between water and salts and between acids and bases.

Another renal function is gluconeogenesis, a role undertaken only during prolonged fasting. At such times the kidneys can supply approximately one-fifth as much glucose as the liver. The kidneys also act as endocrine glands. They produce the enzyme renin, which helps regulate blood pressure and kidney function and hormone erythropoietin which stimulates red blood cell production in bone marrow. The kidneys also metabolize vitamin D to its active form.

Besides the urine forming, kidneys, the urinary system includes the urinary bladder which provides a temporary storage reservoir, for urine and three tube like organs, the paired ureter and urethra. The two kidneys produce urine, a liquid containing water, ions and small soluble compounds. Urine leaving the kidneys travels along the paired ureters to the urinary bladder for temporary storage. When urination or micturition occurs, contraction of the vascular bladder forces the urine, through the urethra and out of the body.

The Organs of Excretion

The skin, liver and large intestine play a minor role in the excretion of metabolic wastes from the body. The primary organs of excretion are the lungs and the kidneys. The lungs excrete carbon dioxide and water vapour. The kidneys excrete the ions of salts such as Na^+, K^+, Cl^-, Mg^{2+} and Ca^{2+}. In addition they excrete the nitrogenous waste, urea creatinine and uric acid along with small amounts of other substances that may vary depending on diet and general health. These substances together with water form the excretion product called urine. Hence the kidney is a regulatory as well as an excretory organ.

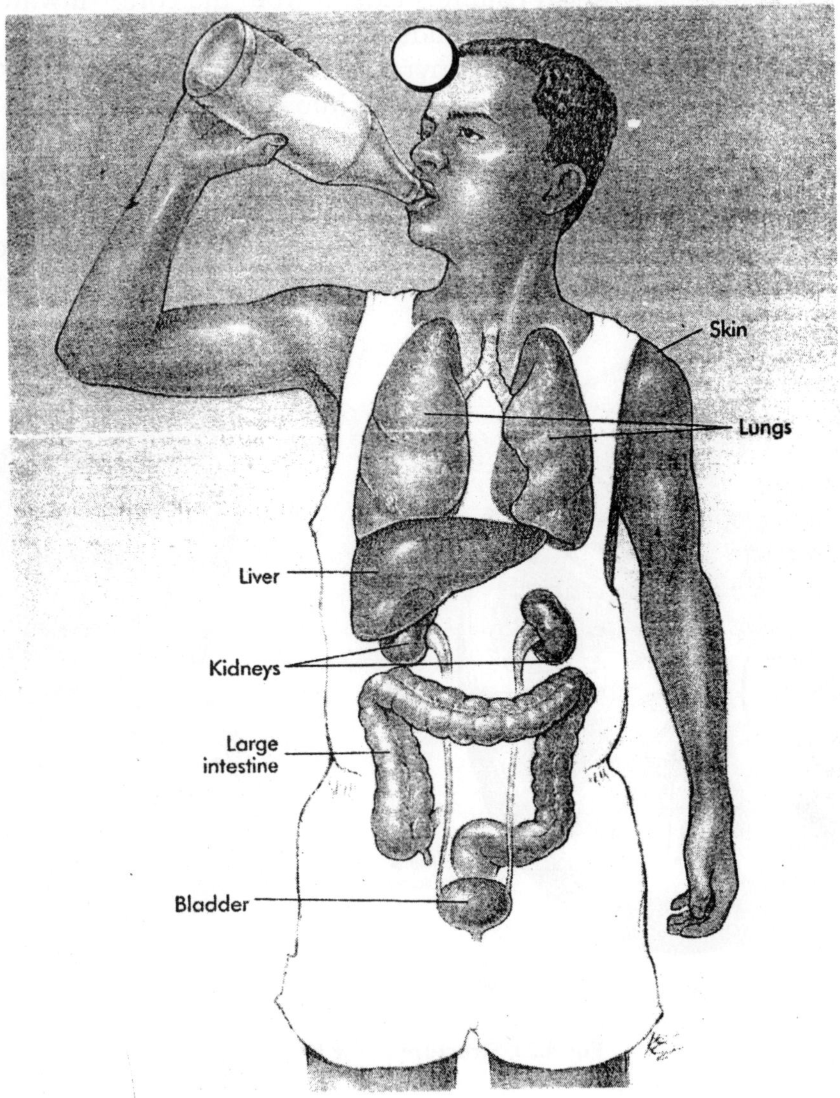

Fig. 4.1 : Organs that Carry Out Excretion

The two kidneys are located on either side of the vertebral column between the last thorasic and third lumber vertebrae. The right kidney often sits slightly lower than the left and both lie between the muscles of the dorsal body wall. Each kidney is bean-shaped. An indentation, called the hilus, is the point of entry for the renal artery and exit for the renal vein and ureter. The surface of the organ is covered by a dense fibrous renal capsule. The inner portion of the capsule folds inward at the hilus and lines an internal cavity, the renal sinus. The kidney can be divided into an outer renal cortex and an inner renal medulla. The medulla contains 6 to 18 conical renal pyramids, whose tips or papillae projects into the renal sinus. Renal columns extend from the cortex inward toward the renal sinus between adjacent renal pyramids.

Urine production begins in the renal pyramids and overlying areas of renal cortex. Ducts within each renal papilla discharge urine into cup-shaped drain, called a minor calyx. Four or five minor calyxes merge to form the major calyxes, both of which combine to form a large funnel-shaped chamber called the renal pelvis. The renal pelvis is connected to the ureter at the hilus of the kidney. The kidney is made up of two main types of tissues, an outer cortex and an inner medulla. These tissues are composed of microscopic filtering units called nephrons, their collecting ducts and blood vessels.

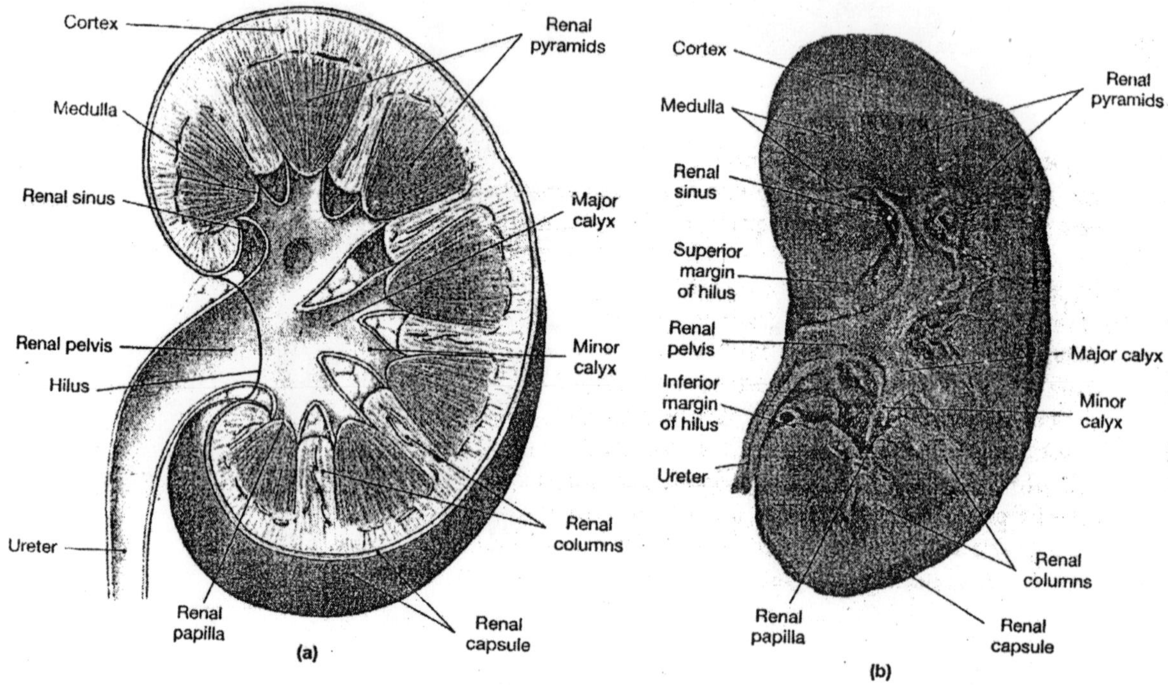

Fig. 4.2 : Structure of the Kidney

The Nephron

Urine production begins in the cortex at microscopic structures called nephrons, the basic functional unit in the kidney. Each nephron consists of a renal tubule. The tubule has two convoluted segments separated by simple U-shaped tube. The convoluted segments are in the cortex and the tube extends partially or completely into the medulla.

The nephron begins at a renal corpuscle that contains a capillary knot, or glomerulus within an expanded chamber. Blood arrives at the glomerulus by the afferent arteriole and departs in the efferent arteriole. Filtration occurs in the renal corpuscles as blood pressure forces fluid and dissolved solutes out of the capillaries and into the surrounding chamber. This movement produces a protein free solution known as a filtrate.

From the renal corpuscle, the filtrate enters the renal tubule that is subdivided into different regions. Major segments include the proximal convoluted tubule, the loop of Henle and the distal convoluted tubule. As the filtrate travels along the tubule, its composition is gradually changed and it is called tubular fluid. The changes that occur and the urine that results depend on the specialized activities under way in each segment of nephron.

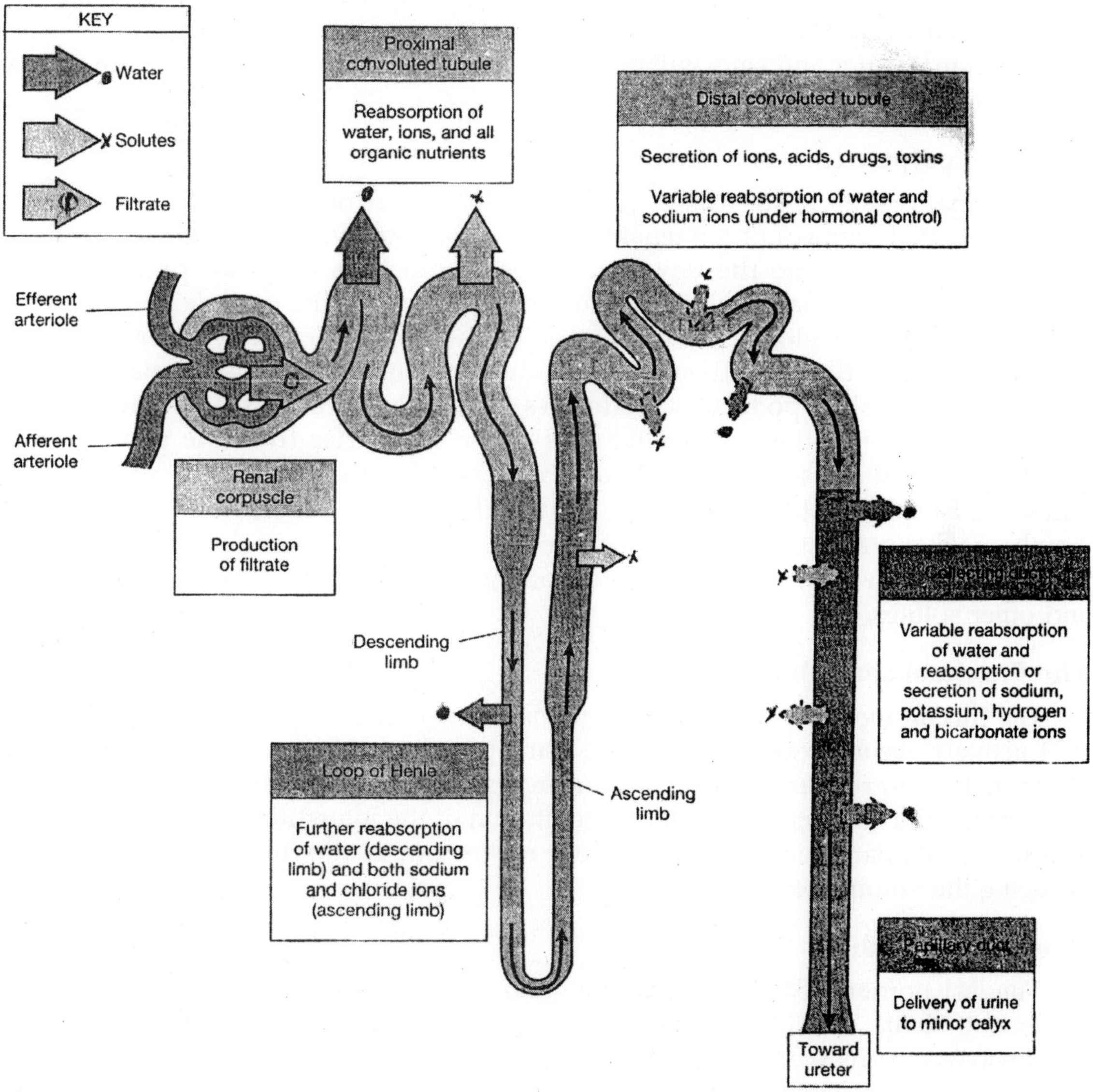

Fig. 4.3 : A Representative Nephron

Each nephron empties into a collecting duct, the start of collecting system. The collecting duct leaves the cortex and descends into the medulla, carrying tubular fluid from many nephrons toward a papillary duct that delivers the fluid now called urine, into the renal pelvis.

Urine is very different from the filtrate produced at the renal corpuscle. The role of each segment of the nrephron in the conversion of filtrate to urine is as, the renal corpuscle is the site of filtration. During filtration, blood pressure forces water and small solutes across the glomerular walls. The functional advantage of this process is that it is passive and does not require an expenditure of energy. The segments of the renal tubule are responsible for reabsorbing all of the useful organic molecules from the filtrate, reabsorbing over 90 per cent of the water in the filtrate and secreting into the tubular fluid any waste products that were missed by the filtration process.

Additional water and salts will be removed in the collecting system before the urine is released into the renal sinus.

The renal corpuscle

The renal corpuscle consists of (1) the capillary knot of the glomerulas and (2) the expanded initial segment of the renal tubule, a region known as Bowman's capsule. The glomerulus projects into the Bowman's capsule much as the heart projects into the pericardiac cavity. A capsular epthelium lines the wall of the capsule and glomerular epithelium covers the glomerular capillaries. The two are separated by the capsular space, which relieves the filtrate and empties into the renal tubule. The glomerular epithelium consists of cells called podocytes, podocytes have cellular processes. A thick basement membrane separates the endothelial cells of the capillaries from the podocytes. The glomerular capillaries are called fenestrated because their cells contain pores. The fenestrated capillary, basement membrane and podocyte processes create a filtration membrane that prevents the passage of blood cells and most plasma proteins but persuits the movement of water, metabolic wastes, ions, glucose, fatty acids, amino acids, vitamins and other solutes.

The Proximal convoluted tubules

The filtrate moves into the proximal convoluted tubule (PCT). The cells lining the PCT actively absorb organic nutrients plasma proteins and ions from the tubular fluid. These materials are then released into the interstitial fluid surrounding the renal tubule. As this transport occurs, the solute concentration of the interstitial fluid increases, while that of the tubular fluid decreases. Water moves out of the tubular fluid by osmosis, reducing the volume of tubular fluid.

The Loop of Henle

The last portion of the proximal convoluted tubule bends sharply and connects to the loop of Henle. This loop can be divided into descending limb that travels toward the renal pelvis and an ascending limb that returns to the cortex. The ascending limb, which is impermeable to water and solutes, actively transports sodium and chloride ions out of the tubular fluid. As a result, the interstitial fluid of the medulla contains an unusually high solute concentration. The descending limb is permeable to water and as it descends into the medulla water moves out of the tubular fluid by osmosis.

The Distal Convoluted Tubule

The ascending limb of the loop of Henle ends where it bends and comes in close contacts with the glomerulus and its vessels. At this point, the distal convoluted tubule (DCT) begins and it passes between the afferent and efferent arterioles.

The distal convoluted tubule is an important site for (1) the active secretion of ions, acids and other materials, and (2) The selective reabsorption of sodium ions from the tubular fluid. In the final portions of the DCT an osmotic flow of water may assist in concentrating the tubular fluid.

The cells of the DCT closest to the glomerulus are unusually tall and their nuclei are clustered together called the macula densa. The cells of the macula densa are closely associated with unusual smooth muscle fibres, the juxtaglomerular cells in the wall of the afferent arteriole. Together the macula densa and juxtaglomerular cells form the juxtaglomerular apparatus, an endocrine structure that secretes two hormones, renin and erythropoietin.

The Collecting System

The distal convoluted tubule, the last segment of the nephron opens into the collecting system. The collecting system consists of collecting ducts and papillary ducts. Each collecting duct receives tubular fluid from many nephrons, and several collecting ducts merge to form a papillary duct that deliverse urine to a minor calyx. In addition to transporting tubular fluid from the nephron to the renal pelvis, the collecting system can make final adjustments to the composition of the urine by reabsorbing water and reabsorbing or secreting sodium, potassium, hydrogen and bicarbonate ions.

The Blood Supply to the Kidneys

In normal individuals about 1200 ml of blood flows through the kidneys each minute or some 20-25 per cent of the cardiac output. This is a phenomenal amount of blood for organs with a combined weight of less than 300 g. Each kidney receives blood from a renal artery that originates from the abdominal aorta. As the renal artery enters the renal sinus, it divides into branches that supply a series of interlobar arteries that radiate outward between the lobes. They then turn, arching along the boundary lines between the cortex and medulla as the arcuate arteries. Each of the arcuates gives rise to a number of interlobular arteries supplying portions of the adjacent lobe.

Blood reaches each glomerulus through an afferent arteriole and leaves in an efferent arteriole. It then travels to the peritubular capillaries that supply the proximal and distal convoluted tubules. The peritubular capillaries a route for the pickup or delivery of substances that are reabsorbed or secreted by these portions of the nephron.

The efferent arterioles and peritubular capillaries are further connected to a series of long slender capillaries that accompany, the loops of Henle into the medulla. These

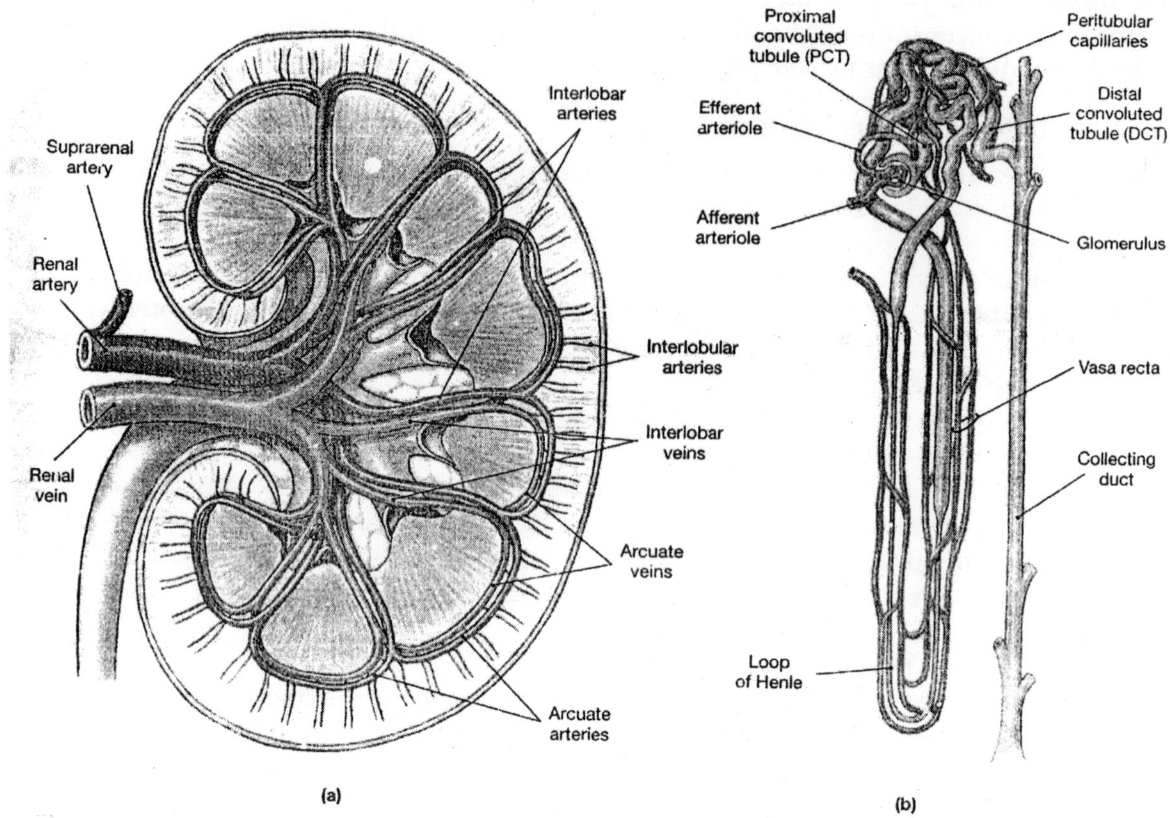

Fig. 4.4 : Blood Supply to the Kidneys

capillaries known as the vasa recta, absorb and transport solutes and water reabsorbed by the loops of Henle or collecting ducts. Under normal conditions, the removal of solutes and water by the vasa recta balances the rates of solute and water reabsorption in the medulla.

Blood from the peritubular capillaries and vasa recta enters a network of venules and small veins that converge on the interlobular veins. In a mirror image of the arterial distribution, blood continues to coverage and empty into the arcuate, interlobar and renal veins.

Basic principles of urine production

The primary goal in urine production is maintaining homeostasis by regulating the volume and composition of the blood. This process involves the excretion and elimination of dissolved solutes. Specifically the following metabolic waste products.

1. Urea : This is the most abundant organic waste and roughly 21 grams of urea are generated each day. Most of it is produced during the breakdown of amino acids.

2. Creatinine : Creatinine is generated in skeletal muscle tissue through the breakdown of creative phosphate a high energy compound that plays an important role in muscle contraction. The body roughly generates 1.8 g of creatinine each day.

3. Uric Acid : Approximately 480 mg of uric acid are produced each day during the breakdown and recycling of RNA.

Since these waste products must be excreted in solution, their elimination is accompanied by an unavoidable water loss. The kidney can minimize this water loss by producing a urine that is four to five times more concentrated than normal body fluid. To produce more concentrated urine kidneys rely on three distinct processes.

1. Filtration : In filtration blood pressure forces water across a filtration membrane solute molecules small enough to pass through the membrane are carried along by the surrounding water molecules.

2. Reabsorption : Reabsorption is the removal of water and solute molecules from the filtrate after it enters the renal tubule. This is a selective process, whereas filtration occurs on the basis of size. Solute reabsorption may involve simple diffusion or the activity of carrier proteins in the tubular epithelium water reabsorption occurs passively through osmosis. Reabsorbed water and solutes recenter the circulation at the peritubular capillaries and vasa recta.

3. Secretion : Secretion is the transport of solutes across the tubular epithelium and into the filtrate. Secretion is necessary because filtration does not force all of the dissolved materials out of the plasma and blood entering the peritubular capillaries may contain undesirable substances.

All segments of the nephron and collecting system participate in the process of urine formation. Most regions perform a combination of reabsorption and secretion, but the balance between the two shifts from one region to another :

- Filtration occurs exclusively in the renal corpuscle, across the capillary walls of the glomerulus.
- Nutrient reabsorption occurs primarily at the distal convoluted tubule.
- Active secretion occurs primarily at the distal convoluted tubule.
- The loop of Henle and the collecting system interact to regulate the amount of water and the number of sodium and potassium ions lost to the urine.

Filtration at the glomerulus filtration pressure

Blood pressure at the glomerulus tends to force water and solutes out of the bloodstream and into the capsular space. For filtration this outward force must exceed any opposing pressures. Such as the osmotic pressure of the blood. The net force promoting filtration is called the filtration pressure. The filtration pressure is very low and kidney filtration coil stop if glomerular blood pressure falls significantly. Reflexive changes in the diameters of the afferent arterioles, the efferent arterioles and the glomerular capillaries can compensate for minor variations in blood pressure. These changes can occur automatically or in response to sympathetic stimulation. More serious declines in systemic blood pressure can reduce or even stop glomerular filtration.

The glomerular filtration rate

Glomerular filtration is the process of filtrate production at the glomerular, it is driven by the filtration pressure. The glomerular filtration rate (GFR) is the amount of filtrate produced in the kidneys each minute. Each kidney contains around 6 square meters of filtration surface, and the GFR average is 125 ml per minute. This means that 20 per cent of the fluid delivered to the kidneys by the renal arteries leaves the bloostream and enters the capsular spaces. In a single day the glomeruli generate about 180 liters of filtrate, roughly 70 times the total plasma volume. But as the filtrate passes through the renal tubules over 99 per cent of it is reabsorbed.

Hormonal regulation of the glomerular filtration rate

The renin-angiotensin system changes the glomerular filtration rate by its effects on blood pressure and volume, When glomerular blood pressure declines, So does the GFR. Under these conditions, the juxtaglomerular apparatus releases the enzyme renin into the blood. Renin starts a chain reaction that ultimately involves many different systems, bringing about a coordinated increase in blood volume and blood pressure. As glomerular blood pressure rises the filteration pressure and the GFR also increases.

Reabsorption and secretion along the renal tubule

Reabsorption and secretion at the kidney involve a combination of diffusion. Osmosis and carrier mediated transport. In carrier mediated transport a specific substrate binds to a carrier protein that facilitates its movement across the cellular membrane. This movement may or may not require ATP.

The proximal convoluted tubule

The cells lining the PCT actively absorb organic nutrients plasma proteins and ions from the filtrate and transport them into the interstitial fluid. As these materials are absorbed and transported osmotic forces pull water across the wall of PCT and into the surrounding interstitial fluid. The PCT usually 60-70 per cent of the volume of the filtrate produced at the glomerulus, along with glucose amino acids, and other organic nutrients. The PCT actively reabsorbs ions, including sodium, potassium, calcium, magnesium, bicarbonate, phosphate and sulfate ions.

Although reabsorption represents the primary function of PCT, a few substances, such as hydrogen ions, can be actively secreted into the tubular fluid. Active secretion can play an important role in the relation of blood pH. As water and other nutrients are removed, the concentration of these waste products gradually rises in the tubular fluid.

The Loop of Henle

Roughly 60-70 per cent of the volume of the filterate produced at the glomerulus has been reabsorbed before the tubular fluid reaches the loop of Henle. In the process, the useful organic molecules, along with mineral ions have been reabsorbed. The loop of Henle will reabsorb more than half of the remaining water as well as two-thirds of the sodium and chloride ions remaining in the tubular fluid.

The descending and ascending limbs of the loop of Henle have different functions. The ascending limb reabsorbs sodium and chloride ions and the descending linb reabsorbs water. The ascending limb, which is impermeable to water, pumps sodium and chloride ions out of the tubular fluid as it flows by and dumps them into the interstitial fluid. Over time, a concentration gradient is created in the medulla, with the highest concentration of solutes near the bend in the loop of Henle. The descending limb is permeable to water but not to solutes. As tubular fluid flows along the descending limb it passes through this concentration gradient. The result is an osmotic flow of water out of the tubular fluid and into the interstitial fluid.

Roughly half the volume of filterate that enters the loop of Henle is reabsorbed in the descending limb, the most of the sodium and chloride ions are removed in the ascending limb with the loss of the sodium and chloride ions, the solute concentration of the filtrate declines to about one-third that of plasma. However, waste products such as urea now make up a significant percentage of the remaining solutes. In essence, most of the water and solutes have been removed, leaving the waste products behind.

The distal convoluted tubule and the collecting system

When the filtrate reaches the distal convoluted tabule roughly 80 per cent of the water and 85 per cent of the solutes have already been reabsorbed. The distal convoluted tubule is connected to a collecting duct that drains into the renal pelvis.

As filtrate passes through the DCT and collecting duct final adjustments are made in its composition and concentration. Composition depends on the type of solutes present,

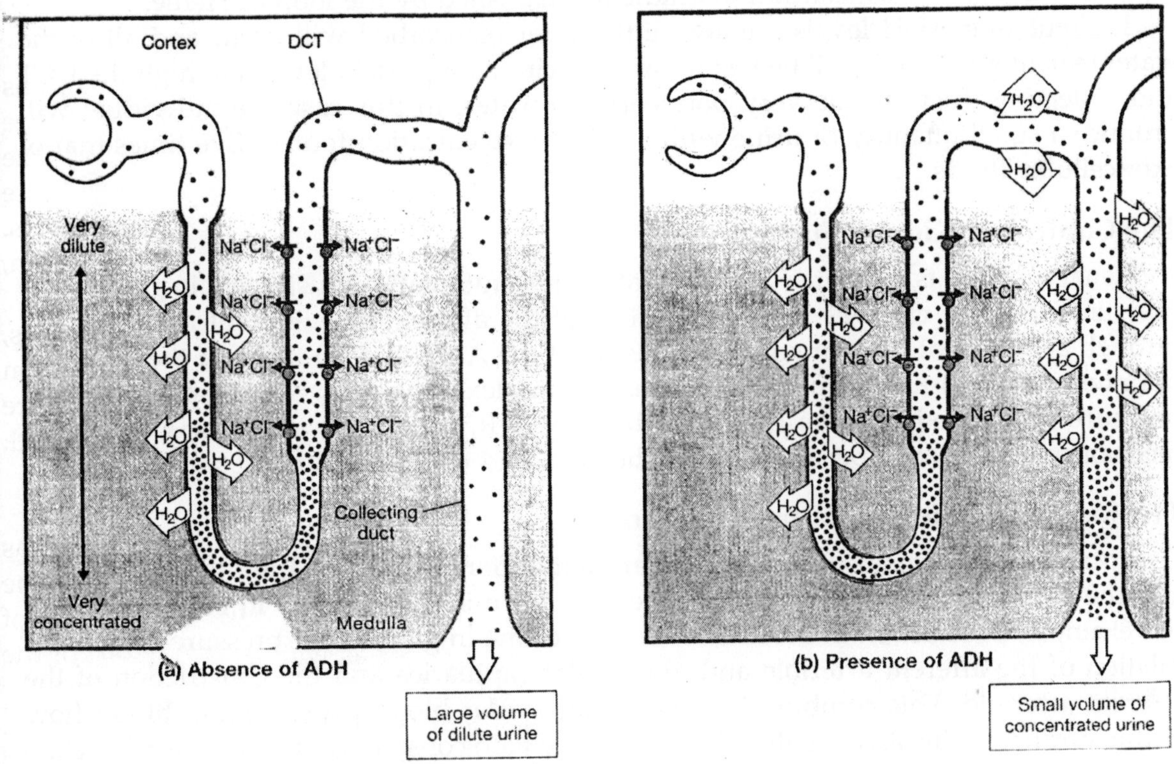

Fig. 4.5 The Effects of ADH on the DCT and Collecting Duct

concentration depends on the volume of water in which they are dissolved. Because the DCT and collecting duct are impermeable to solutes changes in filtrate composition can occur only through active reabsorption or secretion. The DCT is primarily concerned with active secretion.

Through out most of the DCT the tubular cells actively transport sodium ions out of the tubular fluid in exchange for potassium ions or hydrogen ions. The DCT and collecting ducts contain ion pumps that regulate the rates of sodium ion reabsorption and potassium ion secretion in response to the hormone aldosterone. Aldosterone secretion occurs (1) in response to circulating ACTH from the anterior pituitary and (2) in response to elevated potassium ion concentrations in the extracellular fluid. The higher the aldosterone levels, the more sodium ions are reabsorbed and the more potassium ions are lost.

The amount of water reabsorbed along the DCT and collecting duct is controlled by circulating levels of antidiuretic hormone (ADH). In the absence of ADH the distal convoluted tubule and collecting ducts are impermeable to water. The higher the level of circulating ADH, the greater the water permeability and the more concentrated the urine water moves out of the DCT and collecting duct because in each case the tubular fluid contains fewer solutes than the surrounding interstitial fluid. As noted above, the fluid arriving at the DCT has a solute concentration only around one-third, that of the cortex, because the ascending limb of loop of Henle has removed most of the sodium and chloride ions. The fluid passing along the collecting duct travels into the medulla, where it passes through the concentration gradient established by the loop of Henle.

If circulating ADH levels are low, little water reabsorbed will occur and all of the water reaching the DCT will be lost in urine. If circulating ADH levels are high the DCT and collecting duct will be very permeable to water. In this case the individual will produce a small quantity of urine with a solute concentration four to five times that of extracellular fluids.

The Control of Kidney Function

Renal function is regulated in three ways (1) by automatic adjustments in glomerular pressures through changes in the diameters of the afferent and efferent arterioles, (2) through activities of the sympathetic division of the ANS, and (3) through the effects of hormones. The hormonal mechanisms make complex, long-term adjustments in blood pressure and blood volume that stabilize the GFR, in part by regulating transport mechanisms and water permeability of the DCT and collecting duct.

The local regulation of Kidney function

Local automatic changes in the diameters of the afferent arteriols, the efferent arterioles and the glomerular capillaries can compensate for minor variations in blood pressure. For example, a reduction in blood flow and a decline in glomerular pressure trigger the dilation of the afferent arteriole and glomerular capillaries and the constriction of the efferent arteriole. This combination keeps glomerular blood pressure and blood flow within normal limits. As a result filtration rates remain constant despite a general decline in arterial blood pressure.

Sympathetic activation and Kidney function

Sympathetic activation has different effects on kidney function. It lowers the glomerular filtration rate by constricting the afferent arterioles and reducing blood flow to the glomerular capillaries.

Sympathetic activation of the vasomotor centre changes the regional pattern of blood circulation and this change can further reduce the GFR. For example, the dilation of superficial vessels in warm weather shunts blood away from the kidneys and glomerular filtration declines temporarily. As the blood flow increases to the skin and skeletal muscles, it decreases to the kidneys. At maximal levels of excretion, renal blood flow may be less than one-quarter of normal resting levels.

Over the long term, sympathetic activation stimulates an increase in blood pressure and blood volume by triggering the release of renin by the juxtaglomerular apparatus.

The Hormonal Control of Kidney Function

The major hormones involved in regulating kidney function are angiotensin II, aldosterone, ADH and ANP. The secretion of angiotensin II, aldosterone and ADH is integrated by the renin-angiotensin system.

The Renin-angiotensin system

If the glomerular pressures remain low because of a decrease in blood volume, a fall in systemic pressures or a blockage in the renal artery or its tributaries, the juxtaglomerular apparatus releases renin into the circulation. Renin converts inactive angiotensinogen to angiotensin I, which is a converting enzyme activates to angiotensin II.

Angiotensin II has the following effects:

1. In peripheral capillary beds it comes a brief but powerful vasoconstriction elevating blood pressure in the renal arteries.
2. At the nephron, it triggers the contraction of the efferent arterioles elevating glomerular pressures and filtration rates.
3. In the CNS, it triggers the release of ADH, which in turn stimulates the reabsorption of water and sodium ions and causes the sensation of thirst.
4. At the adrenal gland it stimulates the secretion of aldosterone by the cortex and epinephrine and norepinephrin (NE) by the adrenal medullae. The result is a sudden, increase in systematic blood pressure. At the kidneys, aldosterone stimulates sodium reabsorption along the DCT and collecting system.

ADH

Antidiuretic hormone (1) increases the water permeability of the DCT and collecting duct, stimulating the reabsorption of water from the tubular fluid and (2) Causes the sensation of thirst leading to the consumption of additional water. ADH release occurs under angiotensin II stimulation, it also occurs independently, when hypothalamic neurons are stimulated by a fall in blood pressure or an elevation in the solute concentration of the circulating blood.

Aldosterone

Aldosterone secretion stimulates the reabsorption of sodium ions and the secretion of potassium ions along the DCT and collecting duct. Aldosterone secretion primarily occurs (1) Under angiotensin II stimulation and (2) in response to a rise in the potassium ion concentration of the blood.

Atrial nutriuteric peptide

The actions of atrial nutriuretic peptide (ANP) oppose those of the renin-agiotensin system. ANP is released by atrial cardiac muscle cells when blood volume and pressure are too high. The action of ANP that affect the kidneys include (1) a decrease in the rate of sodium ion reabsorption in the DCT leading to increased sodium ion loss in the urine,

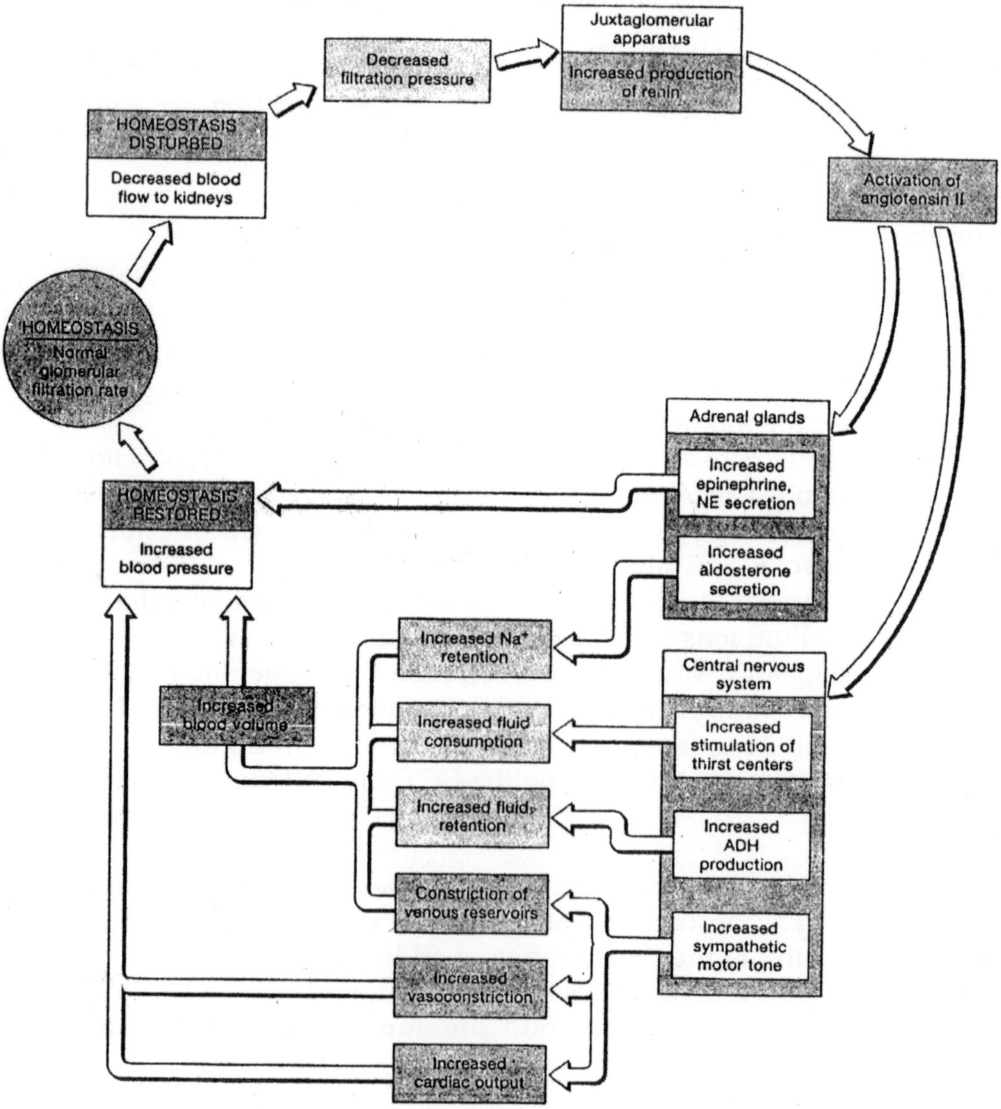

Fig. 4.6 The Renin-Angiotensin System

(2) dilation of the glomerular capillaries which results in increased glomerular filtration and urinary water loss, and (3) inactivation of the renin-angiotensin system through inhibition of renin, aldosterone, and ADH secretion. The net result is an accelerated loss of sodium ions and an increase in the volume of urine produced. This combination lowers blood volume and blood pressure.

Urine transport, storage and elimination

Filtrate modification and urine production end when the fluid enters the renal pelvis. The rest of the urinary system is responsible for the transport, storage and elimination of the urine.

The Ureter and urinary bladder

The ureter extend from the kidneys to the urinary bladder. Like the kidneys, the ureters are retroperitoneal and they penetrate the posterior wall of the bladder without entering the peritoneal cavity. Under normal conditions peristaltic contractions begin at the apex of the renal papillae and sweep along the minor and major calyces toward the renal pelvis. Similar contractions move urine out of the renal pelvis and along the ureter to the bladder.

In the male, the base of the urinary bladder lies between the rectum and the pubic symphysis. In the female the urinary bladder sits inferior to the uterus and anterior to the vagina. The area surrounding the urethral entrance called the neck of the urinarry bladder, contains a muscular sphincter, that also extends along the proximal portions of the urethra. This internal urethral sphincter provides involuntary control over the discharge of urine from the bladder. The bladder wall contains both longitudinal and circular smooth muscle layers that form the powerful destrusor muscle of the bladder. Contraction of this muscle compresses the urinary bladder and expels its contents into the urethra.

The Urethra

In female the urethra is very short from the bladder to the vestibule. In the male, the urethra extends from the neck of the urinary bladder to the tip of the penis. In both sexes as the urethra passes through the urogenital diaphragm forms the external urethral sphincter.

The micturition reflex and urination

Urine reaches the urinarv bladder by the peristaltic contractions of the ureters. The process of urination is coordinated by the micturition reflex. Stretch receptors in the wall of the urinary bladder are stimulated as it falls with urine. Afferent sensory fibres in the pelvic nerves carry the resulting impulses to the sacral spinal cord. The increased level of activities by the sensory receptors and the sensory fibres (1) facilitates parasympathetic motor neurons in the sacral spinal cord, and (2) stimulates interneurons that relay sensations to the cerebral cortex. As a result, we become consciously aware of the fluid pressure in the urinary bladder.

The urge to urinate usually appears when the bladder contains about 200 ml of urine. The micturition reflex begins to function when the stretch receptors have provided adequate stimulation to the parasympathetic motor neurons. At this time the motor neurons stimulate the smooth muscle in the bladder wall. These commands travel over the pelvic nerves and produce a sustained contraction of the urinary bladder.

This contraction elevates fluid pressures inside the bladder but urine ejection cannot occur unless both the internal and external sphincters are relaxed. If external sphincter does not relax the internal sphincter remains closed and the bladder gradually relaxes. A further increase in bladder volume begins the cycle again usually within an hour. Once the volume of the urinary bladder exceeds 500 ml the micturition reflex may generate enough pressure to force open the internal sphincter. This opening leads to a reflexive relaxation in the external sphincter and urination occurs. Normally, after micturition less than 10 ml of urine remain in the bladder.

Fluid electrolyte and acid-base balance

In our body water accounts for up to 99 per cent of the volume of extra-cellular fluid (ECF) and it is essential ingredient of cytoplasm. All of a cell's operations rely on water as a diffusion medium for the distribution of gases nutrients and waste products. If the water content of the body changes, cellular activities are also changed. For example, when the water content of the body reaches very low levels, proteins denature, enzymes cease functioning and cell die.

The ionic concentrations and pH of the body's water are as important as its absolute quantity. If concentrations of calcium or potassium ions in the ECF become too high, cardiac arrhythmias develop and the individual's life is in danger. Low pH is especially dangerous because hydrogen ions break chemical bonds, change the shapes of complex molecules, distrupt cell membranes and impair tissue functions.

Fluid and electrolyte balance

Nearly two-thirds of the total body water content is found inside living cells as intracellular fluid (ICF). The extracellular fluid (ECF) contains the rest of the body. Water exchange between the ECF occurs across the endothelial lining of capillaries. Fluid way also travel from the interstitial spaces to the plasma by the lymphatic system. The principal ions in the ECF are sodium, chloride and bicarbonate. The ICF contains an abundant of potassium, magnesium and phosphate ions plus large numbers of negatively charged proteins.

Despite these differences in the concentration of specific substances, the intracellular and extracellular osmolarities are identical.

Fluid Balance

Water circulates freely within the extracellular fluid compartments. Capillary blood pressure forces water out of the plasma and into the interstitial space. Some of that water is reabsorbed along the distal portion of the capillary bed, and the rest circulates into lymphatic vessels for transport to the venous circulation.

Water moves back across the epithelial surface lining the peritoneal, pleural and pericardial cavities. The flow rate is significant roughly 7 liters of peritoneal fluid are produced and reabsorbed each day. Water also moves between the blood and the cerebrospinal fluid, the aqueous and vitreous humous of the eye, and the perilymph and endolymph of the inner ear.

Roughly 2500 ml of water are lost each day through urine faeces and perspiration. The losses due to perspiration vary depending on the activities undertaken, but the additional deficits can be considerable, reaching well over 4 liters an hour. Water losses are normally balanced by the gain of fluids through eating (48 per cent) drinking (40 percent) and metabolic generation (12 per cent).

Fluid Shifts

Water movement between the ECF and ICF is called the fluid shift. Fluid shifts occur rapidly, reaching equilibrium within a period of minutes to hours. These shifts occur in response to changes in the osmolarity of the extracellular fluid.

If the ECF becomes more concentrated with respect to the ICF, water will move from the cells into the ECF until osmotic equilibrium is restored.

If the ECF becomes more dilute with respect to the ICF, water will move from the ECF into the cells and the volume of the ICF will increase.

In summary, if the osmolarity of the ECF changes a fluid shift between ICF and ECF will tend to oppose the change. Because the volume of the ICF is much greater than that of the ECF, the ICF acts as a "water reserve". In effect, instead of a large change in the composition of the ECF there are smaller changes in both the ECF and ICF.

Electrolyte Balance

An individual is in electrolyte balance when the rates of gain and loss are equal for each of the individual electrolytes in the body. Electrolytes balance is important for the following reasons:

1. A gain or loss of electrolytes can cause a gain or loss in water.
2. The concentrations of individual electrolytes affect a variety of cell functions.

Two cations, sodium and potassium merit special attention (1) they are major contributors to the osmolarities of the ECF and ICF and (2) they have direct effects on the normal functioning of living cells. Sodium is the dominant cation within the extracellular fluid, because more than 90 per cent of the osmolarity of the ECF results from the presence of sodium salts, principally sodium chloride (NaCl) and Sodium bicarbonate ($NaHCO_3$) alternations in the osmolarity of extracellular fluids usually reflect changes in the concentration of sodium ions. Potassium is the dominant cation in the intracellular fluid, extracellular potassium concentrations are normally low.

The most common problems with electrolyte balance are caused by an imbalance between sodium gains and losses.

Problems with potassium balance are less common but significantly more dangerous than those related to sodium balance.

Sodium Balance

The amount of sodium in the ECF represents a balance between sodium ion absorption at the digestive tract and sodium ion excretion at the kidneys and other sites. The rate of uptake varies directly with the amount included in the diet. The kidneys are responsible for regulating sodium ion losses, in response to circulating levels of aldosterone (decreased sodium loss) and ANP increased sodium loss.

Whenever the rate of sodium intake or output changes, there is a corresponding gain or loss of water that tends to keep the sodium concentration constant. For example, eating a heavily salted meal will not raise the sodium ion concentration of body fluids because as sodium chloride crosses the digestive epithelium, osmosis brings additional water into the body. This is why, individuals with high blood pressure are told to restrict their salt intake, dietary salt will be absorbed and because 'water follows salt' the blood volume and blood pressure will increase.

Potassium Balance

Potassium ions are the primarily cations of the intracellular fluid. Roughly 98 per cent of the potassium content of the body lies within the ICF. The potassium concentration of the ECF, which is relatively low represents a balance between (1) the rate of entry across the digestive epithelium and (2) the rate of loss into the urine. The rate of entry is proportional to the amount of potassium in the diet. Urinary potassium losses are controlled by adjusting the rate of active secretion along the distal convoluted tubules of the kidneys. The secondary rate is primarily determines by aldosterone levels. The ion pumps sensitive to this hormone reabsorb sodium ions from the filtrate is exchange for potassium ions from the interstitial fluid. When potassium levels rise in the ECF, aldosterone levels climb and additional potassium ions are lost in the urine. When potassium levels fall in the ECF aldosterone levels fall, and potassium ions are conserved.

Acid-Base Balance

The pH of body fluids represents a balance between the acids and bases and salts in solution. This pH normally remains within narrow limits, usually from 7.35 to 7.45. Any deviation outside the normal range is extremely dangerous because changes in hydrogen ion concentrations disrupt the stability of cell membranes, after protein structure and change the activities of important enzymes.

When pH falls below 7.35 a state of acidosis exist. Alkalosis exists if the pH increases above 7.45. These conditions affect all systems, but the nervous system and cardiovascular system are particularly sensitive to pH fluctuations. For example, severe acidosis can be deadly because (1) CNS function deteriorates and the individual becomes comatose, (2) cardiac contractions grow weak and irregular and symptoms of heart failure develop, and (3) peripheral vasodilation produces a drop in blood pressure, and circulatory collapse may occur.

Acids in the body

Carbon dioxide concentration is the most important factor affecting the pH in body tissues. In solution carbon dioxide interacts with water to form molecules of carbonic acid (H_2Co_3). The carbonic acid molecules dissociate to produce hydrogen ions and bicarbonate ions. The complete reactions is :

$$CO_2 + H_2O \rightleftharpoons H_2CO_3 \rightleftharpoons H^+ + HCO_3^-$$

The reaction occurs spontaneously in body fluids, but it occurs very rapidly in the presence of carbonic anhydrase, an intracellular enzyme found in red blood cells, liver and kidney cell, parietal cells of the stomach and in other cell types.

Because most of the carbon dioxide in solution is converted to carbonic acid and most of the carbonic acid dissociates, there is a direct relationship between the Pco_2 and the pH. When carbon dioxide concentrations rise, additional hydrogen ions and bicarbonate ions are released and the PH goes down.

At the alveoli, carbon dioxide diffuses into the atmosphere, the number of hydrogen ions and bicarbonate ions declines and the pH rises. Metabolic acids are generated during normal metabolism. Some are generated during the catabolism of amino acids, carbohydrates or lipids.

Buffers and Buffer Systems

The acids produced in the course of normal metabolic operations must be controlled by the buffers and buffer systems in body fluids. Buffers are dissolved compounds that can provide or remove hydrogen ions and thereby stabilize the pH of a solution. Buffers include weak acids that can donate hydrogen ions and weak bases that can absorb them. A buffer system consists of a combination of a weak acid and its association products, a hydrogen ion (H^+) and an anion. There are three major buffer systems, each with slightly different characteristics and distribution.

Protein buffer systems contribute to the regulation of pH in the ECF and ICF protein buffer systems, depend on the ability of amino acids to respond to alterations in pH by accepting or releasing hydrogen ions. If the pH climbs, the carboxyl group (–COOH) of the amino acid can dissociate, releasing a hydrogen ion. If the pH drops, the amino group ($-NH_2$) can accept an additional hydrogen ion forming an $^-NH_3^+$ group.

The plasma proteins and hemoglobin in red blood cells make substantial contributions to the buffering capabilities of the blood. In the interstitial fluids, extracellular protein fibres and dissolved amino acids also help to regulate pH. In the intracellular fluids of active cells structural and other proteins provide an extensive buffering capability that prevents destructive pH changes when organic acids are produced by cellular metabolism.

The carbonic acid-bicarbonate buffer system is an important buffer system in the ECF. Carbon dioxide generation occurs in all living tissues, most of it is converted to carbonic acid, which then dissociates into a hydrogen ion and bicarbonate ion. The net effect is that $CO_2 + H_2O + \rightleftharpoons H^+ + HCO_3^-$. The carbonic acid and its dissociation products form the carbonic acid-bicarbonate buffer system. If hydrogen ions are removed, they will be replaced through the combination of water and carbon dioxide, if hydrogen ions are added, most will be removed through the formation of carbon dioxide and water.

The primary rôle of the carbonic acid-bicarbonate buffer system is to prevent pH changes caused by metabolic acids. The hydrogen ions released through the dissociation of these acids combine with bicarbonate ions, producing water and carbon dioxide. The carbon dioxide can then be excreted at the lungs. This buffering system can cope with large amounts of acid because body fluids contain an abundance of bicarbonate ions, primarily in the form of dissolved molecules of sodium bicarbonate, $NaHCO_3$. This readily available supply of bicarbonate ions is known on the bicarbonate reserve when hydrogen ions enter the ECF, the bicarbonate ions that combine with them are replaced by the carbonate reserve.

The phosphate buffer system consists of an anion H_2PO_4, that is a weak acid. In solution it reversibly dissociates into a hydrogen ion and HPO_4^-. In the ECF, the phosphate buffer system plays only a supporting role in the regulation of pH, primarily because the concentration of bicarbonate ions far exceeds that of phosphate ions. However, the phosphate buffer system is quite important in buffering the pH of the intracellular fluids, where the concentration of phosphate ions is relatively high.

Maintenance of acid-base balance

The maintenance of acid-base balance involves controlling hydrogen ions losses and gains. In this process, the pulmonary and renal mechanisms support the buffer system by (1) secreting or absorbing hydrogen ions, (2) controlling the excretion of acids and bases, and when necessary (3) generating additional buffers. It is the combination of buffer systems and these pulmonary and renal mechanisms that maintains pH within narrow limits.

Pulmonary contributions to pH regulation

The lungs contribute to pH regulation by their effects on the carbonic acid-bicarbonate buffer system. Increasing or decreasing the rate of respiration can have an effect on the buffering capacity of body fluids by lowering or raising the PCO_2 changes, PCO_2 have a direct effect on the concentration of hydrogen ions in the plasma. Since the additional carbon dioxide molecules will form carbonic acid which immediately dissociates.

A rise in PCO_2 stimulates chemoreceptors in the carotid and aortic bodies and within the CNS a fall in the PCO_2 inhibits them. Stimulation of the chemoreceptors leads to an increase in the respiratory rate. As the rate of respiration increases more CO_2 is lost at the lungs and the PCO_2 returns to normal levels. When the PCO_2 of the blood or CSF declines, respiratory activity becomes depressed, the breathing rate falls and the PCO_2 in the extracellular fluids rises.

Changes in respiratory rate affect pH because when the PCO_2 rises, the pH declines and when the PCO_2 decreases, the PH increases. A change in the respiratory rate that helps stabilize PH is called respiratory compensation.

Renal contributions to pH regulation

Glomerular filtration puts hydrogen ions, carbon dioxide and the other components of the carbonic acid-bicarbonate and phosphate buffer systems into the filtrate. The kidney tubules then modify the pH of the filtrate by secreting hydrogen ions or reabsorbing bicarbonate ions. A change in the rates of hydrogen ion and bicarbonate ion secretion or absorption in response to changes in plasma pH is called renal compensation.

(5)

Muscular System

The three types of muscle tissue are skeletal, cardiac and smooth. These muscle tissues differ in the structure of their cells, their body location their function and the means by which they are activated to contract. Skeletal and smooth muscle cells are elongated, for this reason are called muscle fibres. Muscle contraction depends on two kinds of myofilaments, actin or myosin.

Skeletal muscle tissue is packaged into the skeletal muscles that attach to and cover the bony skeleton. Skeletal fibres are the largest of the muscle cell types have stripes called striations and can be controlled voluntarily. Although it is often activated by reflexes without our willed "command" skeletal muscle is called voluntary muscle. Skeletal muscle can contract rapidly, but it tires easily and must rest after short periods of activity.

Cardiac muscle tissue occurs only in the heart, where it constitutes the bulk of the heart walls. Like skeletal muscle, cardiac muscle is striated, but it is not voluntary. Cardiac muscle usually contracts at a steady rate set by the heart's pacemaker.

Smooth muscle tissue is found in the wall of hollow visceral organs such as on the stomach, urinary bladder, and respiratory passages. Its role is to force fluids and other substances through internal body channels. It has no striations and like cardiac muscle it is not subject to voluntary control.

Muscle Functions

All movements of the human body and its parts are a result of muscle contraction. Skeletal muscles are responsible for all locomotion and manipulation and they enable to respond quickly to changes in the external environment.

The coursing of blood through body reflects the work of the rhythmically beating cardiac muscle of heart and the smooth muscle in the walls of blood vessels, which helps to maintain blood pressure. Smooth muscle in organs of the digestive, urinary and reproductive tracts propels substances through the organs and along the tract.

Maintaining Posture : Skeletal muscle maintain body posture that enables us to maintain an erect or seated posture despite the never ending downward pull of gravity.

Stabilizing Joints : Even as muscles pull on bones to cause movements, they stabilize the joints of the skeleton.

Generating Heat : Muscles generate heat as they contract. This heat is important in maintaining normal body temperature.

Support Soft Tissues : The abdominal wall and the floor of the pelvic cavity consist of layers of muscle that support the weight of visceral organs and shield internal tissues from injury.

Guard Entrances and Exits : Skeletal muscles guard openings to the digestive and urinary tracts and provide voluntary control over swallowing, defaecating and urination.

Functional characteristics of Muscle

1. Excitability or Irritability : It is the ability to receive and respond to a stimulus. A stimulus is an environmental change, it may arise either inside or outside the body. In the case of muscle the stimulus is usually a chemical for example a neurotransmitter released by a nerve cell, a hormone or a local change in pH. The response is generating of an electrical impulse that passes along the sarcolemma and causes the muscle cells to contract.

2. Contractility : It is the ability to shorten actively when adequately stimulated. This property sets muscle apart from all other tissue types.

3. Extensibility : It is the ability to be stretched or extended. Muscle fibres shorten when contracting, but they can be stretched, even beyond their resting length, when relaxed.

4. Elasticity : It is the ability of a muscle fibre to recoil and resume its resting length after being stretched.

The anatomy of Skeletal Muscle

Each skeletal muscle is made up of several kinds of tissues. A skeletal muscle contains blood vessels, nerve fibres, connective tissues and skeletal muscle tissues.

Connective tissue organization

The individual muscle fibres are held together by several different layers of connective tissue.

1. Epimysium : "An overcoat" of dense irregular connective tissue surrounds the whole muscle. This coat is the epimysium, a layer of collagen fibres that separates the muscle from surrounding tissues and organs.

At each end of the muscle, the epimysial fibres come together to form tendons that attach skeletal muscles to bone. Any contraction of the muscle will exert a pull on its tendon and in turn on the attached bone.

2. Perimysium and Fascicles : Within each skeletal muscle, the muscle fibres are grouped into fascicles that resemble bundles of sticks. Surrounding each fascicle in a layer of fibrous connective tissue called perimysium. In addition to collagen and elastic fibres, the perimysium contains blood vessels and nerves that supply the fascicles.

3. Endomysium : Within a fascicle, each muscle fibre is surrounded by a fine sheath of connective tissue consisting mostly of reticular fibres. This is the endomysium. The endomysium surrounds each skeletal muscle fibres and lies adjacent muscle fibres together.

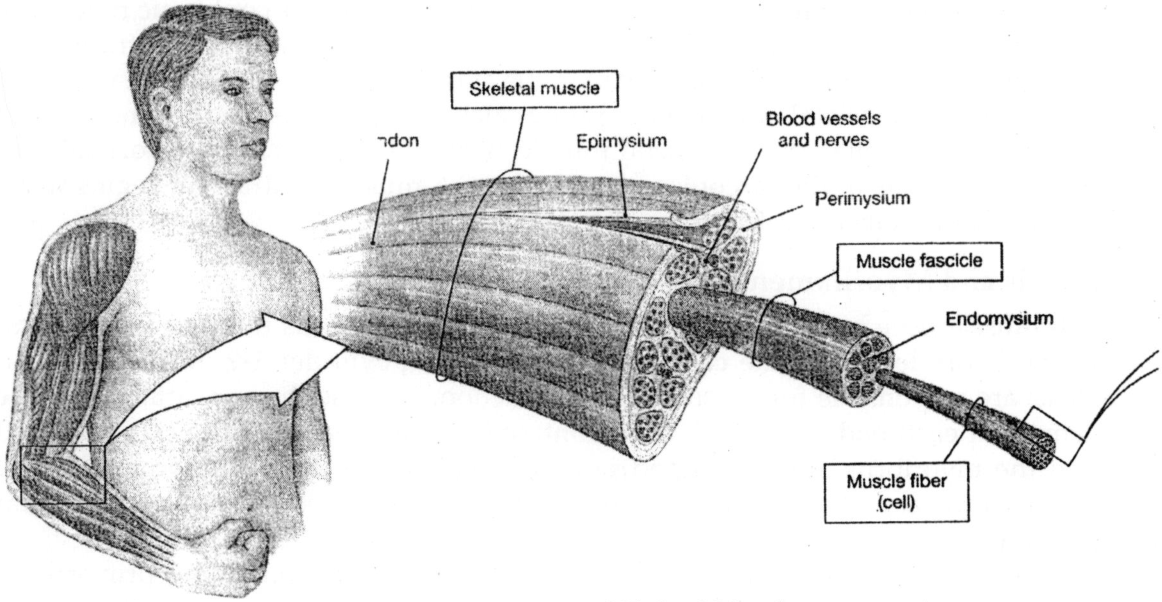

Fig. 5.1 : Organization of Skeletal Muscles

Nerve and blood supply

The normal activity of a skeletal muscle is absolutely dependent on nerves and its rich blood supply. In general, each muscle is served by one nerve, an artery and one or more veins, all of which enter or exit near the central part of the muscle and branched through its connective tissue septa. Each skeletal muscle fibre is controlled by a motor neuron whose cell body lies within the central nervous system. Axons, or nerve fibres of the motor neurons involved with a particular skeletal muscle penetrate the epimysium, branch through the perimysium and enter the endomysium to control individual muscle fibres. Since muscle contraction requires a tremendous amount of energy, network of blood vessels delivers the oxygen and nutrients needed for the production of ATP in active skeletal muscles.

A skeletal muscle fibre from a leg muscle could have a diameter of 100 μm and a length equal to that of the entire muscle (30-40 cm or 10-16 in). Each skeletal muscle fibre is multinucleate, containing hundreds of nuclei just beneath the cell membrane. The cell membrane or sarcolemma of a muscle fibre surrounds the cytoplasm, or sarcoplasm openings scattered across the surface of the sarcolemma lead into a network of narrow tubules called transverse tubules or T tubules. They are filled with extracellular fluid and they form passage ways through the muscle fibre like a series of tunnels. The T tubules play a major role in coordinating the contraction of the muscle fibre.

The sarcoplasm contains unusual large amounts of glycosomes, (stored glycogen) and oxygen-binding protein called myoglobin that is not found in other cell types. Myoglobin a red pigment that stores oxygen within the muscle cells is similar to hemoglobin. The usual organelles are present, as well as some are highly modified in muscle fibres. These are myofibrils and sarcoplasmic reticular. As a T tubule encircles a myofibril it makes close contact with expanded chambers of the sarcoplasmic reticulum. These chambers are called cisternae. These cisternae contain high concentrations of calcium ions. The calcium ion concentration in the cytoplasm of all cells is kept very low. Most cells, including skeletal muscle fibres pump calcium ions across their cell membranes and into the extracellular fluid. Skeletal muscle fibres, also actively transport calcium ions into the cisternae of the sarcoplasmic reticulum. A muscle contraction begins when the stored calcium ions are released by the cisternae.

Myofibrils and Myofilaments

Each muscle fibre contain large number of rod like myofibrils that run parallel and extend the entire length of the cell. Each myofibril is a cylinder 1-2 μm in diameter, myofibrils are responsible for muscle fibre contraction. Because they are attached to the sarcolemma at each end of the cell, their contraction shortens the entire cell. Scattered between the myofibrils are mitochondria and glycogen granules. The breakdown of glycogen and the activity of mitochondria provide the ATP needed to power muscular contraction.

Myofibrils are bundles of myofilaments, protein filaments containing primarily of proteins actin and myosin. Actin molecules are found in thin filaments and the myosin molecules are found in thick filaments. Myofilaments are organized in repeating functional units called sarcomeres.

Sarcomere Organization

The arrangement of thick and thin filament within a sarcomere produces a bonded appearance. All of the myofibrils are arranged parallel to the long axis of the cell, with their sarcomeres lying side by side. As a result the entire muscle fibre has a banded, or striated, appearance corresponding to the bonds of the individual sarcomeres.

Each myofibril consists of a linear series of approximately 10,000 sarcomeres. The sarcomere is the smallest functional unit of the muscle fibre, interactions between the thick and thin filaments of sarcomeres are responsible for muscle contraction. A repeated series of dark A bands and light I bands are evident along the length of each myofibril. In an intact muscle fibre, the A and I bands are perfectly aligned with one another and this gives the cell as a whole its striped (striated) appearance.

Each A band has a lighter stripe in its mid-section called the H zone (H stands for helle which means bright). The H zones are visible only in relaxed muscle fibres. Each H zone is bisected by a dark line called M line. The I bands also have a midline interruption a darker area called the Z disc. A sarcomere is the region of a myofibril between two successive Z discs. Thus the functional units of skeletal muscle are very minute portions of the myofibrils.

The banding pattern of a myofibril at the molecular level have arrangement of two types of smaller structures called filaments or myofilaments within the sarcomeres. The central thick filaments extend the entire length of the A band. The more lateral thin filaments extend across the I band and pathway into the A band. The Z disc also called Z-line composed of proteins called connection. The Z disc anchors the thin filaments and also connects each myofibril to the next throughout the width of the muscle cell. The H zone of the A band appears less dense because the thin filaments do not overlap the thick ones in this region. The M line in the centre of the H zone is slightly darker because of the presence of fine protein (desmin) strands that hold adjacent thick filaments together in that area.

Ultrastructure and Molecular Composition of the Myofilaments

Thick filaments are composed primarily of the protein myosin. Each myosin molecule has a rod like tail terminating in two globular heads. The tail consists of two heavy polypeptide chains, its heads are the ends of the heavy chains, each made of "fat" by the attachment of two smaller light polypeptide chains. Sometimes called cross- bridges. The heads of myosin link the thick and thin myofilaments together during contraction. Each thick filament within a sarcomere contains about 200 myosin molecules. The myosin molecules are bundled together with their tails forming the central part of the filament and their heads facing outward and in opposite directions at each end. As a result, the central portion of a thick filament is smooth. The heads of myosin molecules contain ATP to generate energy for muscle contraction.

The thin filaments are composed chiefly of actin. The polypeptide sub-units of actin, called globular actin or G actin, bear the active sites to which the myosin cross-bridges attach during contraction. The G actin monomers are polymerized into long actin filaments. The backbone of each thin filament appears to be formed by an actin filament that coils back on itself. Forming a helical structure several regulatory proteins are also present in the thin filament. In a resting muscle, the active sites along the thin filaments are covered by strands of the protein tropomyosin. The tropomyosin strands are held in position by molecules of troponin that are bound to the actin strand.

Sliding filament mechanism of contraction

The sliding filament theory of muscle contraction, proposed in 1954 by Hugh Huxley, states that during contraction, the thin filaments slide past the thick ones so that the actin and myosin filaments overlaps to a greater degree. In a relaxed muscle fibre, the thick and thin filaments overlap only slightly. But when muscle fibres are stimulated adequately by the nervous system the cross bridges made on to myosin binding sites on actin in the thin filaments and the sliding begins. The sliding occurs through interactions between the thick and thin filaments. It begins when the myosin heads of thick filaments bind to active sites on thin filaments. When they connect thick filaments and thin filaments, the myosin heads are called cross-bridges. When cross-bridge binds to an active site, it pivots toward the centre of the sarcomere, pulling the thin filament in that direction. The cross-bridge then detaches and returns to its original position, ready to repeat a cycle of "attach, pivot, detach, and return". Overall, the distance between successive Z discs is reduced, the I bands shortens, the H zones disappear and the A bands move closer together but do not change in length.

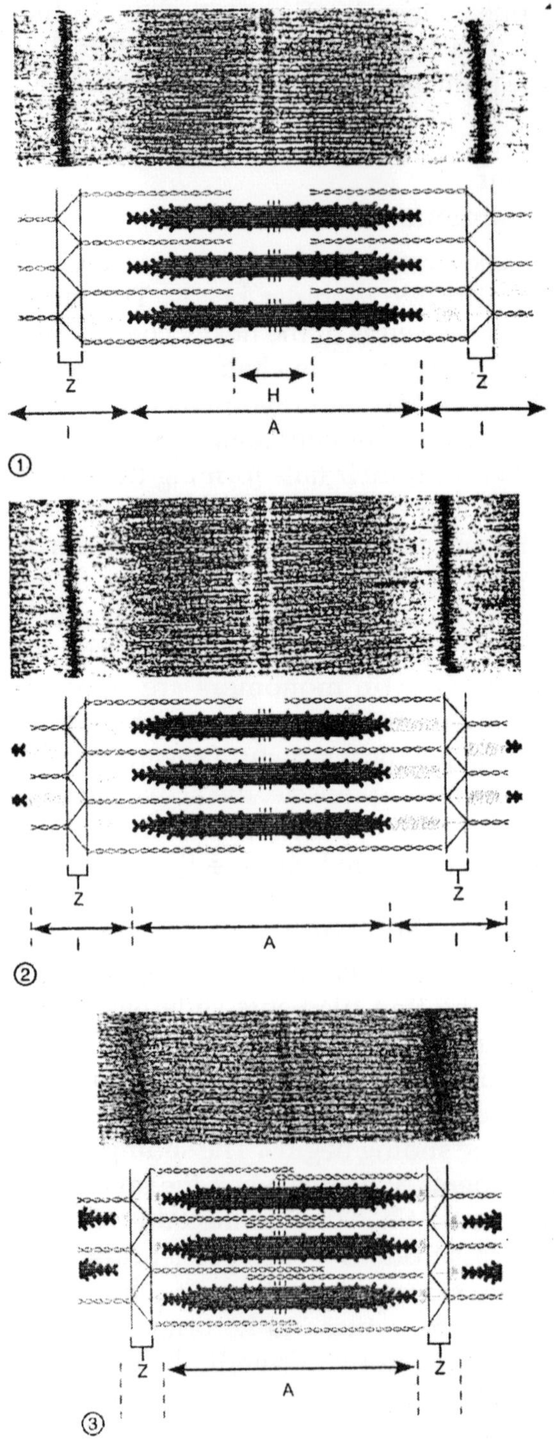

Fig. 5.2 Sliding Filament Model of Contraction

Cross-bridge attachment to actin requires calcium ions, and the nerve impulse leading to contraction causes an increase in calcium ions within the muscle cell. When intracellular calcium levels are low, the muscle cell is relaxed, and the active (myosin binding) sites on actin once physically blocked by troptomyosin molecules. As calcium ions become available they bind to regulatory sites on troponin, coming it to change shape. This event moves tropomyosin deeper into the groove of the actin helix and away from the myosin binding sites. Thus, the tropomyosin "blockage" is removed when calcium is present.

Once binding sites on actin are exposed, the following events occur in rapid succession:

1. Cross-Bridge Attachment : The activated myosin heads are strongly attracted to the exposed binding sites on actin and cross-bridge attachment occurs.

2. The Working (Power) Stroke : As a myosin head binds it pivots, changing from its high energy configuration to its bent low-energy shape, which pulls on the thin filament,

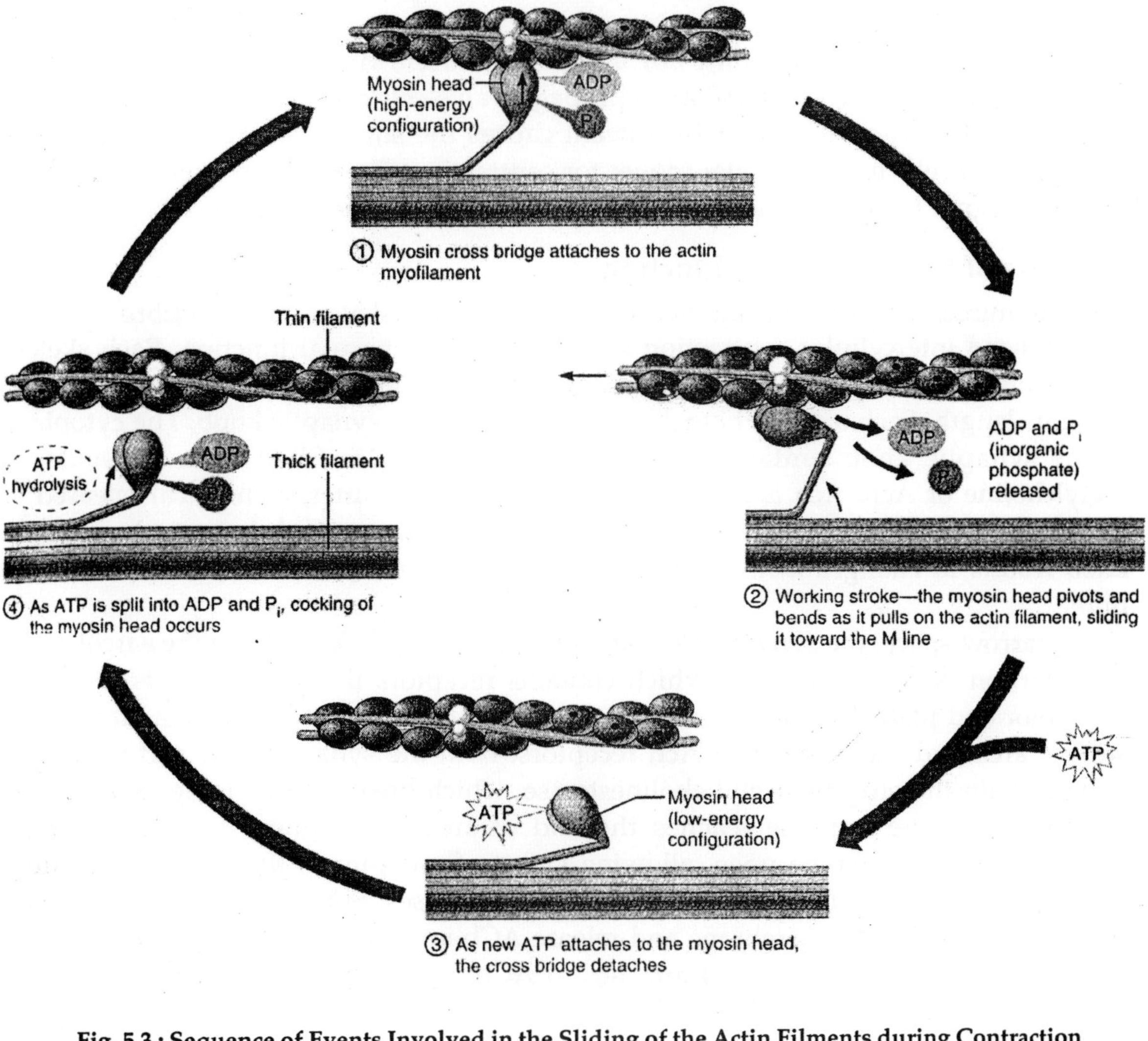

Fig. 5.3 : Sequence of Events Involved in the Sliding of the Actin Filments during Contraction

sliding it toward the centre of the sarcomere. At the same time ADP and inorganic phosphate (Pi) generated during the prior contraction cycle are released from the myosin head.

3. Cross-Bridge detachment : As a new ATP molecule binds to the myosin head, myosin's hold on actin loosen and cross-bridge detaches from actin.

4. "Cocking" of the Myosin head : Hydrolysis of ATP to ADP and Pi by ATPase provides the energy needed to return the myosin head to its high energy or "cocked" position. This provides the potential energy needed for its next sequence of attachment and working stroke. At this point the cycle is back where it started. The myosin head is in its upright high energy configuration, ready to take another "step" and attach to an actin site along the thin filament. Some myosin heads are always in contact with actin so that the thin filaments cannot slide backward as this cycle is repeated again and again during contraction.

Regulation of Contraction : For a skeletal muscle fibre to contract, it must be stimulated by a nerve ending and must propagate an electrical current or action potential along its sarcolemma. This electrical event causes the short-lived rise in intracellular calcium ion levels that is the final trigger for contraction. The series of events linking the electrical signal to contraction is called excitation- contraction coupling.

Structure of Neuromuscular Junction

Communication between the nervous system and a skeletal muscle fibre occurs at a specialized intercellular contraction known as neuromuscular junction. Each skeletal muscle fibre is controlled by a motor neuron at a single neuromuscular junction midway along its length. Each axon or branch of an axon ends at a synaptic knob. The cytoplasm of the synaptic knob contains mitochondria and vesicles filled with molecules of acetylcholine or Ach. Ach is an example of a neurotransmitter, a chemical released by a neuron to change the activities of other cells. The release of Ach from the synaptic knob results in changes in the sarcolemma that trigger the contraction of the muscle fibre.

A narrow space, the synaptic cleft separates the synaptic knob from the sarcolemma. This portion of the membrane, which contains receptors that bind Ach, is known as the motor end plate. The motor end plate has deep creases that increase the membrane surface area and the number of Ach receptors. Both the synaptic cleft and moter end plate contain the enzyme acetyl cholinesterase, which breaks down molecules of ACh.

When a nerve impulse reaches the end of an axon voltage regulated calcium channels in its membrane open, allowing Ca^{2+} to flow, inform the extracellular fluid. The presence of calcium inside the axon terminal causes. Some of the synaptic vesicle to fuse with the axonal membrane and release ACh into the synaptic cleft by exocytosis ACh diffuses across the left and attaches to ACh receptors on the Sarcolemma.

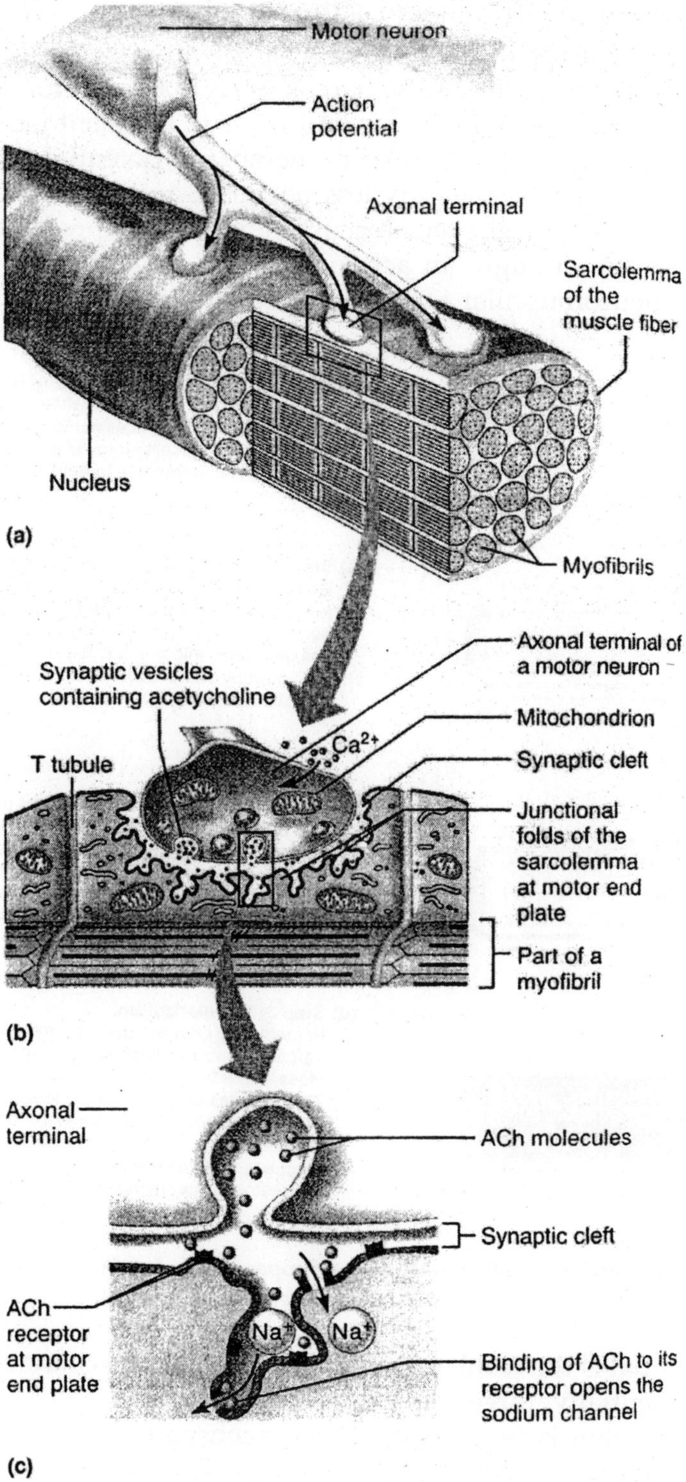

Fig. 5.4 : The Neuromuscular Junction

Generation of an action potential across the sarcolemma

Like plasma membranes of all cells, a resting sarcolemma is polarized. The binding of ACh molecules to ACh receptors on the Sarcolemma opens chemically regulated Na^+ channels housed within the ACh receptors and leads to transient permeability changes in the Sarcolemma. The result is a change in membrane potential. (voltage). Such that the muscle cell interior becomes slightly less negative, an event called depolarization. Initially depolarization is a local event (occurring only at the receptor site), but if the nerve stimulus is strong enough, an action potential is generated that passes in all directions from the neuromuscular junction across the Sarcolemma.

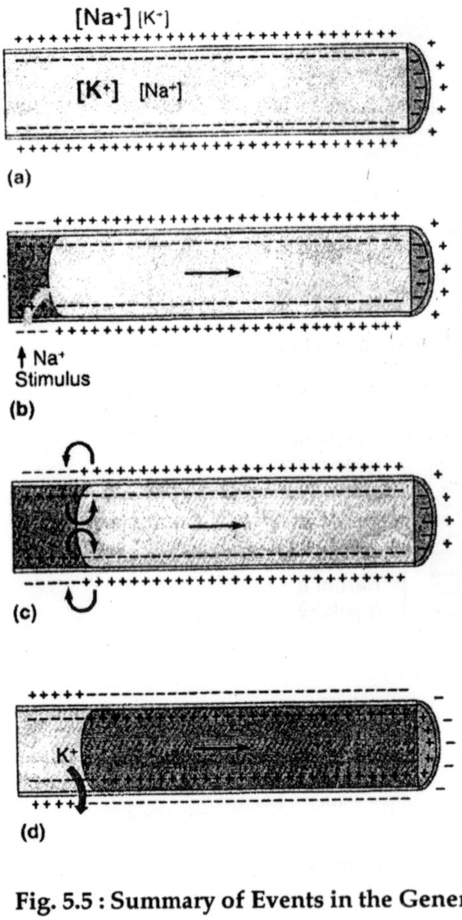

(a) Electrical conditions of a resting (polarized) sarcolemma. The outside face is positive, while the inside face is negative. The predominant extracellular ion is sodium (Na^+); the predominant intracellular ion is potassium (K^+). The sarcolemma is relatively impermeable to both ions.

(b) Step 1: Depolarization and generation of the action potential. Stimulation by a motor nerve fiber (via the release of acetylcholine) causes that patch of sarcolemma to become permeable to sodium (sodium channels open). As sodium ions diffuse rapidly into the cell, the resting potential is decreased (i.e., depolarization occurs). If the stimulus is strong enough, an action potential is initiated.

(c) Step 2: Propagation of the action potential. The positive charge inside the initial patch of sarcolemma changes the permeability of an adjacent patch, opening voltage-regulated Na^+ channels there. Consequently the membrane potential in that region decreases and depolarization occurs there as well. Thus, the action potential travels rapidly over the entire sarcolemma.

(d) Step 3: Repolarization. Immediately after the depolarization wave passes, the sarcolemma's permeability changes once again: Na^+ channels close and K^+ channels open, allowing K^+ to diffuse from the cell. This restores the electrical conditions of the resting (polarized) state. Repolarization occurs in the same direction as depolarization, and must occur before the muscle fiber can be stimulated again. The ionic concentrations of the resting state are restored later by the sodium-potassium pump.

Fig. 5.5 : Summary of Events in the Generation and Propagation of an Action Potential in a Skeletal Muscle Fibre

The action potential is the result of a sequence of electrical changes that occurs along the sarcolemma. Essentially, three steps are involved :

1. First, the membrane is depolarized. This is a consequence of sodium (Na^+) channels opening and Na^+ entering the cell.
2. During step 2, the action potential is propogated as the local depolarization wave

spreads to the adjacent areas of the sarcolemma and opens voltage regulated sodium channels there. Sodium ions, normally restricted from entering, now diffuse into the cell following their electrochemical gradient.

3. Step 3 is repolarization, which restores the sarcolemma to its initial polarized state. The repolarization wave, which quickly follows the depolarization wave, is a consequence of Na^+ channels closing and K^+ channels opening. Since the potassium ion concentration is higher inside the cell than in the extracellular fluid, K^+ diffuses rapidly out of the muscle fibre.

During repolarization, a muscle fibre is said to be in a refractory period, because the cell cannot be stimulated again until repolarization is complete. Notice that repolarization only restores electrical conditions of the resting (polarized) state. The ATP dependent Na^+ K^+ pump must be "revived up" to restore the ionic conditions of the resting state, but Several contractions can occur before ionic imbalance interfere with contractile activity.

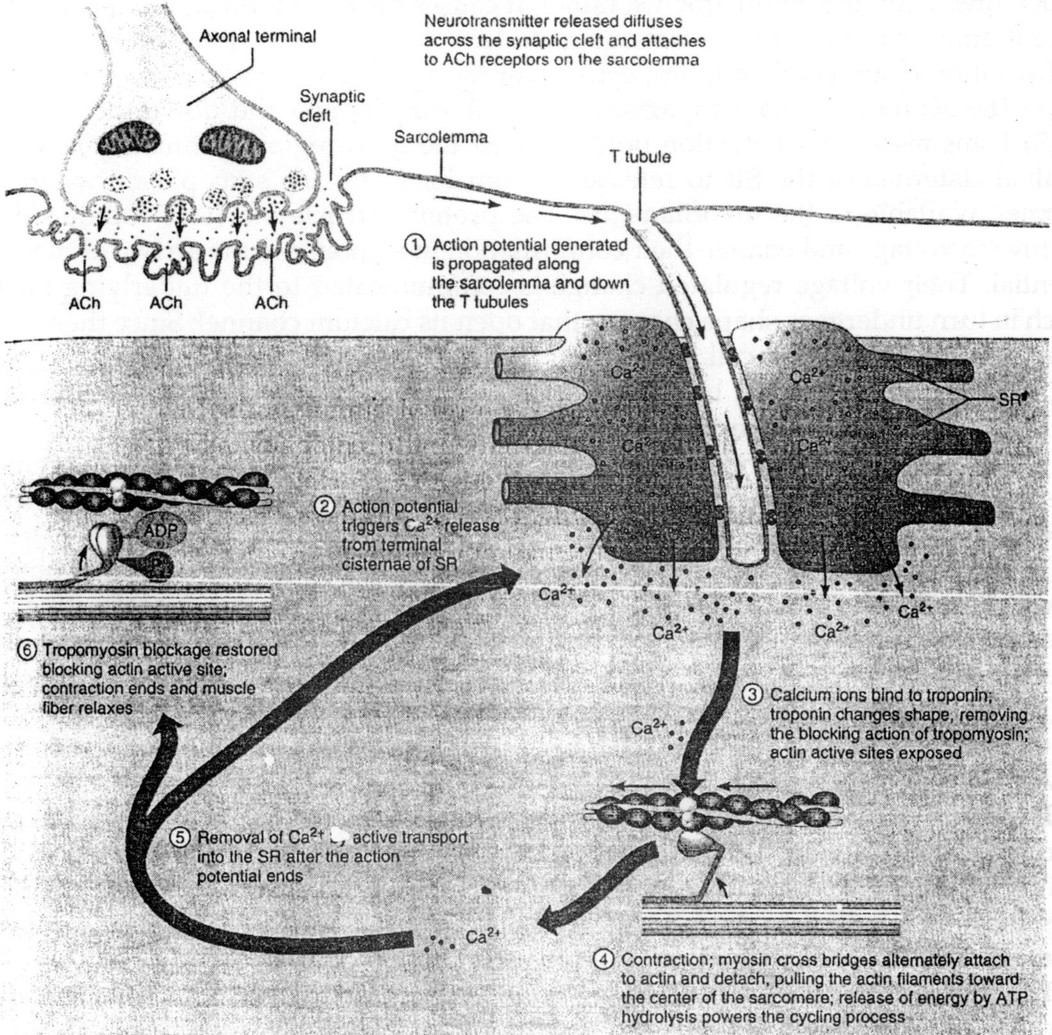

Fig. 5.6 : Sequence of Events in Excitation-Contraction Coupling

Once initiated, the action potential is instoppable and ultimately results in contraction of the muscle cell.

Destruction of acetylcholine : After ACh is released from the motor neuron and binds to the ACh receptors, it is swiftly destroyed by acetylcholinesterase or AChE, an enzyme located on the sarcolemma at the neuromuscular junction and in the synaptic cleft. This prevents continued muscle fibre contraction in the absence of additional nervous system stimulation.

Excitation-Contraction coupling : Excitation contraction coupling is the sequence of events by which transmission of an action potential along the sarcolemma leads to the sliding of myofilaments. The action potential is very brief and ends well before any signs of contraction are obvious. The period from action potential initiation to the beginning of mechanical activity (shortening) is called the latent period (laltent=hidden). The events of excitation-contraction coupling occur during this period. As, the electrical signal does not act directly on the myofilaments, rather, it causes the rise in intracellular calcium ion concentration that allows the filaments to slide.

Excitation contraction coupling consists of the following steps:

(1) The action potential propagates along the sarcolemma and down the T tubules.

(2) Transmission of the action potential part the triad regions ultimately causes the terminal cisternae of the SR to release calcium ions into the sarcoplasm, where Ca^{2+} becomes available to the myofilaments. The protein particle on the T tubule side are sensitive to voltage and change their conformation in response to the arrival of the action potential. Their voltage regulated change is communicated to the underlying SR foot, which in turn undergoes shape changes that open its calcium channel. Since these events occur at every triad in the cell.

(3) Some of this calcium binds to troponin, which changes shape and removes the blocking action of tropomyosin.

(4) The myosin cross-bridges attach and pull the thin filaments toward the center of the sarcomere. This occurs when the intracellular calcium is present at a concentration of 10^{-5}M.

(5) The short-lived calcium signal ends usually within 30 ms after the action potential is over. The fall in calcium levels reflects the operation of a continually active, ATP dependent calcium pump that moves calcium back into the tubules of the SR to be stored once again.

(6) When intracellular calcium levels drop too low to allow contraction, the tropomyosin blockade is re established and myosin ATPases are inhibited. Cross-bridge activity ends and relaxation occurs.

The entire sequence of events is repeated when another nerve impulse arrives at the neuromuscular junction. When the impulses are delivered very rapidly, intracellular calcium levels, increase greatly due to successive release of calcium from the SR. In such cases, the muscle cells do not completely relax between successive stimuli and contraction is stronger and more sustained until serious stimulation ceases.

The Motor Unit : Each muscle is served by at least one motor nerve, which contains hundreds of moter neuron axons. As an axon enters a muscle, each of which forms a neuromuscular junction with a single muscle fibres it supplies is called a motor unit when a moter neuron transmits an electrical impulse, all the muscle fibres, that it innervates respond by contracting. The number of muscle fibres per motor unit may be as high as several hundred or as few as four muscles that exert very fine control (such as the muscles controlling movements of the fingers and eyes) have small motor units. Otherwise large, weight bearing muscles, whose movements are less precise (such as the hip muscles), have large motor units. The muscle fibres in a single motor unit are not clustered together but are spread throughout the muscle. As a result, stimulation of a single motor units causes a weak contraction of the entire muscle.

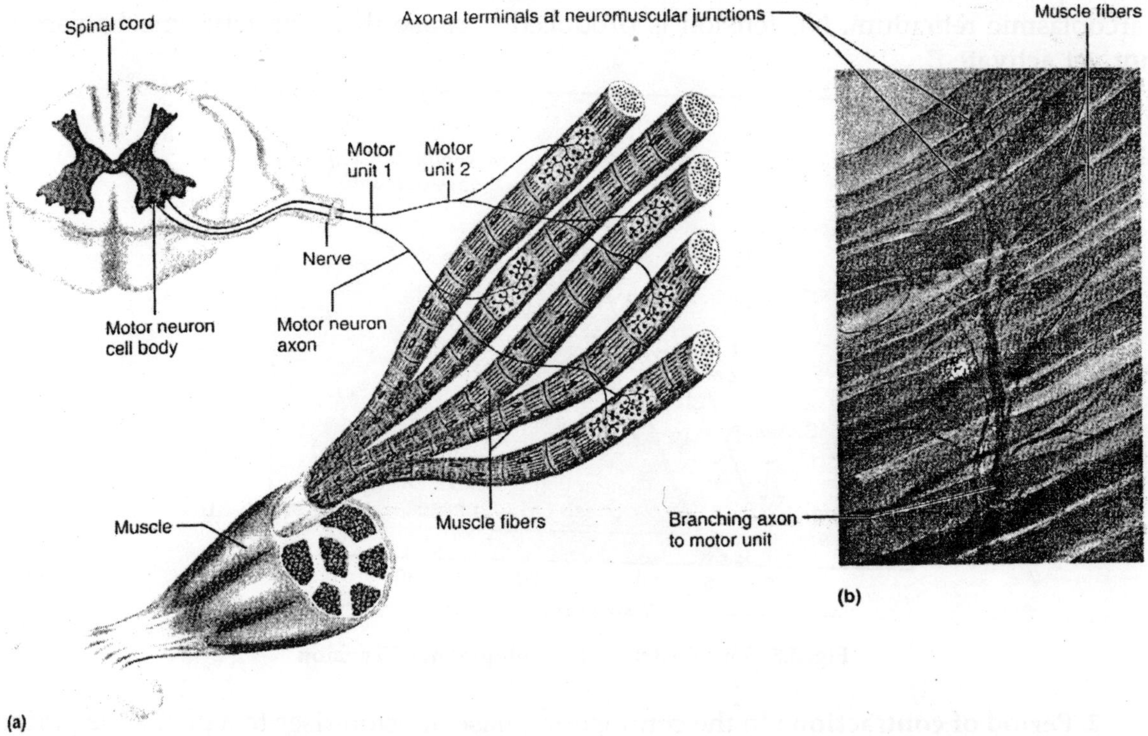

Fig. 5.7 : Motor Units

Muscle mechanics

The amount of tension produced by an individual muscle fibre depends on the number of cross-bridge interactions. If a muscle fibre at a given resting length is stimulated to contract, it will always produce the same amount of tension. There is no mechanism to regulate the amount of tension produced in that contraction. The muscle fibre is either "ON" (producing tension) or "OFF" (relaxed). This is known as the all-or-none principle.

An entire skeletal muscle contracts when its component muscle fibres are stimulated. The amount of tension produced in the skeletal muscle as a whole is determined by (1) the frequency of stimulation and (2) the number of muscle fibres activated.

The Muscle twitch and development of muscle tension

A muscle twitch is a single stimulus-contraction-relaxation sequence in a muscle fibre, i.e. the response of a muscle to a single brief threshold stimulus is called a muscle twitch. The muscle contracts quickly and then relaxed. A twitch may be strong or weak, depending on the number of motor units activated, but in any twitch myogram or graph three phases are seen.

1. Latent period : The latent period is the first few milliseconds following stimulation when excitation-contraction coupling is occurring. During this period, muscle tension is beginning to increase but no response is seen on the myogram. Over this period the action potential sweeps across the sarcolemma, and calcium ions are released by the sarcoplasmic reticulum. No tension is produced because the contractile mechanism is not yet activated.

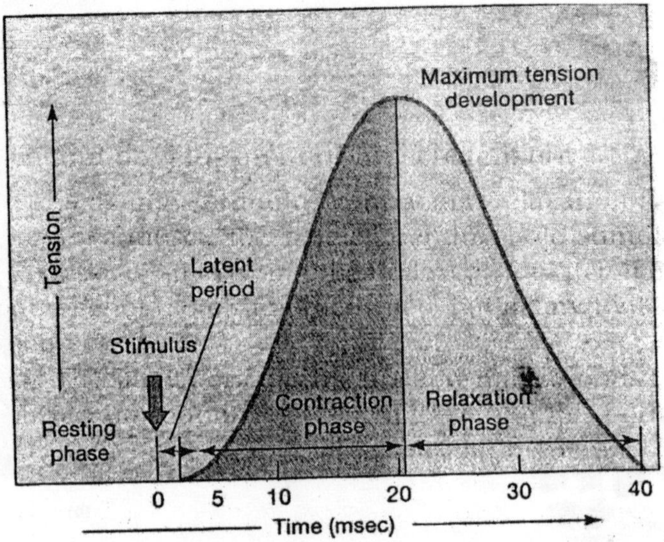

Fig. 5.8 : The Twitch and Development of Tension

2. Period of contraction : In the contraction phase, tension rises to a peak. The period of contraction is when cross-bridges are active, from the onset to the peak of tension development. Throughout this period the cross-bridges are interacting with the active sites on the actin filaments.

3. Period of relaxation : The period of contraction is followed by the period of relaxation. During the relaxation phase the muscle tension falls to resting levels as the cross-bridges detach.

Muscle response to frequency of stimulation wave summation and tetanus : If two identical stimuli (electrical shocks or nerve impulses) are delivered to a muscle in rapid succession the second twitch will be stranger than first. On the myogram it will appear to ride on the shoulders of the first contraction. This phenomenon, called wave, or temporal, summation occurs because a second contraction occurs before the muscle has completely relaxed. Since the muscle is already partially contracted and more calcium

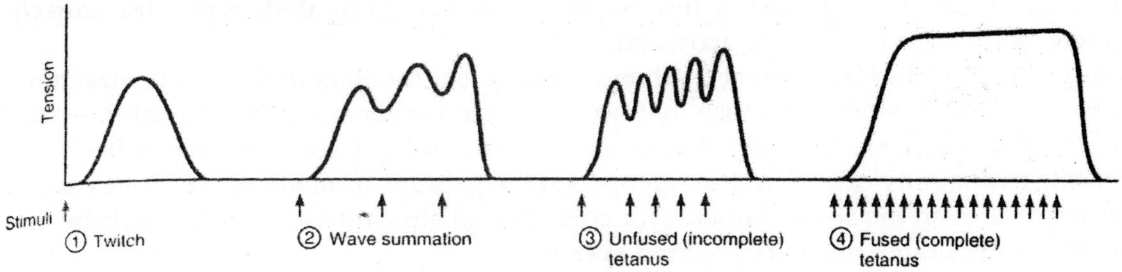

Fig. 5.9 : Wave Summation and Tetanus

is being released to replace tension produced during the second contraction causes more shortening than first. In other words, the contractions are summed. If the stimulus strength or voltage is held constant and the muscle is stimulated at an increasingly faster rate, the relaxation time between the twitches become shorter and shorter, the concentration of Ca^{2+} in the sarcoplasm higher and higher and the degree of summation greater and greater, progressing to a sustained but quivering contraction referred to as unfused or incomplete tetanus. Finally, all evidence of muscle relaxation disappears and the contractions fuse into a smooth, sustained contraction, called fused or complete tetanus.

Complete tetanus can be obtained by increasing the rate of stimulation until the relaxation phase is completely eliminated. In complete tetanus the action potentials are arriving so fast that the sarcoplasmic reticulum does not have time to reclaim the calcium ions. The high calcium ion concentration in the cytoplasm prolongs the state of contraction, making it continues. Mostly all normal muscular contractions involve the complete tetanus of the participating muscle units.

Muscle response to stronger stimuli-multiple motor unit summation : We have a remarkable ability to control the amount of tension exerted by our skeletal muscles. During a normal movement, our muscles contract smoothly, not jerkily, because activated muscle fibres are responding in complete tetanus. The total force exerted by the muscle as a whole depends on how many muscle fibres are activated.

A typical skeletal muscle contains thousands of muscle fibres. Although some motor neurons control a single muscle fibre most control hundreds or thousands of muscle fibres through multiple synaptic knobs. All of the muscle fibres controlled by a single motor neuron constitute a motor unit.

The size of a motor unit indicates how fine the control of movement can be, when a decision is made to perform a specific movement a specific groups of motor neurons within the central nervous system are stimulated. The stimulated neurons do not respond spontaneously and overtime the number of activated motor units gradually increases. The smooth but steady increase in muscular tension produced by increasing the number of active motor units is called recruitment. The stimulus at which the first observable muscle contraction occurs is called the threshold stimulus peak tension production occurs when all of the motor units in the muscle are contracting in complete tetanus. Such contractions do not last long, however, because the muscle fibres soon use up their available energy supplies.

In weak muscle contractions, few motor units are stimulated, when the muscle contracts many motor units are activated.

Treppe - The staircase effect : When a muscle begins to contract, its contractions may be only half as strong as those that occur later in response to stimulus of the same strength. Thus the tracing shows a staircase pattern called treppe. Treppe reflects the increasing availability of Ca^{2+} in the sarcoplasm the greater numbers of Ca^{2+} ions expose more active sites on the actin filaments for cross-bridge attachment. As the muscle begins to work and liberates heat, its enzyme systems become more efficient. These factors produce a slightly stronger contraction with each successive stimulus during the initial phase of muscle activity.

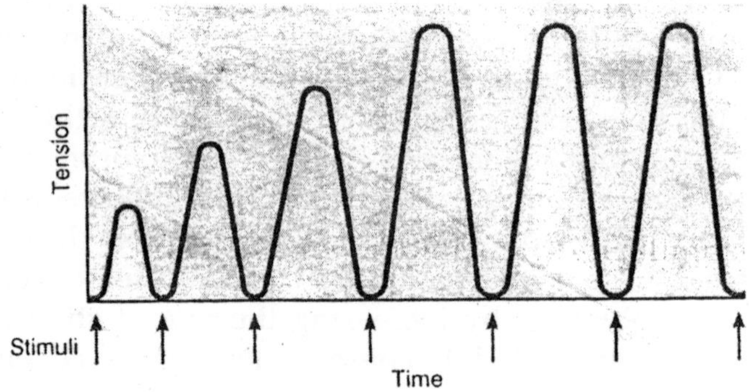

Fig. 5.10 Myogram of Treppe (the Staircase Effect)

Muscle Tone: Some of the motor units within any particular muscle are always active even when the entire muscle is not contracting. Their contractions do not produce enough tension to cause movement, but they do tense and firm the muscle. This resting tension in a skeletal muscle is called muscle tone. A muscle with little muscle tone appears limp and flacid whereas one with moderate muscle tone is quite firm and solid. This is due to spinal reflexes, that activate first one group of motor units and then another in response to activation if stretch receptors in the muscles and tendons. Muscle tone does not produce active movements, but it keeps the muscles firm, healthy and ready to respond to stimulation. Skeletal muscle tone also helps stabilize joints and maintain posture.

Isotonic and isometric contractions

Muscle contractions may be classified as isotonic or isometric on the basis of the pattern of tension production and overall change in shape. In an isotonic contraction tension rises to a level that is maintained until relaxation occurs. During such contractions, the muscle shortens on the tension in the muscle remains constant. Lifting an object of a desk, walking, running involve isotonic contractions of this kind. Once sufficient tension has developed to lift the load, the tension remains relatively constant through the rest of the contractile period.

Isotonic contractions are of two types, concentric and accentric. Concentric contractions in which the muscle shorters and does work pick up a book or kicking a ball are more familiar. However, eccentric contractions, in which the muscle contracts as it lengthens, are equally important for coordination and purposeful movements. Eccentric contractions occur in calf muscle, for example, as you walk up a long, sleep while. Eccentric contractions are about 50 per cent more forceful than concentric ones at the same load and more often cause delayed. Onset muscle soreness just why this is so is unclear, but it may be that the muscle stretching that occurs during such contractions causes microtears in the muscles.

Effective moment also requires isometric (metric = measure) contractions. In isometric contractions tension continues to increase to the muscle's peak tension producing capacity, but the muscle neither shortens or lengthens. Isometric contractions occur when a muscle attempts to move a load that is greater than the force (tension) the muscle is able to develop. Muscles that act primarily to maintain upright posture or to hold joints in stationary positions while movements occur at other joints are contracting isometrically. In our knee bend the anterior thigh muscles contract isometrically, at two points (1) when the squat position is held for a few seconds, both the anterior and posterior thigh muscles, contract isometrically to hold the knee, in the flexed position and (2) as one begins to rise to the upright position the quadriceps muscles contract isometrically until their tension exceeds the load and then muscle shortening begins. So the quadriceps contractile sequence for a deep knee bend from start to finish is (1) knee flex (eccentric), (2) hold squat position (isometric), (3) knee extend (isometric, then concentric).

Electrochemical and mechanical events occurring within a muscle are identical in both isotonic and isometric contractions. However, the result is different. In isotonic contractions, the thin filaments are sliding, in isometric contractions, the cross-bridges are generating force but are not moving the thin filaments.

The energetics of muscular activity

Muscle contraction requires large amounts of energy. For example, an active skeletal muscle fibre may require some 600 trillion molecules of ATP each second not including the energy needed to pump the calcium ions back into the sarcoplasmic reticulum. Although resting skeletal muscle cells contain large energy reserves in the form of ATP and other high energy compounds, the reserves are only enough to sustain a contraction until additional ATP can be generated. Throughout the rest of the contraction the muscle fibre will generate ATP at roughly the same rate as it is used.

ATP and CP reserves : The primary function of ATP is the transfer of energy from one location to another rather than the long-term storage of energy. At rest, a skeletal muscle fibre produces more ATP than it needs, and under these conditions ATP transfers energy to another high-energy compound, creatine phosphate (CP). During a contraction each cross-bridge breaks down ATP, producing ADP and phosphate group. The energy stored in creatine phosphate is then used to "recharge" the ADP back to ATP.

A resting skeletal muscle fibre contains about six times as much creatine phosphate as ATP. But when a muscle fibre is contracting repeatedly, both of these energy reserves will be exhausted in about 30 seconds. At such time, the muscle fibre must then rely on other mechanisms to convert ADP to ATP.

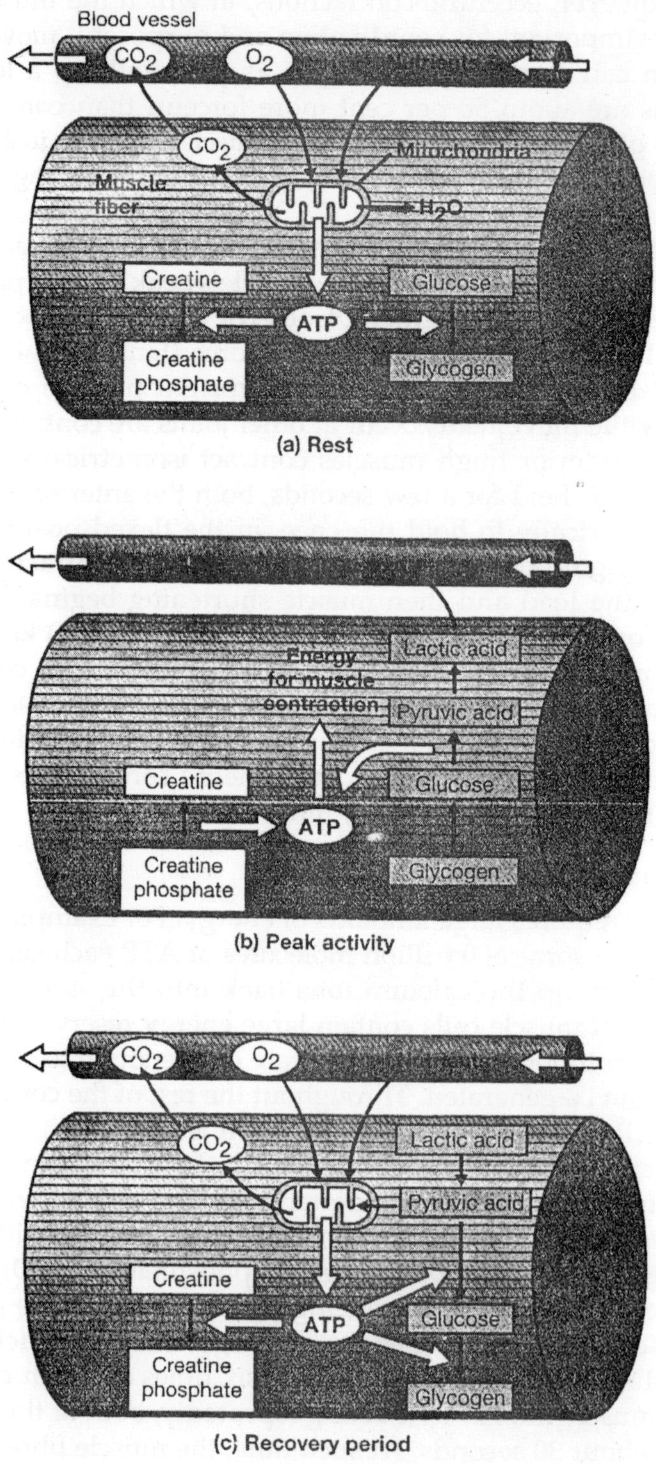

Fig. 5.11 Muscle Metabolism

ATP generation : Most cells in the body generate ATP through aerobic metabolism in mitochondria.

Aerobic metabolism : Aerobic metabolism normally provides 95 percent of the ATP needed by a resting cell. Aerobic respiration occurs in the mitochondria, requires oxygen and involves a sequence of chemical reactions in which the bonds of fuel molecules are broken and the energy released is used to make ATP. These reactions are collectively known as oxidative phosphorylation. The mitochondria absorb oxygen, ADP, phosphate ions and organic substrates from the surrounding cytoplasm. The organic substrates are carbon chains produced by disassembling carbohydrates, lipids or proteins. The absorbed molecules then enter the TCA cycle, where they are completely broken down. The carbon atoms and oxygen atoms are released as carbon dioxide (CO_2). The hydrogen atoms are shuttled to respiratory enzymes on the mitochondrial cristae, and they ultimately combine with oxygen to form water, large amounts of energy are released and used to make ATP. During aerobic respiration, glucose is broken down, yielding water, CO_2 and ATP.

Glucose + Oxygen → Carbondioxide + Water + ATP.

The carbon dioxide released diffuses out of the muscle tissue into the blood and is removed from the body by lungs. The maximum rate of ATP generation within mitochondria is limited by the availability of oxygen. A sufficient supply of oxygen becomes a problem as the energy demands of the muscle fibre increase. If muscle fibre has enough oxygen, a muscle cell will form ATP by aerobic reactions. When exercise demands begin to exceed the ability of the muscle cells to carry out the necessary reactions quickly enough, glycolysis begins to contribute more and more of the total ATP generated. If the anaerobic mechanism is allowed to continue and accelerate, it eventually and typically leads to lactic acid accumulation and muscle fatigue.

Glycolysis : Glycolysis is the breakdown of glucose to pyruvic acid in the cytoplasm of the cell. It is called an anaerobic process because it does not require oxygen. This reaction provides a net gain of 2 ATP and generates 2 molecule of pyruvic acid. The ATP yield of glycolysis is much lower than that of aerobic metabolism, the breakdown of 2 pyruvic acid molecules in mitochondria would generate 34 ATP. However, glycolysis can continue to provide ATP when the availability of oxygen limits mitochandrial activity. During glycolysis, glucose is broken down to two pyruvic acid molecules and some of the energy released is captured to form small amounts of ATP. This pathway occurs in both the presence and absence of oxygen, but since it does not use oxygen, it is an anaerobic. Ordinarily, pyruvic acid then enters the oxygen requiring aerobic pathways in the mitochondria and reacts with oxygen to produce still more ATP. In such cases, since oxygen is ultimately used the respiration process as a whole is described as aerobic. But when muscles contract vigorously and contractile activity reaches about 70 per cent of the maximum possible, the bulging muscles compress the blood vessels within them, impairing blood and hence oxygen delivery. Under these conditions, most of the pyruvic acid produced during glycolysis is converted into lactic acid and the overall process is referred to as anaerobic glycolysis. Thus, during oxygen deficit, lactic acid, rather than carbon dioxide and water is the end product of cellular metabolism of glucose. Most of the lactic acid diffuses out of the muscles into the blood stream and is completely washed out of the muscle tissue within 30 minutes after exercise stops. Subsequently the lactic acid is picked up by liver, heart or kidney cells which can use it as an energy source. Additionally liver cells can reconvert it to pyruvic acid or glucose and release it back into the blood stream for muscle use, a process called "Cori cycle" or convert it to glycogen for storage.

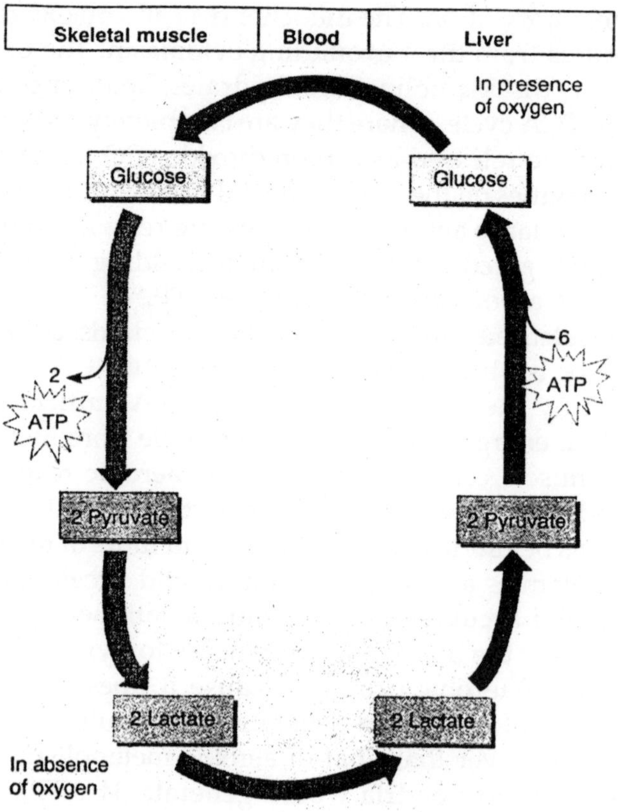

Fig 5.12 : The Cori Cycle

The anaerobic pathway yields only about 5 per cent as much ATP from each glucose molecule as the aerobic pathways, however it produces ATP about 2½ times faster. The anaerobic process of glycolysis enables the cell to continue generating ATP when mitochondrial activity alone cannot meet the demand. However this pathway has its drawbacks.

For example, when glycolysis produces pyruvic acid faster than it can be used by the mitochondria, pyruvic acid levels in the sarcoplasm increase. Under these conditions pyruvic acid is converted to lactic acid. The conversion of pyruvic acid to lactic acid poses a problem because lactic acid is an organic acid whose accumulation can cause dangerous changes in the pH inside and outside of the muscle fibre. Under anaerobic conditions 18 molecules of glucose must be converted to lactic acid molecules to obtain the same amount of energy produced by the aerobic catabolism of a single glucose molecule.

Muscle fatigue : A skeletal muscle fibre is fatigued when it can no longer contract despite continued neural stimulation. Muscle fatigue may be caused by the exhaustion of energy reserves or the build-up of lactic acid. Muscle fatigue is a state of physiological inability to contract. Exercise, accumulation of lactic acid and ionic imbalance also contribute to muscle fatigue. Lactic acid when causes muscle pH to drop, causes extreme fatigue and so limits the usefulness of the anaerobic mechanisms for ATP production. As action potentials are transmitted, potassium is lost from the muscle cells, and excess sodium enters, so long as ATP is available to energize the Na^+ K^+ pump, these slight imbalance of ions are corrected. However, without ATP, the pump is inactive and muscle cells become non-responsive. In general, intense exercise of short duration produces fatigue rapidly but recovery is also rapid. By contrast, the slow developing fatigue of prolonged low intencity exercise may require several hours for complete recovery.

Oxygen debt : Oxygen debt is defined as the extra amount of oxygen that must be taken in by the body for these restorative processes and it represents the difference between the amount of oxygen needed for totally aerobic muscle activity and the amount actually used. All non-aerobic sources of ATP used during muscle activity contribute to this debt.

6

Neural Tissue and the Central Nervous System

The nervous system is the master controlling and communicating system of the body. It is responsible for all behaviour, every thought, action and emotion reflects its activity. Its cells communicate by electrical, signals, which are rapid, specific and usually cause almost immediate responses.

The nervous system has three overlapping functions: (1) It uses its millions of sensory receptors to monitor changes occurring both inside and outside the body. These changes are called stimuli and the gathered information is called sensory input. (2) It processes and interprets the sensory impact and decides what should be done at each moment a process called integration. (3) It causes a response by activating effecter organs our muscles, or glands the response is called motor output.

Nervous system divided into two principal parts: (1) The central nervous system (CNS) consists of brain and spinal cord. The CNS is the integrating and command centre of the nervous system. It interprets incoming sensory information and dictates motor responses boned on past experience, reflexes and current conditions. The peripheral nervous system (PNS), the part of the nervous system outside the CNS, consists mainly of the nerves that extend from the brain and spinal cord. Spinal nerves carry impulses to and from the spinal cord, cranial nerves carry impulse to and from the brain. These peripheral nerves serve as the communication lines that link all parts of the body to the central nervous system.

The peripheral nervous system has two functional subdivisions. The sensory or afferent division consists of nerve fibres that convey impulses to the central nervous system from sensory receptors located throughout the body, sensory fibres conveying impulse from the skin, skeletal muscles and joints are called somatic afferent fibres, whereas those transmitting impulses from the visceral organs are called visceral afferent fibres. The sensory division keeps the CNS constantly informed of events going on both inside and outside the body.

The motor or efferent division transmits impulse from the CNS to effector organs, the muscles and glands. These impulses activate muscles to contract and glands to secrete.

The motor division also has two main parts:

1. The somatic nervous system is composed of somatic motor nerve fibres that conduct impulse from the CNS to skeletal muscle. It is often referred as the voluntary nervous system.
2. The autonomic nervous system (ANS) consists of visceral motor nerve fibres that regulate the activity of smooth muscles, cardiac muscles and glands. The ANS is also referred to as the involuntary system. It has two functional subdivisions, the sympathetic and parasympathetic, which bring about opposite effects on the activity of the same visceral organs, one stimulates and the other inhibits.

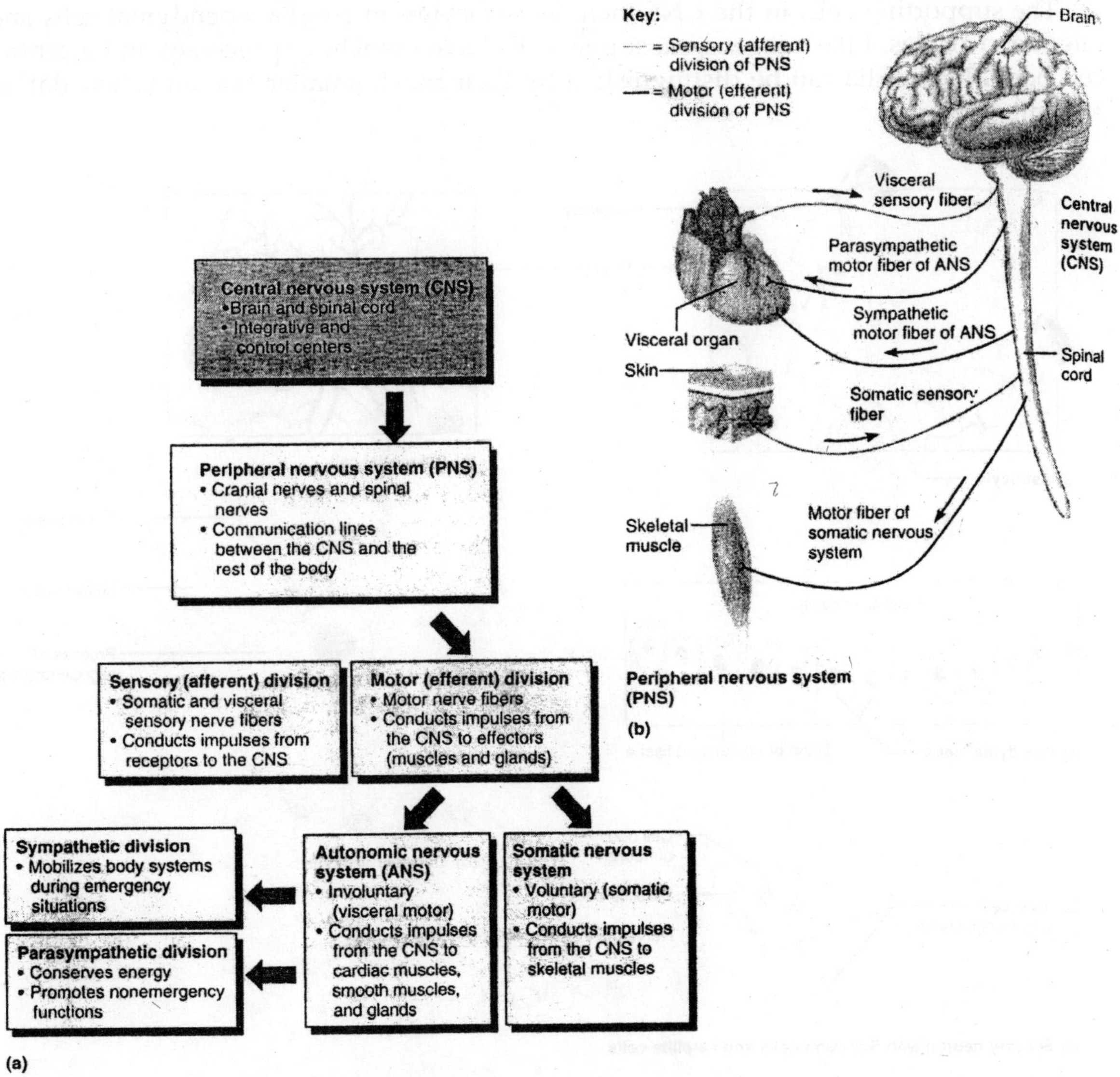

Fig. 6.1 : Organization in the Nervous System

The nervous system consists of two types of cells : (1) neurons the excitable nerve cells, and (2) supporting cells.

Supporting cells (Neuroglia)

All neurons associate closely with non-nervous supporting cells, also called neuroglia. There are six types of neuroglia four in the CNS and two in the PNS. Each type has a unique function, selected supporting cells segregate and insulate neurones so that electrical activities of adjacent neurons don't interfere with each other.

Supporting cells in the CNS

The supporting cells in the CNS include astrocytes, microglia, ependymal cells and oligodendrocytes. Like neurons, most glial cells have branching processes and a central cell body. Neuroglia can be distinguished by their much smaller size and their darker staining nuclei.

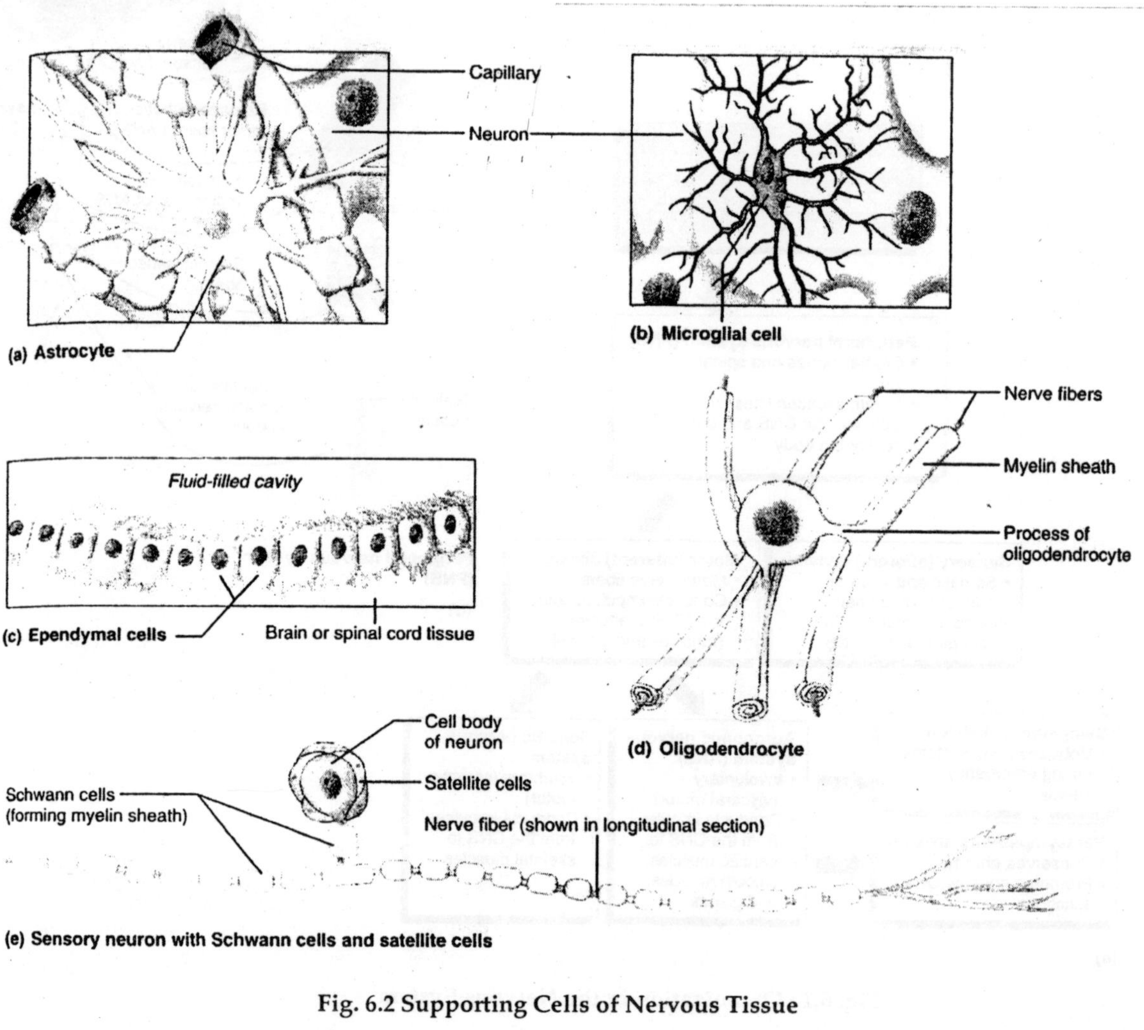

Fig. 6.2 Supporting Cells of Nervous Tissue

The star-shaped astrocytes are the most abundant. Astrocytes play role in making exchanges between capillaries and neurons, guiding the migration of young neurons and helping to determine capillary permeability. Astrocytes also control the chemical environment around neurons, glucose provides the fuel source for producing the ATP needed to carry out their activities. Astrocytes have been shown to signal such other by intracellular calcium pulses.

Microglia are small oval cells with long process. Their branches touch nearby neurons, monitoring their health and when they sense, that certain neurons are injured or in other trouble the microglia round up and migrate toward them. Where invading microorganisms or dead neurons are present, the microglia transform into a special type of macrophage that phagocytizes the microorganisms or neural debris.

Epedymal cells line the central cavities of the brain and the spinal cord. Where they form a permeable barrier between the cerebrospinal fluid that fills those cavities and the tissue fluid bathing the cells of the CNS. The beating of their cilia helps to circulate the cerebrospinal fluid.

Supporting cells in the PNS

The two kinds of supporting cells in the PNS-satellite cells and Schwan cells, differ mainly in location satellite cells surround neuron cell bodies within ganglia, but their function is still unknown.

Schwan cells surround and form myelin sheaths around the larger nerve fibres in the peripheral nervous system. Hence, they are functionally similar to oligodendrocytes.

Neurons : The neurons also called nerve cells are the structural units of the nervous system. Neurons are highly specialized cells that conduct messages in the form of nerve impulses from one part of the body to another. Besides their ability to conduct nerve impulses neurons have some other special characteristics.

1. They have extreme longevity—Given good nutrition, neurons can live and function optimally for a life time (over 100 years).
2. They are amitotic—As neurons assume their roles as communicating links of the nervous system, they lose their ability to divide.
3. They have an exceptionally high metabolic rate and require continuous and abundant supplies of oxygen and glucose, neurons cannot survive for more than a few minutes without oxygen.

Neurons are typically large complex cells. Although they vary in structure, they all have a cell body from which one or more slender processes project. The plasma membrane of neurons is the site of electrical signalling, and it plays a crucial role in cell-to-cell interactions that occur during development. Most neurons have three functional components in common (1) a receptive or input region, (2) a conductive component, and (3) a secretory or output component.

Cell body : The cell body consists of a transparent spherical nucleus with a nucleolus surrounded by cytoplasm. Also called the perikaryon or soma. The cell body is the major biosynthetic centre of a neuron. Except for centrioles, it contains usual organelles.

A neuron's protein consisting of clustered-free ribosomes and rough endoplasmic reticulum (ER). This rough ER referred to as Nissl's bodies or chromatophoristic substance. The Golgi apparatus is also well developed and forms an arc or complete circle around the nucleus Mitochondria are scattered everywhere among the other organelles. Microtubules and neurofibrils, bundles of filaments, which are important in maintaining cell shape and integrity are seen throughout the cell body.

The cell body is the focal point for the outgrowth of neurons processes during embryonic development. In most neurons, the plasma membrane of the cell body also acts as part of the receptive surface that receives information from other neurons.

Most neuron cell bodies are located within the CNS, where they are protected by the bones of the skull and vertebral column. Clusters of cell bodies in the CNS are called nuclei, whereas the far fewer collections of cell bodies that lie along the nerves in the PNS are called ganglia.

Processes : Arm like processes extend from the cell body of all neurons. The brain and spinal cord (CNS) contain both neuron cell bodies and their processes. The PNS, for the most part consists chiefly of neuron processes. Bundles of neuron processes are called tracts in the CNS and nerves in the PNS.

The two types of neurone processes dendrites and axons differ from each other in the structure and function of their plasma membrane.

Dendrides : Dendrites of motor neurons are short tapering, diffusely branching. Typically, motor neurons have hundreds of lacy dendride clustering close to the cell body. All organelles present in the cell body also occur in dendrites. Dendrites correspond to the main receptive or input regions. They provide an enormous surface area for receiving signals from other neurons. Dendrites convey incoming messages toward the cell body. These electrical signals are not nerve impulses (action potentials) but are short distance signals called graded potentials.

The Axon : Each neuron has a single axon. The initial region of the axon arises from a cone-shaped area of the cell body called axon hillock and then narrows to form a slender process that is uniform in diameter for the rest of its length. In some neurons, the axon is very short or absent, in others it is long and accounts for nearly the entire length of the neuron. For example, axons of motor neurons controlling the skeletal muscles of toe extend from the lumbar region of foot a distance of a meter or more making them the longest cells in the body. Any long axon is called a nerve fibre.

Each neuron has only one axon, but axons may give off occasional branches along their length. These rare branches called axon collaterals, extend from the axon is undivided. The knoblike distal endings of the terminal branches are called axonal terminals, synoptic knobs or button.

Functionally, axons are the conducting components of the neuron. They generate nerve impulses and transmit them away from the cell body. In motor neurons the nerve impulses is generated at the junction of the axon hillock and axon and conducted along the axon to the axonal terminals. These terminals represent the secretary component of the neuron, it cames chemicals stored in vesicles there to be released into the extracellular space.Neurotransmitter exite or exhibit neurons with which the axon is in close contact.

An axon contains the same organelles found in the dendrites and cell body with two very important exceptions, it lacks the structures involved with protein synthesis and packaging, Nissls bodies, and a Golgi apparatus. An axon depends on its cell body to renew the necessary proteins and membrane components and an efficient transport mechanisms to distribute them. Axons quickly decay if cut or severely damaged.

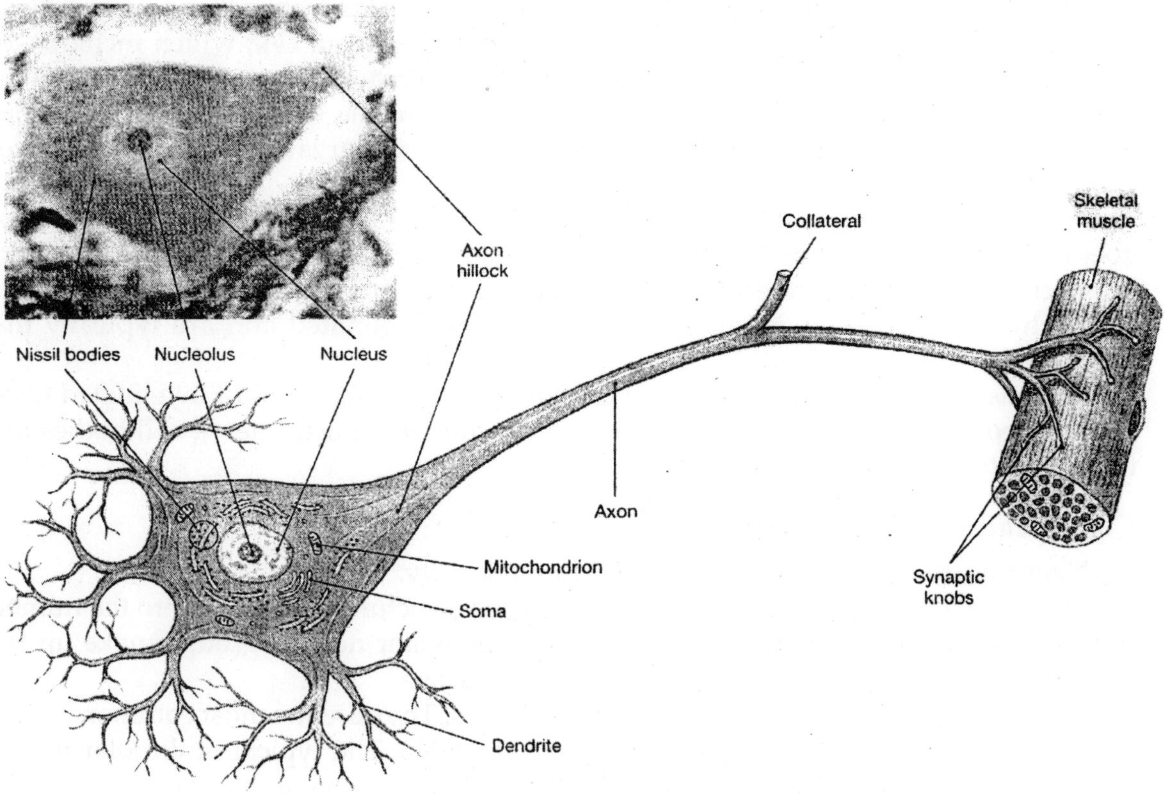

Fig. 6.3 Anatomy of a Multipolar Neuron

Substances travel continuously both away from and toward the cell body along the axon by the several types of cytoskeletal elements (microtubules, actin filaments, etc.). Substances moved toward the axonal terminals include mitochondria, cytoskeletal elements.

Substances transported in the opposite direction are mostly organelles being returned to the cell body for degradation or recycling. The reverse transport process is also an important means of intracellular communication for advising the cell body of conditions at the axonal terminals and for delivering vesicles containing signal molecules to the some.

Myelin sheath and Neurolemma

Many nerve fibres, particularly those that are long, or large in diameter are covered with a whitish, fatty, segmented sheath called myelin sheath. Myelin protects and electrically insulates fibres from one another and it increases the speed of transmission of nerve impulses. Myelinated fibres conduct nerve impulses rapidly, whereas unmyelinated fibres conduct impulses quite slowly.

Myelin sheaths in the peripheral nervous system are formed by Schwan cells. The Schwan cells indent to receive the axon and then wrap themselves around it in a jelly roll fashion. The nucleus and most of the cytoplasm of the Schwan cell end up as a bulge just external of the myelin sheath. This portion of the Schwan cell, which includes the exposed part of its plasma membrane is called neurolemma. Adjacent Schwan cells along an axon do not touch one another. So there are gaps in the sheath. These gaps called nodes of Ranvier or neurofibral nodes, occur at regular intervals along the myelinated axon.

Sometimes Schwan cells surround peripheral nerve fibres but the coiling process does not occur. In such a single Schwan cell can partially enclose 15 or more axons, each of which occupies a separate recess in the Schwan cell surface. Nerve fibres associated with Schwan cells in this manner are said to be unmyelinated and are typically thin fibres.

Regions of the brain and spinal cord containing dense collections of myelinated fibres are referred to as white matter and gray matter contains mostly nerve cell bodies and unmyelinated fibres.

Classification of neurons

Neurons are classified structurally and functionally:

Structural classification : Neurons are grouped structurally according to the number of processes extending from their cell body. Three major neuron groups make up this classification, multipolar, bipolar and unipolar neurons.

Multipolar neurons have three or more processes. They are the most common neuron type in humans and the major neuron type in the CNS. The typical multipolar neuron has numerous branching dendrites and one axon, some neuron of this class lack an axon and have only dendrites.

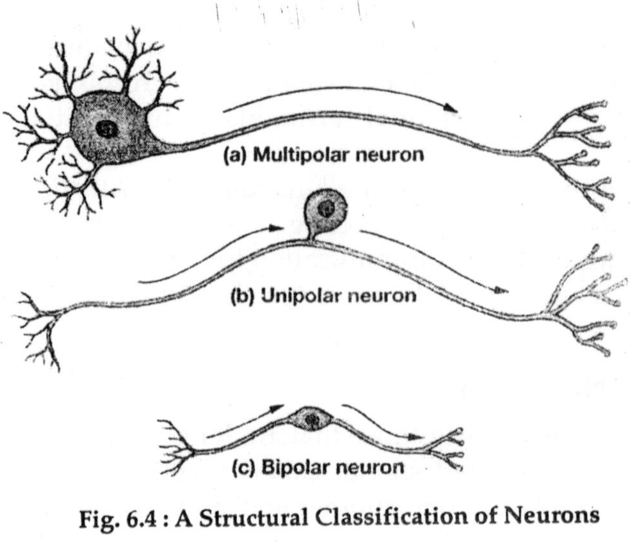

Fig. 6.4 : A Structural Classification of Neurons

Bipolar neurons have two processes, an axon and a dendrite. These rare neurons are found only in some of the special sense organs, where they act as receptor cells for example. Some neurons in the retina of the eye and in the olfactory mucosa.

Multipolar	*Bipolar*	*Unipolar (pseudounipolar)*
Structural Class: Neuron Type According to the Number of Processes Extending from the Cell Body		
Many processes extend from the cell body; all dendrites except for a single axon.	Two processes extend from the cell: one is a fused dendrite, the other is an axon.	One process extends from the cell body and forms central and peripheral processes, which together comprise the axon. Only the distal endings of the peripheral process are dendrites.

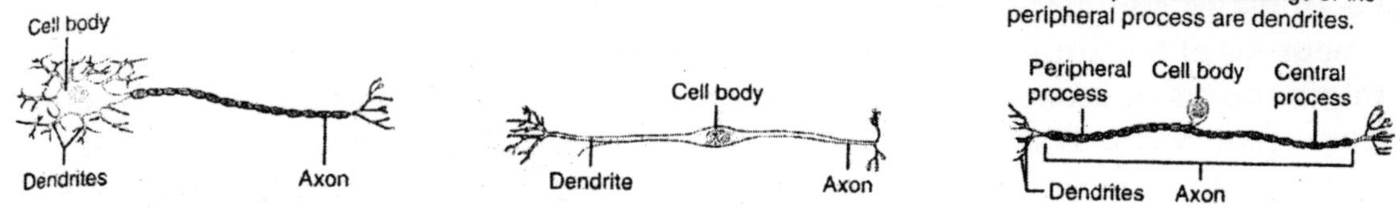

Multipolar	*Bipolar*	*Unipolar (pseudounipolar)*
Relationship of Anatomy to the Three Functional Regions		
☐ = Receptive region (receives stimulus). Plasma membrane exhibits chemically gated ion channels.	▩ = Conducting region (generates/transmits action potential). Plasma membrane exhibits voltage-gated Na^+ and K^+ channels.	▩ = Secretory region (releases neurotransmitters). Plasma membrane exhibits voltage-gated Ca^{2+} channels.

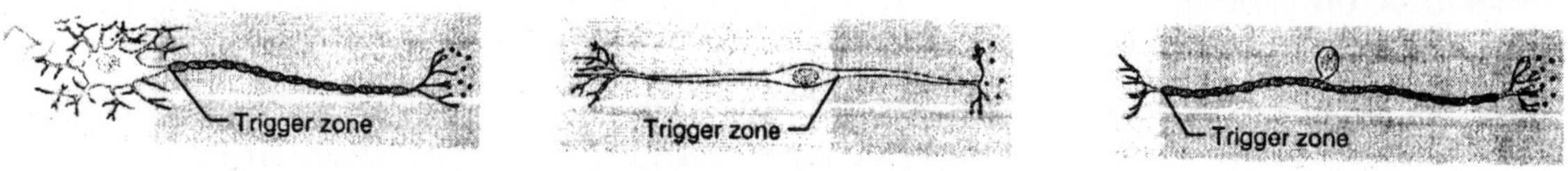

Multipolar	*Bipolar*	*Unipolar (pseudounipolar)*
	(Many bipolar neurons do not generate action potentials and, in those that do, the location of the trigger zone is not universal.)	
Relative Abundance and Location in Human Body		
Most abundant in body. Major neuron type in the CNS.	Rare. Are found in some special sensory organs (olfactory mucosa, eye).	Found mainly in the PNS. Common only in dorsal root ganglia of the spinal cord and sensory ganglia of cranial nerves.
Structural Variations		

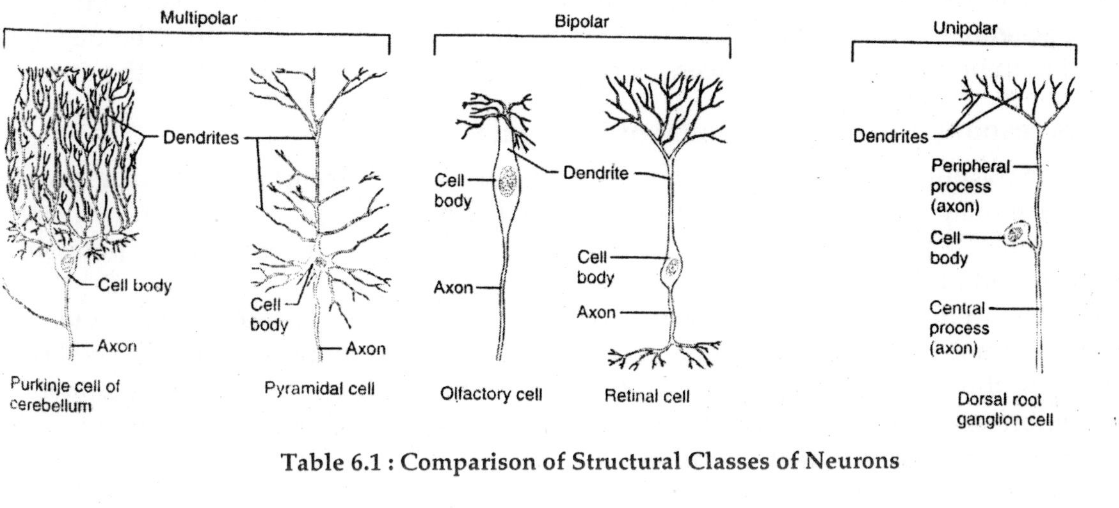

Table 6.1 : Comparison of Structural Classes of Neurons

Unipolar neurons have a single short process that emerges from the cell body.

Functional classification : There are sensory neurons, motor neurons and inter neurons.

Sensory or afferent neurons : They transmit impulses from sensory receptors in the skin or internal organs toward or into the central nervous system. Except for the bipolar neurons found in some of the special sense organs, all sensory neurons of the body are unipolar. Functionally, only the most distal parts of these unipolar neurons act as impulse receptor sites and the peripheral processes are very long.

Motor or efferent neurons : They carry impulses away from the CNS to the effector organs (muscles and glands) of the body. Motor neurons are multipolar and except for some neurons of the autonomic nervous system, their cell bodies are located in the CNS.

Interneurons or associated neurons : They lie between motor and sensory neurons in neural pathways. They are located entirely within the brain and spinal cord. All interneurons are multipolar. They are responsible for the analysis of sensory inputs and the coordination of motor outputs. The Purkinje and pyramidal cells are examples of this type.

Neurophysiology : Neurons are highly irritable (responsive to stimuli). When a neuron is adequately stimulated, an electrical impulse is conducted along the length of its axons. This response, called the action potential (nerve impulse) is always the same regardless of the source on type of stimulus and it underlies all functional activities of the nervous system.

Basic Principles of Electricity : The human body as a whole is electrically neutral it has the same number of positive and negative charges. However, there are areas where one type of charges predominates, making such regions positively or negatively charged.

The cell membrane of an undisturbed cell has an excess of positive charges on the outside and an excess of negative charges on the inside. Such an uneven distribution of charges is known as a potential difference and the size of the potential difference is measured in terms of volts. Because the charges are separated by a cell membrane, the potential difference across the cell membrane of a living cell is called as membrane potential. The resting potential or membrane potential of an undisturbed cell is very small. For example, the resting potential of a neuron averages about 0.07 volts. The resting potential of a neuron is –70 mv, with the minus sign indicating that the inside of the cell membrane contains an excess of negative charges as compared with the outside.

Factors responsible for the membrane potential

The extracellular and intracellular fluids differ in ionic composition. For example, the extracellular fluid contains relatively high concentrations of sodium ion (Na^+) and chloride ions (Cl^-) whereas the intracellular fluid contains high concentration of potassium ions (K+) and negatively charged proteins (Pr^-).

The intracellular and extracellular fluids are separated by the cell membrane. The proteins cannot cross the membrane at all, and the ions can enter or leave the cell only by passing through membrane channels. There are many different types of channels in the membrane some are always open (leak channels) and others open or close under specific circumstances (gated channels).

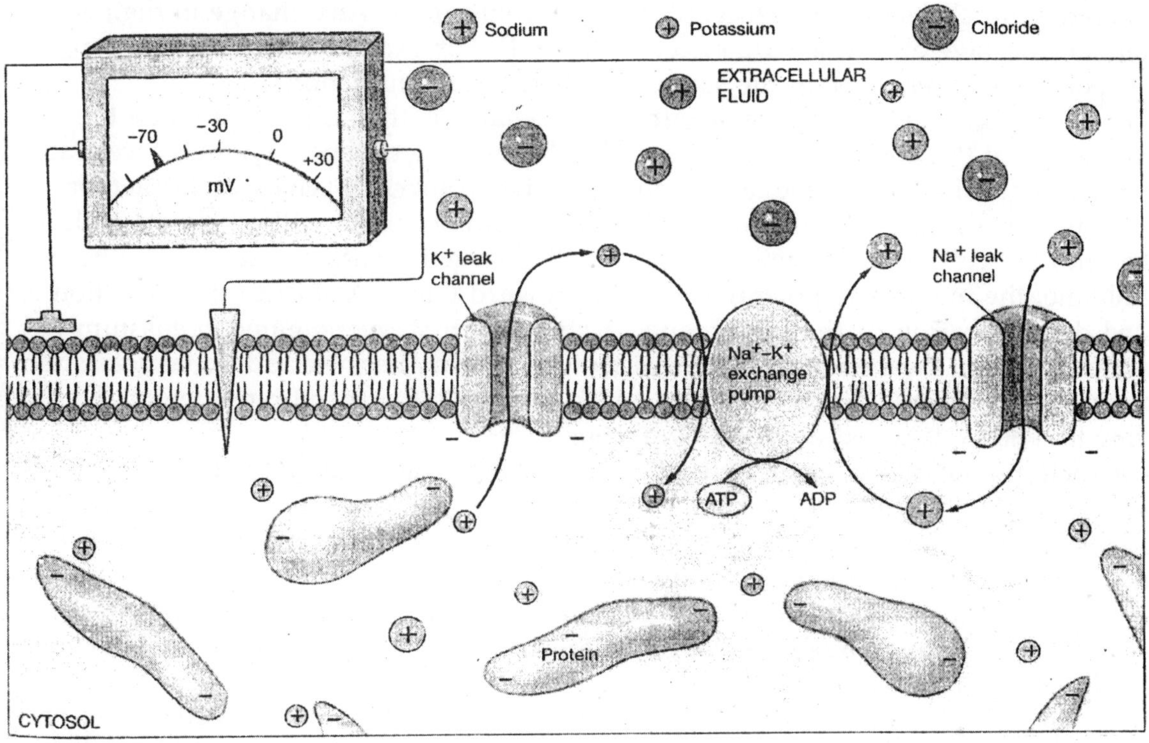

Figure 8-6
The Cell Membrane at the Resting Potential

Fig. 6.5 : The Cell Membrane at the Resting Potential

Because the intracellular concentration of potassium ions is relatively high, potassium ion tend to diffuse out of the cell. This movement is driven by the concentration gradient for potassium ions. Similarly, the concentration gradient for sodium ions tends to promote their movement into the cell. However, the cell membrane is significantly more permeable to potassium ions than to sodium ions. As a result, potassium ions diffuse out of the cell faster than sodium ions enter the cytoplasm. The cell therefore experiences a net loss of positive charges, and as a result the interior of the cell membrane contains an excess of negative charges, primarily from negatively charged proteins.

The resting potential remains stable over time because the cell membrane contains the sodium-potassium exchange pump, an ion pump. At a membrane potential of –70 mv, the rate of sodium entry to potassium loss can be balanced by the sodium-potassium exchange pump.

Changes in the membrane potential

Every living cell has a resting potential. Any stimulus that (1) alters membrane permeability to sodium or potassium or (2) alters the activity of the exchange pump will disturb the resting potential of a cell. Examples of stimuli that can affect the membrane potential include exposure to specific chemicals, mechanical pressure, changes in temperature, or shifts in the extracellular ion concentrations. Any change in the resting potential can have an immediate effect on the cell. For example, in a skeletal muscle fibre, permeability changes in the sarcolemma trigger a contraction.

In most cases, a stimulus opens gates of ion channels that are closed when the cell membrane is at the normal resting potentials. The opening of these channels accelerates the movement of ions across the cell membrane and this movement changes the membrane potential. For example, the opening of gated sodium channels will accelerate sodium entry into the cell. As the number of positively charged ions increases inside the cell membrane, the membrane potential will shift toward OmV. A shift in this direction is called depolarization of the membrane. A stimulus that opens gated potassium ion channels will shift the membrane potential away from OmV because additional potassium ions will leave the cell. Such a change which may take the membrane potential from –70mv to –80mv is called a hyperpolarization.

An action potential is a conducted change in the permeability of the cell membrane. Skeletal muscle fibres and axons have membranes that will conduct action potentials. In a skeletal muscle fibre, the action potential begins at the neuromuscular junction and travels across the entire membrane. Surface, including the T tubules. The resulting ion movements trigger a contraction. In an axon an action potential usually begins near the axon hillock and travels along the length of the axon toward the synaptic knobs, where arrivals activates the synapses.

Action Potentials : The principal way neurons communicate by generating and propagating action potentials (APs) and for the most part, only cells with excitable membranes-neurons and muscle cells can generate action potentials.

The events of action potential generation and transmission are identical in skeletal muscle cells and neurons. However, in a neuron, a transmitted action potential is also called a nerve impulse. A neuron transmits a nerve impulse only when it is adequately stimulated. The stimulus changes the permeability of the neuron's membrane by opening specific voltage-gated channels that are located on axons. Only axons are capable of generating action potentials. These channels open and close in response to changes in the membrane potential and are activated by local currents (graded potentials) that spread toward the axon along the dendritic and cell body membranes. In many neurons, the transition from the local graded potential to the action potential takes place at the axon hillock. In sensory neurons the action potential is generated by the peripheral (axonal) process proximal to the receptor region.

Generation of an action potential

Generating an action potential involves three overlapping changes in membrane permeability due to opening and closing of active ion gates, all induced by depolarization of the axonal membrane. These permeability changes are first a transient increase in Na^+ permeability followed by restoration of Na^+ impermeability, and then a short lived increase in K^+ impermeability. The first two permeability changes occur during the depolarization phase of action potential generation. The third permeability change is responsible for both the repolarization and undershoot phases. Each of these phases will start with a neuron in the resting state.

1. Resting state-voltage-gated channels closed : In the resting state, all the voltage-gated Na^+ and K^+ channels are closed. Small amounts of K^+ are passing by leakage channels and even smaller amounts of Na^+ are diffusing in.

Each Na^+ channel has two voltage sensitive gates, an activation gate that is closed when resting and responds to depolarization by opening rapidly and an inactivation gate that is open at rest and responds to depolarization by closing slowly. Thus, depolarization opens and then closes the sodium channels. Both gates must be open for the channel to allow Na^+ entry, but the closing of either gate effectively closes the channels. Each active potassium channel has a single voltage sensitive gate, it is closed. When

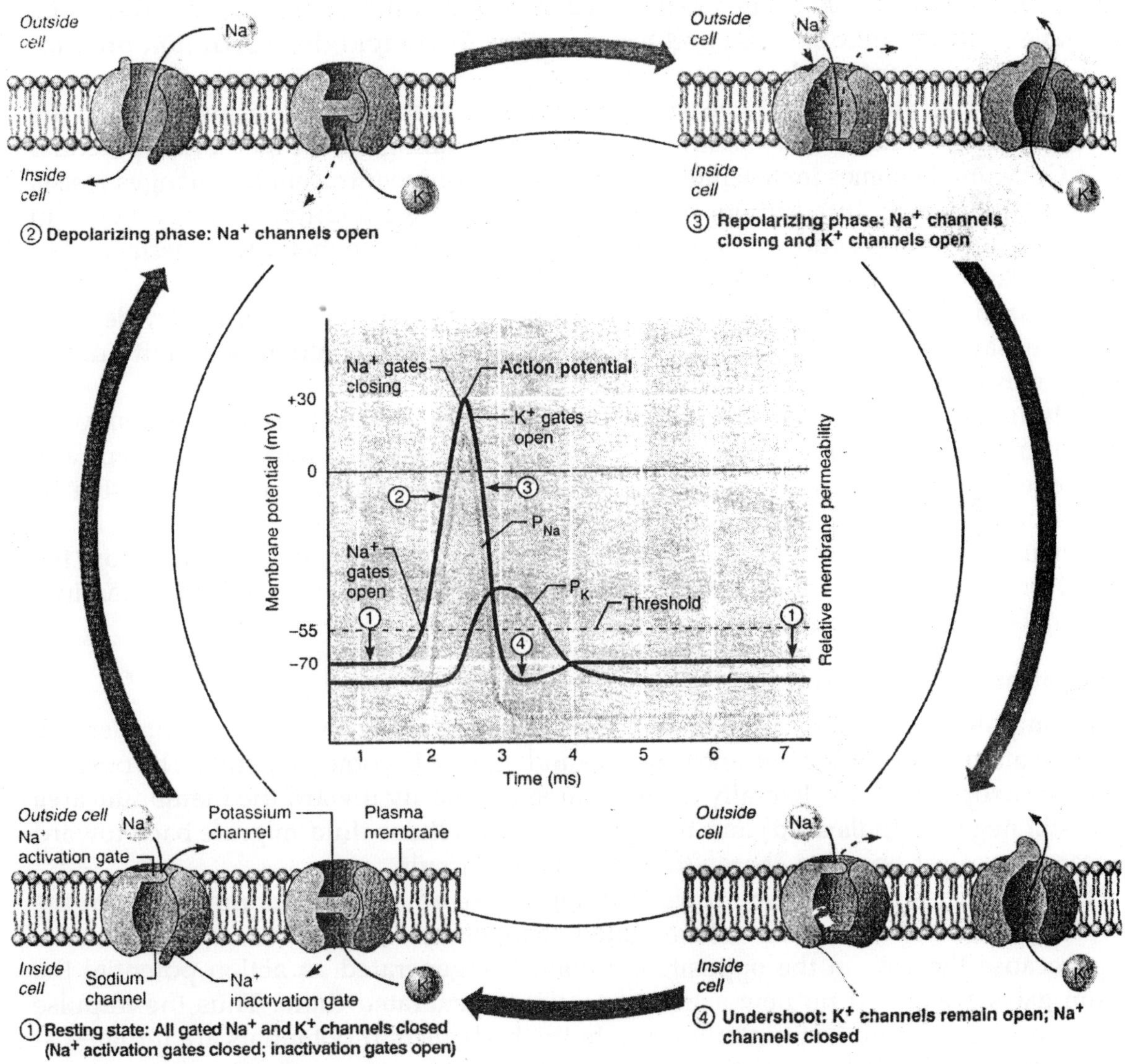

Fig 6.6 The phases of the action potential and the role of gated ion channels in those phase.

resting and opens slowly in response to depolarization.

2. Depolarization phase–increase in sodium permeability and reversal of the membrane potential : As the axonal membrane is depolarized by local currents, the sodium channel activation gates open quickly and sodium rushes into the cell at the point of depolarization. This influx of positive charge depolarizes that local "patch" of membrane still further, opening more activation gates so that the cell interior becomes progressively less negative. When depolarization of the membrane at the stimulation site reaches a certain critical level called threshold depolarization becomes self-generating. After being initiated by the stimulus, depolarization is driven by the ionic currents created by sodium ion influx. As more sodium enters, the membrane depolarizes further and opens more activation gates until all sodium channels are open. At this point, Na+ permeability is about 1000 times greater than it is in a resting neuron. As a result the membrane potential becomes less and less negative. This rapid depolarization produce rising of the action potential.

3. Repolarization phase : decrease in sodium permeability–The rising phase of the action potential persists for only about 1 ms and is self-limiting. As the membrane potential passes OmV and becomes increasingly positive, the positive intracellular changes resists further sodium entry. In addition, inactivation gates of the sodium channels begin to close after a few milliseconds of depolarization. As a result, the membrane permeability to sodium declines to resting levels.

Repolarizing phase–increase in potassium permeability–As sodium entry declines potassium dates open and potassium rushes out of the cell. Internal negativity of the resting neuron is restored, called repolarization.

4. Undershoot potassium permeability continues–Potassium gates are slow to respond to the depolarization signal the period of increased K^+ permeability typically lasts longer than to restore the resting polarized state. As a result of the excessive K^+ efflux, an after hyperpolarization called the undershoot.

Although, repolarization restores resting electrical conditions, it does not restore the original ionic distributions of the resting state. The redistribution is the sodium potassium pump following repolarization.

Propagation of an action potential

Action potential must be propagated or transmitted along the axon's entire length. In action potential, the inside becomes positive and outside becomes negative. The positive ions in the axoplasm move laterally from the area of polarity toward the membrane area that is still negative (polarized) and those in the extracellular fluid migrate back toward the area of greatest negative charge to complete the circuit.

This establishes local current flows that depolarize adjacent membrane areas in the forward direction which opens voltage gated channels and triggers an action potential there, because the area in the opposite direction has generated an action potential the sodium gates are closed no new action potential is generated there. Thus the impulse propagates among from its point of origin. In the body, action potentials are initiated at one end of the axon and conducted away from that point toward the axon's terminals.

One initiated, an action potential is self-propagating process that continues along the axon at a constant velocity.

Following depolarization each segment of axonal membrane repolarizes, which restores the resting membrane potential in that region.

The Synapse

In the nervous system, information moves from one location to another in the form of action potentials by synapses. A synapse from the Greek Syn, meaning "to clasp or join" is a unique junction that mediates information transfer from one neuron to the next or from a neuron to an effector cell.

Most synapses occur between the axonal endings of one neuron and the dendrites or the cell bodies (soma) of other neurons and are called axodendritic or axosomatic synapses. Less common are the synapses between axons (axoaxonic) between dendrites (dendrodendritic) or between dendrites and cell bodies (dendrosomatic).

The neuron conducting impulses toward the synapse is called the presynaptic neuron. The neuron that transmits the electrical signal away from the synapse is called the postsynaptic neuron. At a given synapse, the presynaptic neuron is the information sender and the postsynaptic neuron is the information receiver. Most neurons function both as presynaptic and postsynaptic neurons.

Communication between neurons and other cells occurs in one direction only across a synapse from the synaptic knob of the presynaptic neuron to the postsynaptic neuron or other cell type. The opposing cell membranes are separated by a narrow synaptic cleft.

Each synaptic knob contains mitochondria synaptic vesicles and areas of endoplasmic reticulum. Every synaptic vesicle contains several thousand molecules of a specific neurotransmitters and on stimulation many of these vesicles release their contents into the synaptic cleft. The neurotransmitter then diffuses across the synaptic cleft and binds to receptors on the postsynaptic membrane.

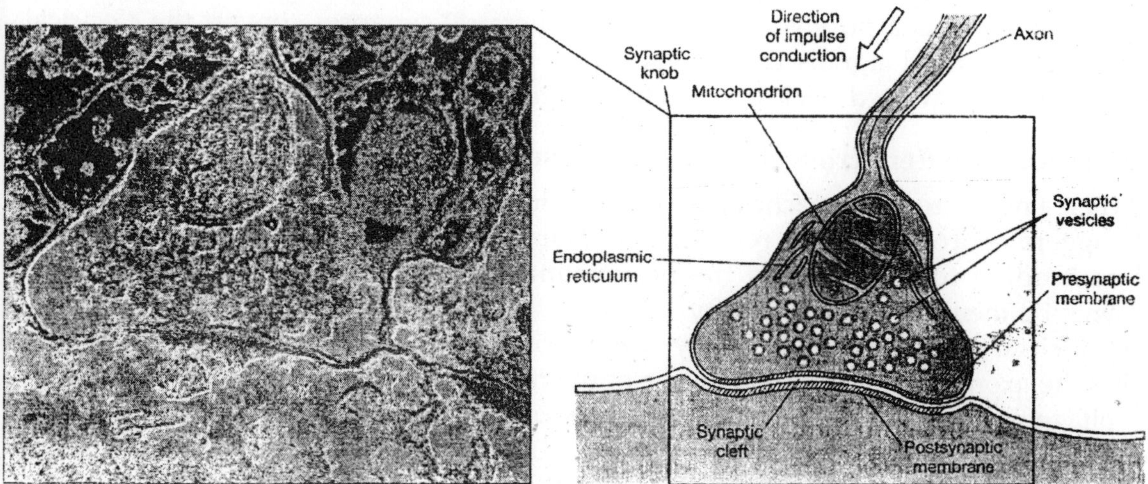

Fig 6.7

There are two varieties of synapses, electrical and chemical.

Electrical Synapses : These are less common found between certain other bodies. They contain protein channels that interconnect the cytoplasm of adjacent neurons and allow the current carrying ions to flow directly from one neuron to the next. Neurons joined in this way are said to be electrically coupled and transmission across these synapses is very rapid. Depending on nature of the synapse, communication may be unidirectional or bidirectional.

In adults, electrical synapses are found in regions of the brain responsible for certain stereotyped movement, such as the normal jerky movements of the eyes. They are more abundant in embryonic nervous tissue, where they permit exchange of guiding clues during early neuronal development. So that neurons can connect properly with one another. As neurons system development continues, most electrical synapses are replaced by chemical synapses.

Chemical Synapses : In contrast to electrical synapses, which are specialized to allow the flow of ions between neurons, chemical synapses are specialized for release and reception of chemical neurotransmitters. Neurotransmitters act to open or close ion channels that influence membrane permeability and membrane potential.

A typical chemical synapse is made up of two parts: (1) a knoblike axonal terminal of the presynaptic (transmitting) neuron, which contains many tiny, membrane bounded sacs called synaptic vesicles, each containing thousands of neurotransmitter molecules, and (2) a receptor region on the membrane of a dendrite or the cell body of the postsynaptic neuron, which bears neurotransmitter receptors.

The presynaptic and postsynaptic membranes are always separated by the synaptic cleft a fluid filled space. Because the current from the presynaptic membrane enters in the fluid filled cleft, chemical synapses effectively prevent a nerve impulse from being directly transmitted from one neuron to another. Instead transmission of signals across these synapses is a chemical event that depends on the release, diffusion and receptor binding of neurotransmitter molecules and results in unindirectional communication between neurons. Thus, while transmission of nerve impulses along an axon and across electrical synapses is a purely electrical event, chemical synapses convert the electrical signals into chemical signals that travel across the synapse to the postsynaptic cells, where they are converted back into electrical signals.

Information transfer across chemical synapses

When a nerve impulse reaches the axon terminal, it sets into motion a chain of events that triggers neurotransmitter release. The neurotransmitter crosses the synaptic cleft and on binding to receptors on the postsynaptic membrane, causes changes in the postsynaptic membrane permeability.

1. Calcium gates open in the presynaptic axonal terminal : When the nerve impulse reaches the axon terminal, depolarization of the membrane opens not only Na^+ channels but voltage regulated Ca^{+2} channels as well. During the brief time the calcium gates are open Ca^{2+} floods into the terminal from the extra-cellular fluid.

2. Neurotransmitter is released by exocytosis : The free calcium into the axonal terminal acts as an intracellular messenger, directing synaptic vesicles to fuse with the axonal membrane and empty their contents by exocytosis into the synaptic cleft. The Ca^{2+} is then quickly removed either taken up into the mitochondria or ejected to the outside by an active calcium membrane pump.

3. Neurotransmitter binds to postsynaptic receptors : The neurotransmitter diffuses across the synaptic cleft and binds reversibly to specific protein receptors that are densely clustered on the postsynaptic membrane.

4. Ion channels open in the Postsynaptic membrane : As the receptor proteins bind neurotransmitter molecules, their three-dimensional shape changes. This causes ion channels to open, and the resulting current flows produce local changes in the membrane potential. Depending on the receptor protein to which the neurotransmitter binds and the type of channel the receptor controls, the postsynaptic neuron may be excited or inhibited.

For each nerve impulse reaching the presynaptic terminal many vesicles are empties into the synaptic cleft. The higher the frequency of impulses reaching the terminals, the greater the total number of synaptic vesicles that fuse and spill their contents, and the greater than effect on the postsynaptic cell.

Termination of neurotransmitter effects

As long as a neurotransmitter is bound to a postsynaptic receptor, it continues to produce its effects on membrane permeability and blocks reception of additional "messages" from presynaptic neurons. Thus some means of "wiping the postsynaptic state clean" is necessary. The effects of neurotransmitters last a few milliseconds before being terminated by one of the three mechanisms:

1. Degradation by enzymes associated with the postsynaptic membrane or present in the synapse.
2. Removal from the synapse by reuptake by astrocytes or the presynaptic terminal where it is stored or destroyed by enzymes, as with norepinephrine.
3. Diffusion of the neurotransmitter away from the synapse, ending its effects there.

Postsynaptic potentials and synaptic integration

Many receptors present on postsynaptic membranes at chemical synapses are specialized to open at ion channels, thereby converting chemical signals into electrical signals. However, unlike the voltage gated ion channels responsible for action potentials, these chemically gated channels are relatively insensitive to changes in membrane potential. Channel opening at postsynaptic membranes cannot possibly become a self-amplifying or self-generating event. Instead neurotransmitter receptors mediate local changes in membrane potential that are graded according to the amount of transmitter released and the time it remains in the area.

Chemical synapses are divided into two types, excitatory and inhibitory, according to how they affect the membrane potential of the postsynaptic neuron. Excitatory postsynaptic potentials (EPSPs) occur at excitatory synapses and inhibitory postsynaptic potentials (IPSPs) are generated at inhibitory synapses.

Excitatory synapses and EPSPs

At excitatory synapses neurotransmitter binding causes depolarization of the postsynaptic membrane. However, in contrast to what happen on axonal membranes, only a single type of channel opens on postsynaptic membranes. This channel allows sodium and potassium ions to diffuse simultaneously through the membrane in opposite directions. The electrochemical gradient for sodium is much steeper than that for potassium, hence the influx of Na^+ is greater than the afflux of K^+ and net depolarization occurs.

If enough neurotransmitter binds, depolarization of the postsynaptic membrane can successfully reach. OmV, which is well above an axon's threshold for firing of an action potential. However, postsynaptic membranes do not generate action potentials, only axon have this capability. The polarity reversal seen in axons never occurs in membranes containing only chemically gated channels because the opposite movements of K+ and Na+ prevent accumulation of excessive positive charge inside the cell. Hence instead of action potentials, local graded depolarization events called excitatory postysynaptic potential (EPSPs) occur at excitatory postsynaptic membranes. Each EPSPs lasts a few milliseconds and then the membrane returns to its resting potential. The only function of EPSPs is to help trigger an action potential distally at the axon hillock of the postsynaptic neuron. Although current flows created by individual EPSPs decline with distance, they can and often do spread all the way to the axon hillock. If currents reaching the axon hillock are strong enough to depolarize the axon to threshold, axonal voltage-gated channels open and an action potential is generated.

Inhibitory synapses and IPSPs

Binding of neurotransmitters at inhibitory synapses reduces a postsynaptic neuron's ability to generate an action potential. Most inhibitory neuro-transmitters induce hyperpolarization of the postsynaptic membrane by making the membrane more permeable to potassium ions, chloride ions or both. Sodium permeability is not affected. If potassium gates are opened potassium ions move out of the cell, if chloride gates are opened, chloride ions move in. In either case the charge on the inner surface of the membrane becomes more negative. As the membrane potential increases and is driven further from the axon's threshold the postsynaptic neuron becomes less and less likely to five and larger depolarizing currents are required to induce an action potential. Such changes in potential are called inhibitary postsynaptic potentials (IPSPs).

Neurotransmitters and their receptors

Neurotransmitters, along with electrical signals are the languages of the nervous system, the means by which each neuron communicates with others to process and send messages to the rest of the body. These molecules that chemically connect neurons affect body and brain, sleep, thought, hunger, memory movement, etc. Mosts factors that specifically affect synaptic transmission do so by enhancing or inhibiting neurotransmitter release or destruction or by blocking their binding to receptors.

Neurotransmitters are classified in two ways, chemically and functionally.

Classification of neurotransmitters according to chemical structure.

Neurotransmitters fall into several classes based on molecular structure:

Acetylcholine : Acetylcholine was the first neurotransmitter to be identified. Acetylcholine (Ach) is synthesized and enclosed in synaptic vesicles within the axonal terminals in a recreation catalyzed by the enzyme choline acetyltransferase. Acetic acid is bound to coenzyme A (CoA) to form acetyl – CoA, which in turn is combined with choline. Then the conezyme is released.

Acetyl-CoA + Choline Choline acetyl transferase. Ach + CoA.

After ACh is released by presynaptic terminal it binds to the postsynaptic receptors briefly. Then it is released and degraded to acetic acid and choline by the enzyme acetylcholinesterase (AChE), located in the synaptic cleft and on postsynaptic membranes. The released choline is recaptured by the presynaptic terminals and reused to synthesize more ACh.

ACh is released by all neurons that stimulate skeletal muscles and by some neurons of the autonomic nervous system.

Biogenic amines : The biogenic amines include the catecholamines such as dopamine, norepinephrine and epinephrine, and the indolamine which include seratonin and histamine.

Biogenic amine neurotransmitters are broadly distributed in the brain, where they play a role in emotional behaviour and help to regulate the biological clock. Additionally, catecholamines (particularly norepinephrine) are released by some motor neurons of the autonomic nervous system. Imbalance of these neurotransmitters are associated with mental illness, for example overproduction of dopamine occurs in schizophrenia. Certain psychoactive drugs can bind, to biogenic amine receptors and induce hallucinations.

Amino Acids: It has been more difficult to prove a neurotransmitter role when the suspect is an amino acid. ACh and biogenic amines are found only in neurons, but amino acids occur in all cells of the body and are important in many biochemical reactions. The amino acids for which a neurotransmitter role is certain include gamma (r) aminobutyric acid (GABA), glycine, asparate, and glutamate but there are others. Amino acid neurotransmitters have been found only in the CNS.

Peptides : The neuropeptides, essentially of amino acids include molecules with diverse effects. For example, a neuropeptide called substance P is an important mediator of pain signals. By contrast, endorphins which include beta endorphin dynorphin and enkephalions act as natural opiates, reducing perception of pain under certain stressful conditions. Enkephalin activity increases in pregnant women in labour.

Some neuropeptides, such as somatostatin vasoactive, intestinal peptide and cholecystokinin are also produced by non-nuclear body tissues and are widespread in the gastrointestinal tract. Such peptides are commonly referred to as gut brain peptides.

Novel Messenges : Just a few years ago it would have been scientific suicide to suggest that ATP, nitric oxide, and carbon monoxide, all molecules might be neurotransmitters.

Although it was well known that adenosine triphosphate (ATP), the universal form of cellular energy was stored in synaptic vesicles, its presence promote synthesis or uptake of other neurotransmitters. ATP is now recognized as a major neurotransmitter in both the CNS and PNS. Like glutamate and acetylcholine it produces a fast excitatory response at certain receptors.

Even more preposterous was the idea that nitric oxide (NO), a short-lived toxic gas could be neurotransmitters. It is synthesized on demand and diffuses out of the cells making it, rather than being stored in vesseles and released by exocytosis. Instead of attaching to surface receptors, it zooms through the plasma membrane of nearby cells to bind with a peculiar intracellular receptor iron in guanylyc cyclase, the enzyme that makes the second messenger cyclic GMP. When the neurotransmitter glutamate binds to NMDA receptors, calcium channels open to allow an influx of Ca^{2+} into the cell. The calcium triggers reactions that activate nitric oxide synthase (NOS), the enzyme needed for NO synthesis. Many believe that NO is the retrograde messenger involved in long-term potentiation (learning and memory), that is it may travel back from the postsynaptic neuron to the presynaptic neuron where it activates guanylyl cyclase. Excessive release of NO is responsible for much of the brain damage seen in stroke patients. In the myenteric plexus of the intestine, NO causes relaxation of intestinal smooth muscle.

NO is the first to-be-discovered class of signalling gases that pass swiftly into cells where they bind briefly to metal containing enzymes and then vanish, carbon monoxide (CO) another airy messenger, also stimulates synthesis of cyclic GMP, and some researchers speculate that CO is the main regulator if cyclic GMP levels in the brain. Though NO and CO are found in different brain regions and appear to act in different pathways, their mode of action is very similar.

Classification of neurotransmitters according to function

Effects–excitatory versus inhibitory : Some neurotransmitters are excitatory (cause depolarization), some are inhibitory (cause hyperpolarization) and others exert both effects, depending on the specific receptor types with which they interact. For example, the amino acids GABA and glycine are usually inhibitory, while glutamate is typically excitatory. On the other hand, ACh and NE each bind to at least two receptor types that cause opposite effects. For example, acetylcholine is excitatory at neuromuscular junction with skeletal muscle and inhibitory when released on cardial muscle.

Mechanism of action–direct versus indirect : Neurotransmitters that open ion channels are said to act directly. These neurotransmitters provoke rapid responses in the postsynaptic cells by promoting changes in membrane potential. ACh and the amino acid neurotransmitters are direct acting neurotransmitters.

The indirectly acting neurotransmitters promote broader, longer lasting effects by acting through intracellular second messenger molecules. In this way their mechanism is similar to that of many hormones. The biogenic amines and the peptides are indirect neurotransmitters.

7

Endocrine System

To function effectively, every cell in the body must communicate with its neighbours and with cells and tissues in distant portions of the body. Most of the communication involve, the release and receipt of chemical messages. Each living cell is continually "talking" to its neighbours by releasing chemicals into the extracellular fluid. These chemicals let cells know what their neighbours are doing at any given moment and the result is the coordination of tissue function at the local level.

The nervous system acts like a telephone company carrying specific "messages" from one location to another inside the body. The source and the destination are quite specific, and the effects are short-lived.

In cellular communication hormones are like addressed letters and the circulatory system is the postal service. A hormone released into the circulation will be distributed throughout the body. Each hormone has specific target cells that will respond to its presence. These cell's possess the receptors needed to bind and "read" the hormonal message. Although a cell may be exposed to the mixture of hormones in circulation at any given moment, it will respond only to those hormones it can bind and read.

Because the target cells can be anywhere in the body, a single hormone can alter the metabolic activities of multiple tissues and organs simultaneously. These effects may be slow to appear but they often persist for days. This persistence makes hormones effective in coordinating cell, tissues, and organ activities.

The endocrine system includes all of the endocrine cells and tissues of the body. Endocrine cells are glandular secretory cells that release their secretions internally rather than on epithelial surface. The chemicals released by endocrine cells may affect only adjacent cells. Hormones are chemical messengers that are released in one tissue and transported by the circulation to reach target cells in other tissues. Causing an effect on specific cells on target organs. Some of these organs, such as the pituitary gland have endocrine secretion as a primary function others such as the pancreas, have many other functions in addition to 'endocrine secretion'.

Today most scientists have expanded their definition of hormones to include any chemical produced by one cell that causes as effect in another. Included in this description, then, are substances, such as neurotransmitters, chemicals produced by the axon end of a nerve cell that travel to and bind with the dendrite end of an adjacent nerve cell, contributing to the propagation of the nerve impulse, along that neuron. Such chemicals are often called local hormones because they affect neighbouring target cells.

The 10 different endocrine glands of the human body make over 30 different hormones. Together, these glands are called the endocrine system. The endocrine system works with the nervous system to integrate the functioning of the various tissues, organs, and organ systems of the body. The nervous system sends messages to muscles and glands regulating muscular contraction and glandular secretion. The hormones of the endocrine system carry messages to any type of cell in the body. The messages of the endocrine hormones are varied but can be grouped into four categories:

1. Regulation : Hormones control internal environment of the body by regulating the secretion and excretion of various chemicals in the blood such as salts and acids.

2. Reproduction : Hormones control the female reproductive cycle and other reproductive processes essential to conception and birth control the development of sex cells, the reproductive organs, and secondary sexual characteristics.

3. Response : Hormones help the body respond to changes in the environment and cope with physical and psychological stress.

4. Growth and Development : Hormones are essential to the proper growth and development of the body from conception to adulthood.

Once molecules of a hormone are released into the blood stream, they travel throughout the body. Although hormone molecules may pass billions of cells. Specific hormones only affect specific cells called target cells. Hormones recognize target cells because they bind to receptor molecules embedded within the cell membrane or located within the cytoplasm of the cell. The binding of a hormone molecule to a receptor molecule activates a chain of events in the target cell that results in the effect of the hormone being expressed.

Hormones can be divided into three different groups on the basis of chemical structure, amino acid derivative, peptide hormones and lipid derivative.

1. Amino acid derivatives : Some hormones are relatively small molecules that are structurally similar to amino acids. This group includes epinephrine, norepinephrine, the thyroid hormones and the pineal hormone melatonin.

2. Peptide Hormones : Peptide hormones consist of chains of amino acids. These molecules range from short amino acid chains, such as ADH and oxytocin, to polypeptides such as growth hormones and prolactin. This is the largest class of hormones and includes all of the hormones secreted by the hypothalamous pituitary gland, heart, kidneys, thymus, digestive tract and pancreas.

3. Lipid derivatives : There are two classes of lipid based hormones (1) steroid hormones derived from cholesterol, and (2) those derived from arachidonic acid, a 20 carbon fatty acid. Steroid hormones are lipids structurally similar to cholesterol. Steroid hormones are released by the reproductive organs and the adrenal glands. The fatty acid base compounds which include the prostaglandins, coordinate cellular activities and affect enzymatic processes, such as blood clotting, that occur in extracellular fluid.

Mechanisms of Hormonal Action

All cellular structures and functions are determined by proteins. Structural proteins determine the general shape and internal structure of a cell and enzymes direct its metabolic activities. Hormones alter cellular operations by changing the identities, activities or quantities of important enzymes and structural proteins in various target cells. The sensitivity of a target cell is determined by the presence or absence of a specific receptor complex either on the cell membrane or in the cytoplasm, with which the hormone interacts.

Hormones and the cell membrane

Epinephrine, norepinephrine and peptide hormones cannot diffuse through a cell membrane. These hormones called first messenger, target receptors on the cell membrane. When a first messenger binds to an appropriate receptor, it triggers the appearance of a second messenger in the cytoplasm. The second messenger may function as an enzyme activator or inhibitor, but the net result will be a change in the cell's metabolic activities.

One of the most important second messengers is cyclic-AMP (EAMP) and the enzyme activated by the receptor is called adenylate cyclase. When activated, adenylate cyclase converts ATP to cyclic-AMP. The specific response of the target cell to EAMP depends on the nature of the enzymes already present in the cytoplasm. As a result, a single hormone can have one effect in one target tissue and quite different effects in other target tissues. The effects of EAMP are usually very short-lived, because another enzyme, phosphodiesterase quickly breaks down EAMP.

Cyclic-AMP is one of the most common second messengers, but there are many others.

Hormones and intracellular receptors

The thyroid hormones and steroid hormones cross the cell membrane and bind to intracellular receptors. Steroid hormones diffuse rapidly through the lipid portion of the cell membrane and bind to receptors in the cytoplasm or nucleus. The hormone receptor complex then binds to DNA segments and triggers the activation or inactivation of specific genes. By altering the rate of mRNA transcription in the nucleus, steroid hormones can change the structure or function of the cell. For example, the hormone testosterone stimulates the production of enzymes and proteins in skeletal muscle fibres increasing muscle size and strength.

Thyroid hormones cross the cell membrane through diffusion or carrier-mediated transport. One within the cell these hormones bind to receptors within the nucleus and activate specific genes. The result is an increase in metabolic activity due to changes in the nature or number of enzymes in the cytoplasm.

Control of endocrine activity

Endocrine activity may be controlled directly by a change in the composition of the extra-cellular fluid, or indirectly, by the hypothalamus. Negative feedback mechanisms provide the basis for the control of endocrine activity.

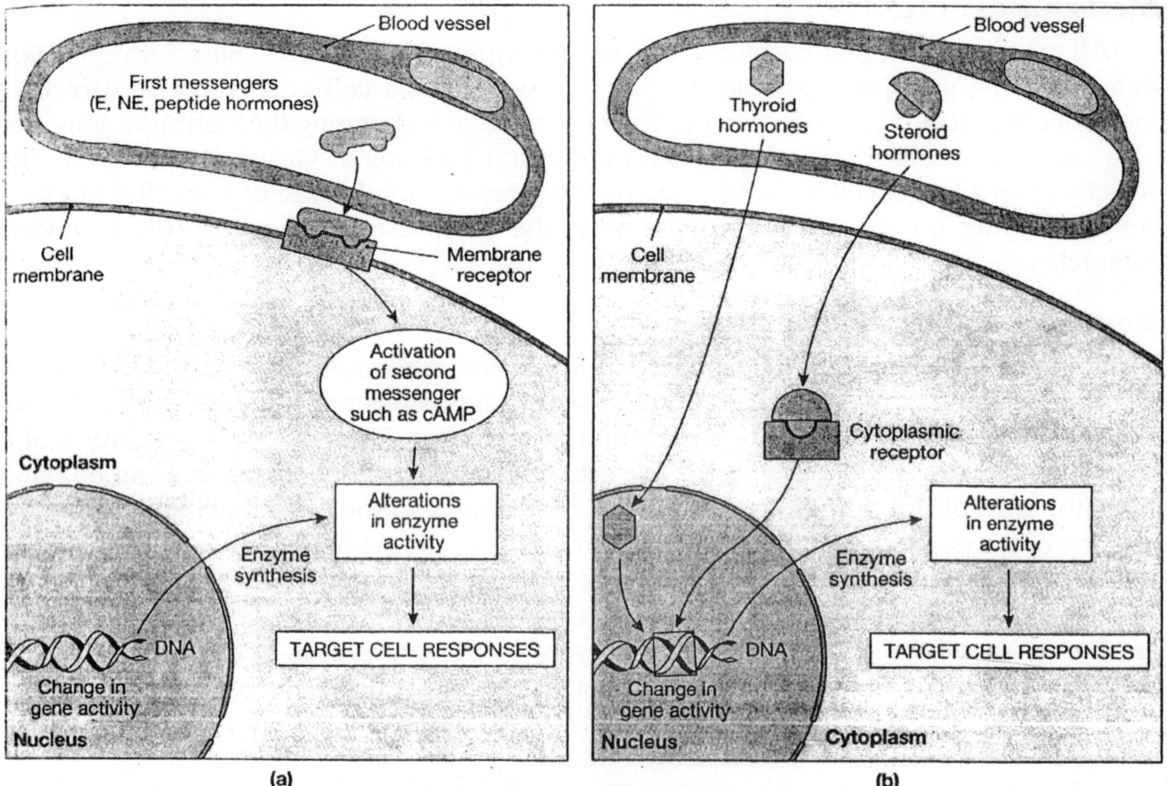

Fig 7.1 : Mechanism of hormone action

Direct negative feedback control

In direct negative feedback control the endocrine cells respond to a change in the composition of the extracellular fluid by releasing their hormone into the circulatory system. The released hormone stimulates target cells to restore homeostasis. For example, control of calcium levels by parathyroid hormone and calcitonin. When circulating calcium levels decline, parathyroid hormone is released and the responses of target cells elevate blood calcium levels. When calcium levels rise, calcitonin is released and responses of target cells lower blood calcium levels.

The hypothalamus and endocrine regulation

Coordinating centres in the hypothalamus regulate the activities of the nervous and endocrine systems in the three ways:

1. The hypothalamus contains autonomic centres that control the endocrine cells of the adrenal medullae through sympathetic innervation. When the sympathetic division is activated, the adrenal medullae release hormones into the bloodstream.
2. The hypothalamus itself acts as an endocrine organ, releasing the hormones ADH and oxytocin into the circulation at the posterior pituitary.
3. The hypothalamus secretes regulatory hormones special hormones that regulate the activities of endocrine cells in the anterior pituitary gland. There are two classes of

regulatory hormones: (1) releasing hormones (RH) stimulate production of one or more hormones in the anterior pituitary, (2) inhibiting hormones (IH) prevent the synthesis and secretion of pituitary hormones.

Major endocrine organs the pituitary gland (Hypophysis)

The pituitary gland or hypophysis secretes nine different hormones. All are peptide hormones that bind to membrane receptors and use cyclic-AMP as a second messenger. This small oval, pea- shaped structure lies nestled within the sella tunica, a depression in the spheroid bone of the skull. The pituitary gland hangs beneath the hypothalamus connected by a slender stalk, the infundibulum. In humans the pituitary gland has two major lobes, one is neural tissue and the other glandular. The posterior lobe is composed largely of pituicytes (glia like supporting cells) and nerve fibres. It releases neurohormones that it receives readymade from the hypothalamus. Thus, the posterior lobe of the pituitary is a hormone storage area and not a true endocrine gland. The posterior lobe plus the infundibulum make up the region called the neurohypophysis. The anterior lobe or adenohypophysis is composed of glandular tissue and it manufactures and releases a number of hormones.

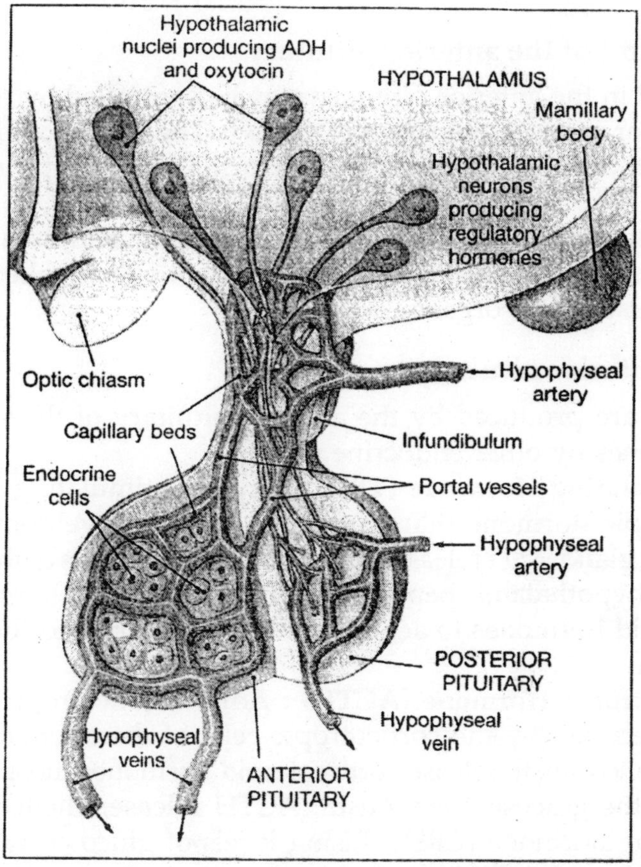

Fig. 7.2 : The Hypophyseal Portal System

The Anterior Pituitary

The anterior pituitary contains endocrine cells surrounded by an extensive capillary network. The capillary network, part of hypophyseal portal system, provides an entry into the circulatory system for the endocrine secretions of the anterior pituitary.

The Hypophyseal portal system : The regulatory hormones produced by the hypothalamus regulate the activities of the anterior pituitary. These hormones released by hypothalamic neurons near the attachment of the infundibulum enter a network of unusually permeable capillaries. Before leaving the hypothalamus, this capillary network unites to form a series of larger vessels that descend to the anterior pituitary and form a second capillary network.

A typical artery usually conducts blood from the heart to the capillary network and a typical vein carries blood from a çapillary network back to the heart. The vessels between the hypothalamus and the anterior pituitary by content carry blood from one capillary network to another. Blood vessels that link two capillary networks are called portal vessels, and the entire complex is termed a portal system.

In the portal system all blood entering the portal vessels will reach the target cells before returning to the general circulation, portal vessels are named after their destinations, so this particular network of vessels represents the hypophyseal portal system.

Hypothalamic control of the anterior pituitary

An endocrine cell in the anterior pituitary may be controlled by releasing hormones inhibiting hormones or some combination of the two. The regulatory hormones released at the hypothalamus are transported directly to the anterior pituitary through the hypophyseal system.

The rate of regulatory hormones secretion by the hypothalamus is regulated through negative feedback mechanisms. Many of these hormones are called trophic, because they activate other tissues and organs.

Hormones of the anterior pituitary

Seven hormones are produced by the anterior pituitary of those four regulate the production of hormones by other endocrine glands.

1. Thyroid Stimulating Hormone (TSH) : Thyroid stimulating hormone (TSH) or thyrotropin, is a tropic hormone that stimulates normal development and secretory activity of the thyroid gland. TSH release from the thyrotropic cells of the anterior pituitary and triggered by the hypothalamic peptide thyrotropin-releasing hormone (TRH). Rising blood levels of thyroid hormones to act on both the pituitary and the hypothalamus to inhibit TSH secretion.

2. Adrenocorticotropic Hormone (ACTH) : Adrenocorticotropic hormone (ACTH) or corticotropin is secreted by the corticotropic cells of the adenohypophysis. ACTH stimulates the adrenal cortex to release corticosteroid hormones most importantly gluco-corticoids that help the glucose metabolism. ACTH release, elicited by hypothalamic corticotropin releasing hormone (CRH), Rising levels of gluco corticoids feedback and block secretion of CRH and ACTH release.

3. Gonadotropins Follicle-Stimulating Harmone (FSH) and Luteinizing Harmone (LH) : These two hormones are referred to collectively as gonadotropins regulate the function of the gonads (ovaries and testes). FSH promotes egg development in women and stimulates the secretion of estrogens, steroid hormone produced by ovarian cells. In men, FSH production supports sperm production in the tests.

LH induces ovulation in women and promotes the ovarian secretion of estrogen and

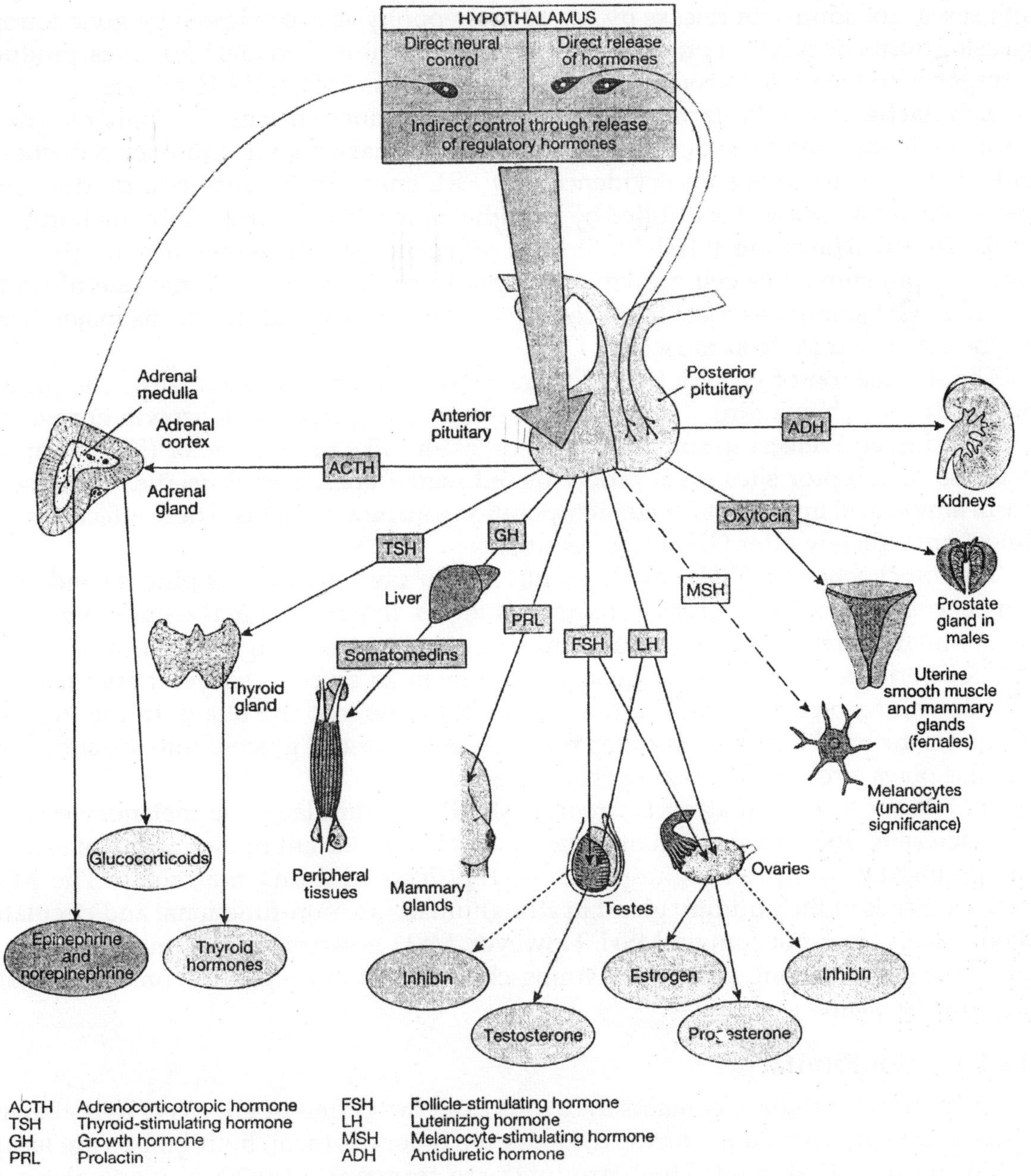

Fig. 7.3 : Pituitary Hormones and Their Targets

the progesterone that prepare the body for possible pregnancy. In men, same hormone is called interstitial-cell-stimulating hormone (ICSH) because it stimulates the interstitial cells of testes to produce sex hormones. These hormones are called androgens, the most important of them is testosterone.

Gonadotropins are absent from the blood of prepubertal boys and girls. However, during puberty, the gonadotropic cells of the adenohypophysis are activated and gonadotropin levels begins to rise causing the gonads to mature to the adult state. In both sexes, gonadotropin release by the adenohypophysis is prompted by gonadotropin releasing hormone (GnRH) produced by the hypothalamus. Gonadal hormones, produced in response to the gonadotropins, feedback to suppress FSH and LH release.

4. Prolactin (PRL) : Prolactin (PRL) is a protein hormone structurally similar to growth hormone. It stimulates the development of the mammary glands and the production of milk. However, there is some evidence that PRL enhances testosterone production in males, prolactin release is controlled by hypothalamic releasing and inhibiting hormones.

5. Growth Harmone (GH) : It is also called human growth hormone (hGH) or somatotropin stimulates cell growth and replication by accelerating the rate of protein synthesis. GH stimulates most body cells to increase in size and divide, its major targets are the bones and skeletal muscles.

The stimulation of growth by GH involves two different mechanisms. The primary mechanism which is indirect. Liver cells respond to the presence of growth hormone by synthesizing and releasing somatomedins or insulin-like growth factor (IGF) hormones that bind to receptor sites on a variety of cell membranes. Somatomedins increase the rate of amino acid uptake and their incorporation into new proteins. These effects develop almost immediately after GH release occurs.

The direct actions of GH usually do not appear until after blood glucose and amino acid concentrations have returned to normal levels. In epithelia and connective tissues, GH stimulates stem cell divisions and the differentiation of daughter cells, GH also has metabolic effects in adipose tissue and in the liver. In adipose tissue, it stimulates the breakdown of stored fats and the release of fatty acids into the blood. In the liver, GH stimulates the breakdown of glycogen reserves and release of glucose into the circulation. GH thus plays a role in mobilizing energy reserves.

6. Melanocyte Stimulating Harmone (MSH) : It stimulates the melanocytes of the skin, increasing their production of melanin. MSH is important in the control of skin and hair pigmentation in fishes, amphibians, reptiles and many mammals. The MSH-producing cells of the pituitary gland in adult humans are non-functional and circulating blood usually does not contain MSH. However, MSH is secreted by human pituitary (1) dutal fetal development, (2) in very young children, (3) in pregnant women, and (4) in some disease state.

The Posterior Pituitary

The posterior pituitary contains the axons from two different groups of hypothalamic neurons. One group manufactures ADH and the other oxytocin, both groups are located within the hypothalamus. Their products are transported within axons along the infundibulum to the posterior pituitary. ADH and oxytocin each composed of nine amino acids are almost identical. They differ in only two amino acids, yet they have very different physiological effects on their target organs. ADH influences body water balance, whereas oxytocin stimulates the contraction of smooth muscle, particularly that of the uterus and breast.

Antidiuretic Hormone (ADH) : Diuresis is urine production. Thus, an antidiuretic is a substance that inhibits or prevents urine formation. ADH is released in response to stimuli such as a rise in the concentration of electrolytes in the blood or a fall in blood volume or pressure. The primary function of ADH is to decrease the amount of water lost at the kidneys with losses minimized, any water absorbed from the digestive tract will be retained, reducing the concentration of electrolytes. ADH also causes the constriction of peripheral blood vessels, which helps to increase blood pressure. Highly specialized hypo thalamic neurons called osmoreceptors, continually monitor the solute concentration of blood. When solute becomes too concentrated the osmoreceptors transmit excitatory impulses to the hypothalamic neurons in the supra-optic nucleus, which synthesize and release ADH. ADH is liberated into the blood by the neurohypophysis, and targets the kidney tubules. The tubule cells respond by reabsorbing more water from the forming urine and returning it to the bloodstream. As a result, less urine is produced and blood volume increases. As solute concentration declines, the osmoreceptors stop depolarizing effectively ending ADH release. Other stimuli triggering ADH release include pain low blood pressure, and certain drugs. Drinking alcoholic beverages inhibits ADH secretion and causes copious urine output. ADH release is also inhibited by drinking excessive amount of water.

At high blood concentrations. ADH causes vasoconstriction. Under certain conditions, such as severe blood loss, exceptionally large amounts of ADH are released. Thus, in turn, causes a rise in systemic blood pressure. The alternative name for this hormone (vasopressin) reflects this particular effect.

Oxytocin—Oxytocin, a strong stimulant of uterine contraction is released in significantly higher amounts during childbirth and in nursing women. The number of oxytocin receptors in the uterus peaks near the end of pregnancy, and uterine smooth muscle becomes more and more sensitive to the stimulatory effects of oxytocin. The hypothalamus responds by synthesizing oxytocin and triggering its release from the neurohypophysis. As blood levels of oxytocin rise the expulsive contractions of labour gain momentum and finally end in birth.

Oxytocin also acts as the hormonal trigger for milk ejection in women whose breasts are actively producing milk in response to prolactin. Suckling causes a reflex-initiated release of oxytocin, which targets specialized myoepithetial cells surrounding the milk producing glands. As these cells contract milk is forced from the breast into the mouth of the suckling infant.

In the male oxytocin stimulates the smooth muscle contraction in the walls of the prostate gland. This action may be important in emission, the ejection of prostatic secretions, spermatozoa and the secretions of other glands into the male reproductive tract before ejaculation occurs.

The Thyroid Gland

The butterfly shaped thyroid gland is located in the anterior neck on the trachea just inferior to the larynx. Its two lateral lobes are connected by a medium tissue mass called the isthmus. The thyroid gland is the largest endocrine gland in the body. It has a deep red colouration because of the large number of blood vessels.

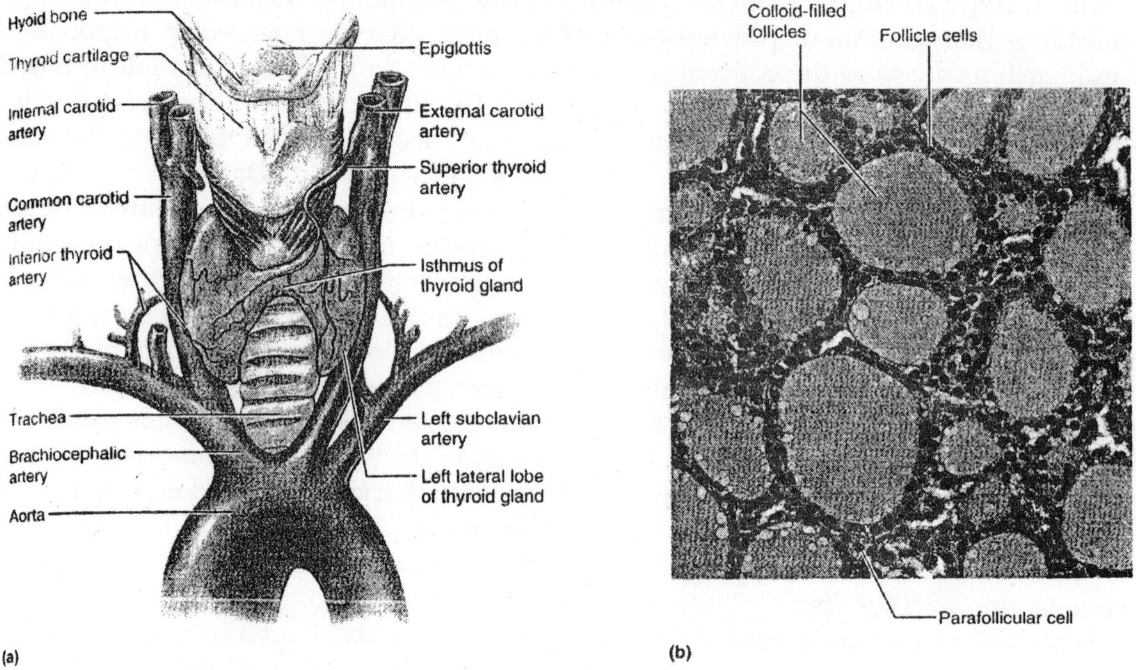

Fig 7.4 Gross and Microscopic Anatomy of the Thyroid Gland

Internally, the thyroid gland has hollow, spherical follicles. The walls of each follicle are formed by cuboidal or squamous epithelial cells called follicle, which produce the glycoprotein thyroglobulin. The central cavity or lumen of follicle stores "colloid" an amber-coloured sticky material consisting of thyroglobulin molecules with attached iodine atoms. Thyroid hormone is derived from this iodinated thyroglobulin. The parafollicular cells another cells found in the thyroid gland produce calcitonin.

Thyroid Hormones (TH)

Thyroid hormones, often referred as the body's major metabolic hormone, is two active iodine-containing hormone, thyroxine or TX contains four atoms of iodine, it is also known as tetraiodothyronine or T4, it accounts for roughly 90 per cent of all thyroid secretions and triiodothyronine or T3 containing three iodine atoms.

Except for the adult brain, spleen, testes, uterus and the thyroid gland itself thyroid hormone affects every cell in the body, because they diffuse through the cytoplasm to reach receptor sites in the nucleus. Thyroid hormones activate genes coding for the synthesis of enzymes involved in glycolysis and energy production, resulting in an increase in cellular rate of metabolism, and oxygen consumption. Because the cell consumes more energy, and energy use is measured in calories, this is called calorigenic effect. When the metabolic rate increases more heat is generated and body temperature rises. Thyroid hormone provokes an increase in the number of adrenergic receptors in blood vessels it plays an important role in maintaining blood pressure. It is also an important regulator of tissue growth and development. It is essential for normal skeletal and nervous system development.

Normal production of thyroid hormones establishes the background rates of cellular metabolism. These hormones exert their primary effects on active tissues and organs, including skeletal muscles liver, heart and kidneys. Overproduction or underproduction of thyroid hormones can cause very serious metabolic problems. Inadequate dietary iodine leads to an inability to synthesize thyroid hormones. Under these conditions, TSH stimulation continues, and the thyroid follicles become distended with non-functional secretions. The result is a swollen and enlarged thyroid gland or goitre.

The 'C' cells of the Thyroid Gland (Calcitonin)

Calcitonin is a polypeptide hormone produced by the parafollicular or C cells of the thyroid gland. Its most important effect is to lower blood calcium levels. The C cells release calcitonin when the calcium ion concentration of the blood rises above normal. The target organs are the bones and the kidneys. Calcitonin reduces calcium levels by inhibiting osteoclasts and stimulating calcium excretion at the kidneys. The resulting reduction in the calcium ion concentrations eliminates the stimulus and "turns off" the C cells.

Calcitocin appears to be important only in childhood, when the skeleton grows quickly and the bones are changing dramatically in mass, size and shape.

Calcium ion has important part in controlling muscle and nerve cell activities. Calcium ion concentration also affect the sodium permeabilities of excitable membranes. At high calcium ion concentrations, sodium permeability decreases and membranes become less responsive. Such problems are prevented by the secretion of calcitonin under appropriate conditions. However, under normal conditions, calcium ion levels seldom rise enough to trigger calcitonin secretion. Most homeostatic adjustments are intended to prevent lower than normal calcium ion concentrations. Low calcium concentrations are dangerous because sodium permeabilities increase and muscle cells and neurons become extremely excitable. If calcium levels fall too far, convulsions or muscular spasms will occur. The parathyroid glands and their hormone secretions are responsible for preventing such disastrous events.

The Parathyroid Glands

Two tiny, yellow-brown pairs of parathyroid glands are embedded in the posterior surfaces of the thyroid gland. The gland cells are separated by the dense capsular fibres of the thyroid. The parathyroids glandular cells are arranged in thick branching cords containing scattered oxyphil cells and large number of the smaller chief cells. The chief cells also called principal cells secrete PTH. The function of oxyphil cells is unclear.

Parathyroid hormone (PTH) or parathormone the protein hormone of these glands is the single, most important hormone controlling the calcium balance of the blood. Its release is triggered by falling blood calcium levels and inhibited by hyper calcemia. PTH increases ionic calcium levels in the blood by stimulating three target organs, the skeleton, the kidneys and the intestine.

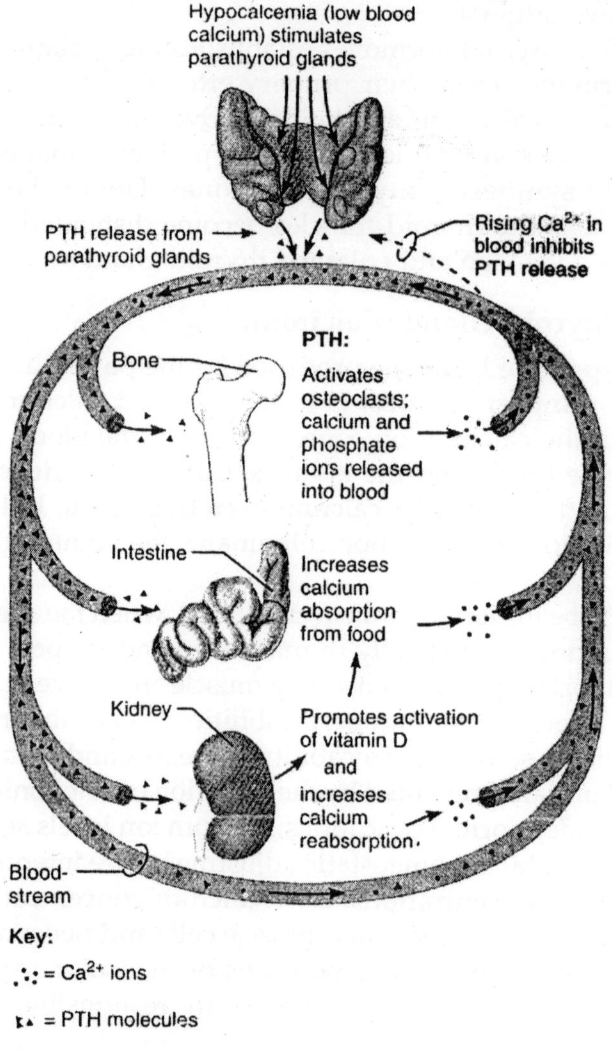

Fig. 7.5 Summary of Parathyroid Hormone's Effects on Bone, the Intestine, and the Kidneys

PTH release (1) stimulates osteoclasts to digest some of bony matrix and release ionic calcium and phosphates to the blood, (2) enhances reabsorption of calcium by the kidneys, and (3) increases absorption of calcium by the intestinal mucosal cells. Calcium absorption by the intestine is enhanced indirectly by PTH's effect on vitamin D activation. Vitamin D is required for absorption of calcium from ingested food.

Since plasma calcium ion homeostasis is essential for so many functions, including transmission of nerve impulses, muscle contraction and blood clotting.

Hyperparathyroidism is rare and usually the result of a parathyroid gland tumour. When it occurs, calcium is leached from the bones and the bones soften and deform as their mineral salts are replaced by fibrous connective tissue. Due to hypercalcemia two main abnormally noted are (1) depression of the nervous system, which leads to abnormal reflexes and weakens of the skeletal muscles, and (2) formation of kidney stone as excess calcium salts precipitate in the kidney tubules. Calcium deposits may also form in soft tissue throughout the body and severely impair vital organ functioning.

Hypoparathyroidism on PTH deficiency most often follows parathyroid gland trauma or removal during thyroid surgery. The deficiency of dietary magnesium can cause functional hypoparathyroidism. The resulting hypocalcemia increases the excitability of neurons and accounts for the classical symptoms of tetany such as loss of sensation muscle twitches, and convulsions. Untreated the symptoms progress to spasms of the larynx, respiratory paralysis and death.

The Adrenal (Suprarenal) Glands

A single adrenal gland caps the superior border of each kidney, because of their location the adrenals are also called suprarenal glands. They are pyramid-shaped, enclosed in a fibrous capsule. Each adrenal gland can be divided into two parts, a superficial adrenal cortex and an inner adrenal medulla. Each adrenal gland is structurally and functionally two endocrine glands in one. The inner adrenal medulla, like a knot of nervous tissue than a gland, acts as a part of the sympathetic nervous system. The outer adrenal cortex encapsulated the medullary region and forming the bulk of the gland is glandular tissue. Each of these regions produces its own set of hormones.

The Adrenal Cortex

The adrenal cortex has a grayish yellow colouration because of the presence of stored lipids, especially cholesterol and various fatty acids. The adrenal cortex produces more than two dozen different steroid hormones collectively called adrenocorticosteriods or simply corticosteroids. These hormones are vital, if the adrenal glands are destroyed or removed, corticosteroids must be administered or the individual will not survive.

The large lipid-laden cortical cells are arranged in three distinct layer or zones. The cell clusters forming the superficial zona glomerulosa mainly produce mineralocorticoids, hormones that help to control the balance of minerals and water in blood. The middle zona fasciculata arranged in more or less linear cords secrete the metabolic hormones called glucocorticoids. The cells of the inner-most zona reticularis, have a netlike arrangement. These cells produce small amounts of adrenal sex hormones or gonadocorticoids.

Mineralocorticoids—The essential function of mineralocorticoids is regulation of the electrolyte (mineral salt) concentrations in extracellular fluids, particularly of sodium and potassium ions. The single most abundant positive ion in extracellular fluid is sodium and while sodium is vital to homeostasis, excessive sodium intake and retention may promote high blood pressure. There are several mineralocorticoids, aldosterone is the most potent, and accounts for over 9 per cent of the mineralocorticoid produced, maintaining sodium ion balance.

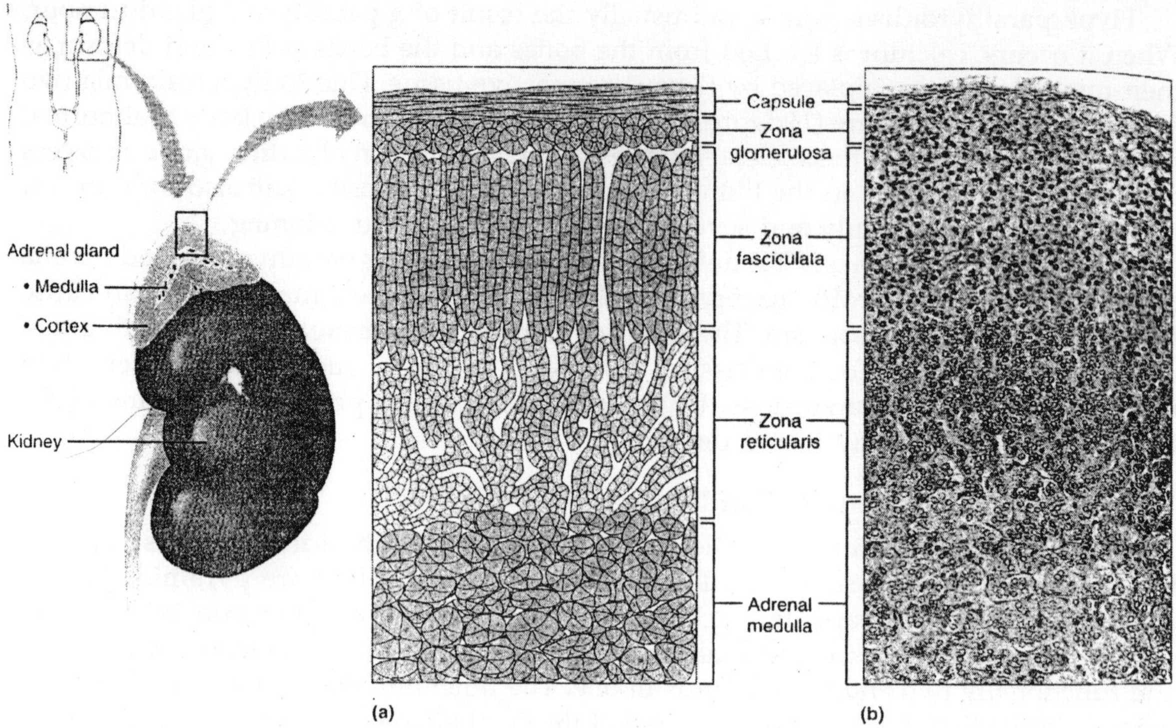

Fig. 7.6 Microscopic Structure of the Adrenal Gland

Aldosterone reduces excretion of sodium from the body. Its primary target is the distal parts of kidney tubules, where it stimulates reabsorption of sodium ions from the forming urine and their return to the bloodstream. Aldosterone also enhances sodium ion reabsorption from perspiration, saliva and gastric juice. The mechanism of aldosterone activity appears to involve the synthesis of an enzyme required for sodium transport.

Aldosterone secretion is stimulated by a number of factors, rising blood levels of potassium ions, low blood levels of sodium and decreasing blood volume and blood pressure. The reverse conditions inhibit aldosterone secretion. Four mechanisms regulate aldosterone secretion, the renin-angiotensin system, plasma concentrations of sodium and potassium ions, controls exerted by ACTH and plasma concentrations of atrial natriuretic peptide.

1. The Renin-angiotensin mechanisms—The renin-angiotensin mechanism, the major regulator of aldosterone release, influences both the electrolyte-water balance of the blood and blood pressure. Specialized cells of the juxtaglomerular apparatus in the kidneys become excited when blood pressure declines or plasma osmolarity drops. They respond by releasing renin into the blood. Renin cleaves off part of the plasma protein angiotensinogen, triggering an enzymatic leading to the formation of angiotension II, a stimulator of aldosterone release by the glomerulosa cells of the adrenal cortex.

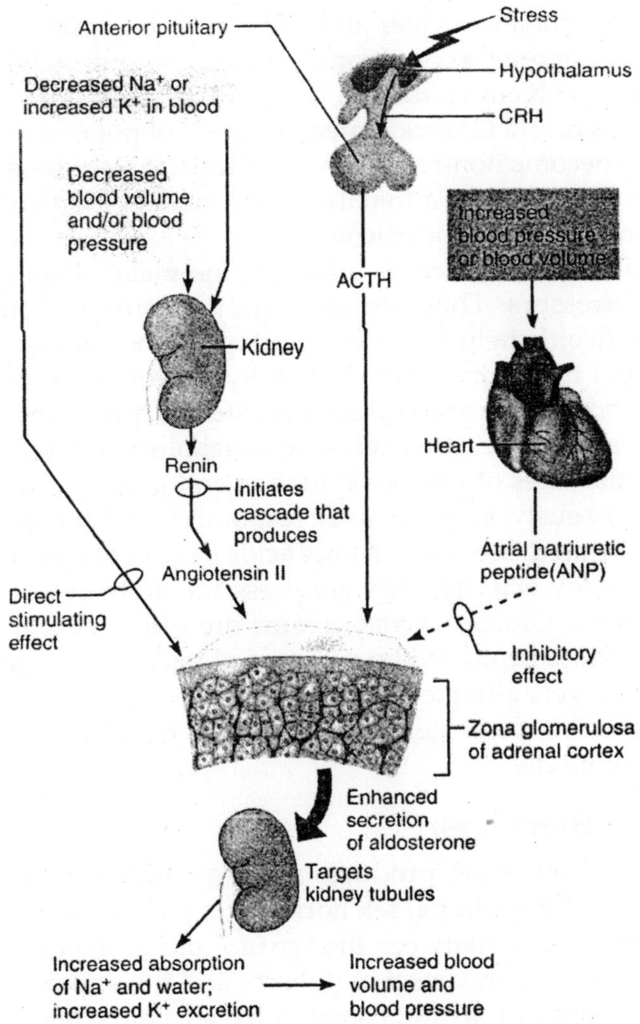

Fig.7.7 : Major Mechanisms Controlloing Aldosterone Release from the Adrenal Cortex

2. Plasma concentration of sodium and potassium ions—Fluctuating blood levels of sodium and potassium ions directly influence the zona glomerulosa cells. Increased potassium and decreased sodium are stimulatory the opposite conditions are inhibitory.

3. ACTH—Under normal circumstances, ACTH released by the anterior pituitary has little or no effect on aldosterone release. When a person is severely stressed the hypothalamus secretes more corticotropin-releasing hormone (CRH) and the rise in ACTH blood levels that follows steps up the rate of aldosterone secretion to a small extent. The rise in blood volume and blood pressure that results helps adequate delivery of nutrients and respiratory gases during the stressful period.

4. Atrial natriuretic peptide (ANP)—Atrial natriuretic peptide, a hormone secreted by the heart, when blood pressure rises. Its major effect is to inhibit the renin-angiotensin mechanism. It blocks renin and aldosterone secretion and inhibit other angiotensin-induced mechanisms that enhance water and sodium reabsorption.

Hypersecretion of aldosterone, a condition called aldosteronism, typically results from adrenal neoplasms. Two problem results (1) hypertension and edema due to excessive sodium and water retention, and (2) accelerated excretion of potassium ions. If potassium loss is extreme, neurons become non-responsive and muscle weakness occurs. Addison's disease a hyposecretary disease of the adrenal cortex, generally involves a deficient output of both mineralocorticoids and glucocorticoids.

Glucocorticoids—The glucocorticoids influence the metabolism of most body cells and help us to resist stressors. They are absolutely essential to life. Under normal circumstances, glucocorticoids help the body to adapt in food intake by keeping blood sugar levels constant and maintain blood volume by preventing the shift of water into tissue cells. Cortisol, corticosterone and cortisone are steroid hormones collectively known as glucocorticoids. These hormones affect glucose metabolism and secreted under ACTH stimulation, accelerate the rates of glucose synthesis and glycogen formation especially within the liver. Simultaneously, adipose tissue responds by releasing fatty acids into the blood and other tissues begin to breakdown fatty acids instead of glucose. Glucocorticoids also have anti-inflammatory activity, they suppress the activities of white blood cells and other immune system. Glucocorticoid creams are often used to control irritating allergic reaches such as those produced by poison and injections of glucocorticoids may be used to control more severe allergic reactions. Because they slow wound healing and suppress immune defenses, topical steroids are used to treat superficial rashes but are never applied to open wounds.

Gonadocorticoids (Sex Hormones)

The adrenal cortex in both sexes produces small quantities of sex hormones called androgens. The exact role of the adrenal sex hormone is still unclear but because adrenal androgen levels rise continuously between the age of 7 and 13 in both boys and girls, it is assumed that they contribute to the onset of puberty and the appearance of axillary and pubic hair during that time. In adult women adrenal androgens are thought to be responsible for the sex drive and they may be converted estrogen after menopause when ovarian estrogens are no longer produced.

The Adrenal Medulla

The adrenal medulla has a reddish brown colouration because of the many blood vessels in this area. It contains large, rounded cells innervated by preganglionic sympathetic fibres.

The adrenal medulla contain two populations of secretory cells, one producing epinephrine (E or adrenaline) and the other norepinephrine (NE or noradrenaline). These hormones are normally released at a low rate, but sympathetic stimulation accelerates the rate of discharge dramatically.

Epinephrine makes up 75-80 per cent of the secretions from the medulla, the rest is norepinephrine. These hormones accelerate cellular energy utilization and mobilize energy reserves. Receptors for epinephrine and norepinephrine are found on skeletal muscle fibres, in adipose tissues, and in the liver, Secretion by the medulla triggers a mobilization of glycogen reserves, in skeletal muscles and accelerates the breakdown of glucose to provide ATP. This combination increases muscular power. In adipose cells, stored fats are broken down to fatty acids and in the liver glycogen molecules are converted to glucose. The fatty acids and glucose are then released into the circulation for use by peripheral tissues. The heart also responds to adrenal medulla hormones with an increase in the rate and force of cardiac contractions.

The Pancrease—The pancreas lies in the J-shaped loop between the stomach and small intestine. It is pink organ, contains both exocrine and endocrine cells. The exocrine pancreas produces large quantities of an alkaline, enzyme-rich fluid that is secreted into the digestive tract.

Cells of the endocrine pancreas form clusters known as pancreatic islets or the islets of Langerhans. The islets are scattered among the exocrine cells. Each islet contains several different cell types. The two most important are alpha cells which produce the hormone glucagon and the beta cells, which secrete insulin. Glucagon and insulin regulate blood glucose concentration.

Regulation of blood glucose concentration

Glucose is the energy source for most cells in the body and under normal conditions the only energy source for neurons. When blood glucose levels rise, beta cells release insulin, and this hormone stimulates glucose transport into its target cells. Almost all cells in the body are affected, the only exceptions are (1) neurons and red blood cells which cannot mobilize other nutrients, and (2) epithelial cells of the kidney tubules and intestinal lining, where glucose is reabsorbed. When glucose is abundant all cells use it as an energy source and stop breaking down amino acids and lipids.

The ATP generated by the breakdown of glucose molecules is used to build proteins and to increase energy reserves, and most cells increase their rates of protein synthesis in response to insulin. A secondary effect is an increase in the rate of amino acid transport across cell membranes. Insulin also stimulates fat cells to increase their rates of triglyceride (fat) synthesis and storage. In the liver and in skeletal muscles, insulin also accelerates the formation of glycogen. In summary, when glucose is abundant insulin secretion stimulates glucose utilization to support growth and to establish glycogen and fat reserves.

When glucose level declines, insulin secretion is suppressed, and so is glucose transport into its target cells. These cells, now shift over to other energy sources, such as fatty acids. At the same time, the alpha cells release glucagon, and energy reserves are mobilized. Skeletal muscles and liver cell breakdown glycogen, a adipose tissue releases fatty acids, and proteins, are brokendown into their component amino acids. The liver takes in the lipids and amino acids and converts them to glucose that can be released into the circulation. As a result, blood glucose concentrations rise toward normal levels. The interplay between insulin and glucagon both stabilizes blood glucose levels and prevents competition between neural tissue and other tissues for limited glucose supplies.

Pancreatic alpha and beta cells are sensitive to blood glucose concentrations and their regulatory activities are not under the direct control of other endocrine or nervous

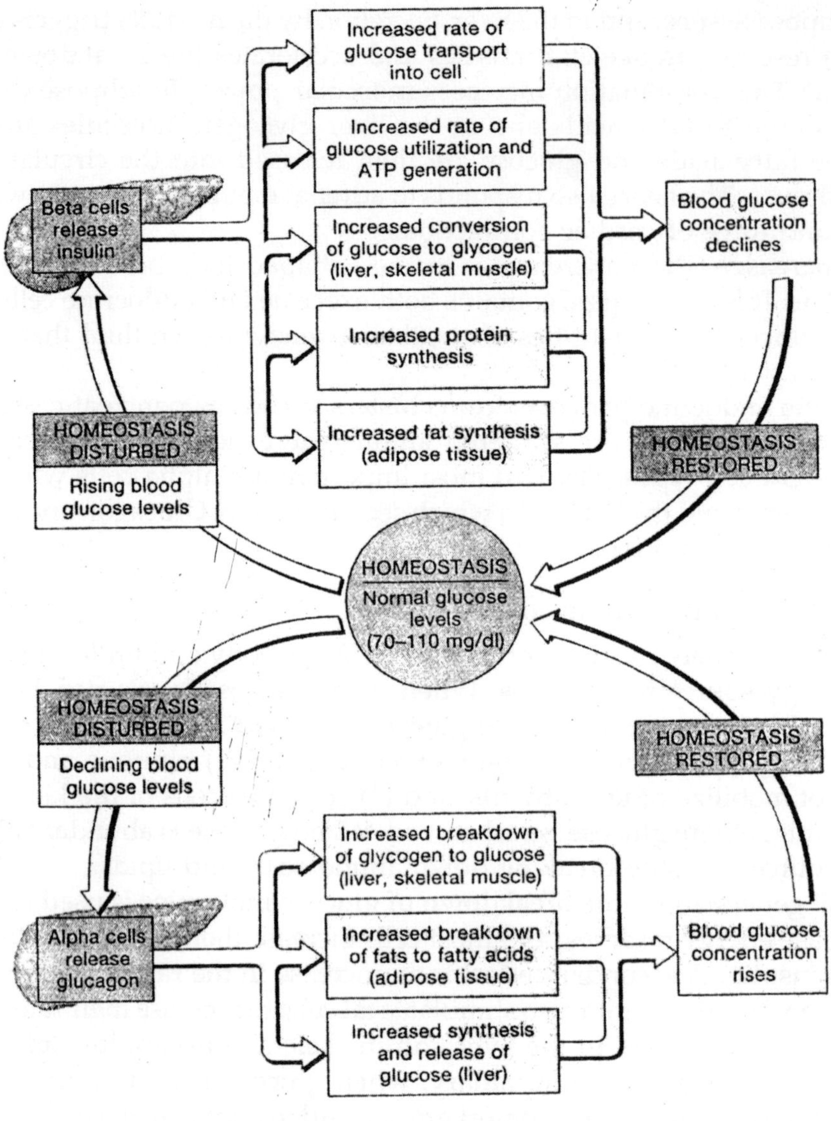

Fig. 7.8 : Regulation of Blood Glucose Concentrations

components. Yet, because the islet cells are extremely sensitive to variations in blood glucose levels, any hormone that affects blood glucose concentrations will indirectly affect the production of insulin and glucagon.

Diabetes mellitus (DM) results from hyposecretion or hypoactivity of insulin. When insulin is absent or deficient, blood sugar levels remain high after a meal because glucose is unable to enter most tissue cells. Ordinarily, when blood sugar levels rise, hyperglycemic hormones are not released, but when hyperglycemia becomes excessive the person begins to feel nauseated. This results, glycogenolysis, lipolysis and gluconeogenesis. Thus already high blood sugar levels higher and excesses of glucose begin to be lost from the body in the urine (glycosuria).

When sugars cannot be used as cellular fuel, more fats are mobilized resulting in high fatty acid levels in the blood a condition called lipidema or lipemia. In severe cases of diabetes mellitus, blood levels of fatty acids and their metabolites rise. The fatty acid metabolites, collectively called ketones or ketone bodies are strong organic acids. When they accumulate faster than they are used or excreted the blood pH drops, resulting in ketoacidosis, and ketones begin to spill into the urine (ketonuria). Ketoacidosis disrupts heart activity and oxygen transport and severe depression of the nervous system leads to coma and finally death.

The three cardinal signs of diabetes mellitus are polyuria, polydispia and polyphagia. The excessive glucose in the kidney filtrate acts as an osmotic diuretic, that is it inhibits water reabsorption by the kidney tubules, resulting in polyuria a huge urine output that leads to decreased blood volume and dehydration. Serious electrolyte, losses also occur as the body rids itself of excess ketones. Ketones are negative charged and carry positive ions out with them, as a result sodium and potassium ions are also lost from the body. Because of the electrolyte imbalance, the person gets abdominal pains and may vomit. Dehydration stimulates hypothalamic thirst centres causing polydispia or excessive thirst. The final cardinal sign polyphagia refers to excessive hunger and food consumption.

Hyperinsulinism or excessive insulin secretion, results in low blood sugar levels or hypoglycemia, which causes anxiety, nervousness and a feeling of weakness. Insufficient glucose delivery to the brain causes disorientation progressing to convulsions, unconsciousness and even death.

The Gonads—The male and female gonads are the endocrine tissue of the reproductive system.

The Testes—In the male the interstitial cells of the testis produce the steroid hormones known as androgens. Testosterone is the most important androgen. This hormone promotes the production of functional sperm, maintains the secretary glands of the male reproductive tract, and determines secondary sexual characteristics such as the distribution of facial hair and body fat. Testosterone also affects the metabolic operations throughout the body, stimulate protein synthesis and muscle growth. During embryonic development, the production of testosterone affects the development of male reproductive ducts, external genitalia and CNS structures that will later affect sexual behaviours.

Sustentacular cells are directly associated with the formation of functional sperms in the testes. These cells also secrete a hormone called inhibin. Inhibin production, which occurs under FSH stimulation depress the secretion of FSH by the anterior pituitary. Throughout adult life, these two hormones interact to maintain sperm production at normal level.

The Ovaries—In the ovaries, female sex cells or ova, develop in specialized structures called follicles under stimulation by FSH. Follicle cells surround the ova produce estrogens. These steroid hormones support the maturation of the eggs and stimulate the growth of the uterine lining. Under FSH stimulation, follicular cells secrete inhibin, which suppresses FSH release through a feedback mechanism. After ovulation has occurred, the follicular cells then begin to release a mixture of estrogen and progesterone, progesterone accelerates the movement of fertilized eggs along the uterine tubes and prepare the uterus for the arrival of a developing embryo progesterone, along with other hormones also causes an enlargement of the mammary glands.

The production of androgens estrogens and progesterone is controlled by regulatory hormones released by the anterior pituitary gland. During pregnancy, the placenta itself functions as an endocrine organ, working together with the ovaries and the pituitary gland to promote normal fetal development and delivery.

The Pineal Gland—The pineal gland lies in the roof of the thalamus. It contains, neurons glial cells and secretory cells that synthesize the hormone melatonin. Melatonin concentrations in the blood rise and fall in diurnal cycle. Peak levels occur during night and make us drowsy, lowest levels occur during day light hours around noon.

In a variety of other mammals melatonin slows the maturation of sperm, eggs and reproductive organs. In some animal mating behaviour and gonadal size vary with changes in the relative lengths of light and dark periods, and melatonin mediate these effects. In children, melatonin may have an antigonadotropic effect, that is it may inhibit too early sexual maturation and thus affect the timing of puberty.

Melatonin is a very effective antioxidant that may protect CNS neurons from free-radicals, such as nitric oxide (NO) or hydrogen peroxide (H_2O_2), that may be generated in active neural tissue. Because of the cyclical nature of its activity, the pineal gland may also be involved with the establishment or maintenance of basic circadian rhythms daily changes in physiological processes that follow a regular pattern. Increased melatonin secretion in darkness has been suggested as a primary cause for seasonal affective disorder. This condition characterized by changes in mood, eating habits and sleeping patterns.

The Thymus—Located deep to the sternum, is the lobulated thymus gland embedded in a mass of connective tissue inside the thoracic cavity. As the child grows, the thymus continues to enlarge slowly, reaching its maximum size just before puberty at a weight of around 40 gm. After puberty, it gradually diminishes in size, by age 50 the thymus may weight less than 12 gm. By old age, it is composed largely of adipose and fibrous connective tissues.

The thymus produces several hormones collectively known as the thymosins. The thymosins play a key role in the development and maintenance of normal immunological defenses. It has been suggested that the gradual decrease in the size and secretory abilities of thymus may make the elderly more susceptible to disease.

Other hormone producing structures—Other hormone producing cells occur within various organs of the body these are the following :

1. Heart—The atria of the heart contain some specialized cardiac muscle cells that secrete atrial natriuretic peptide (ANP). This peptide hormone reduces blood volume, blood pressure and blood sodium concentration when these parameters become elevated.

2. Gastrointestinal Tract—Enteroendocrine cells are hormone secreting cells present within the mucosa of organs of gastrointestinal tract. They release several amine and peptide hormones that help to regulate a wide variety of digestive functions.

3. The placenta secretes several steroid and protein hormones that influence the course of pregnancy. Placental hormones include estrogen and progesterone as well as human chorionic gonado tropin.

4. Kidney—Unidentified cells in the kidney secrete erythropoietin. This protein hormone signals the bone marrow to increase its production of red blood cells.

5. Skin—The skin produces cholecalciferol, an inactive form of vitamin D3 when modified cholesterol molecules in epidermal cells are exposed to ultraviolet radiation. This compound then enters the blood with the dermal capillaries is modified in the liver and becomes fully activated in the kidney. The active form of vitamin D3, is essential part of the carrier system that intestinal cells use to absorb Ca^{2+} from the diet, without this vitamin, the bones become weak and soft.

Adipose Tissue—Adipose cells release leptin following then uptake of glucose and lipids which they store as fat. Leptin binds to CNS neurons concerned with appetite control.

8

Reproduction

Anatomy of Male Reproductive System

The sperm producing testes, or male gonads, lie within the scrotum from the testes, the sperm are delivered to the body through a system of ducts including, epididymis, ductus deferens and urethra, which opens to the outside at the tip of the penis. The accessory sex glands, which empty their secretions into the ducts during ejaculation are the seminal vesicles, prostate gland, and bulbourethral gland.

The Scrotum

The Scrotum (pouch) is a sac of skin that hangs outside the abdominopelvic cavity at the root of penis. The paired testes or testicles, lie suspended in the scrotum. A midline septum divides the scrotum into right and left halves, providing one compartment for each testis. The scrotum provides a temperature about 3°C lower, is an essential adaptation. The scrotum responds to changes in temperature. When it is cold the testes are pulled closer to the warmth of the body wall, and the scrotum becomes shorter and heavily wrinkled to reduce heat loss when it is warm, the scrotal skin is flaccid and loose to increase the surface area for cooling, and the testis hang lower.

The Testes

Each testis is 4 cm long and 2.5 cm in diameter, is surrounded by two tunics. The outer tunic is tunica vaginalis. Deep to this is the tunica albuginea. Septa extending from the tunica albuginea divide the testis into 250 to 300 compartments or tubules. Each lobule, contains one to four tightly coiled seminiferous (sperm carrying) tubules.

The seminiferous tubules of each lobule coverage to form a tubulus rectus, a straight tubule that conveys sperm into the rete testis, a tubular network on the posterior side of testis. From the rete testis sperm leave the testis through the efferent ductules, and enter the epididymis.

Lying in the soft connective tissue surrounding the seminiferous tubules are the interstitial cells or Leydig cells. These cells produce androgens (most importantly testosterone) which they secrete into the surrounding interstitial fluid.

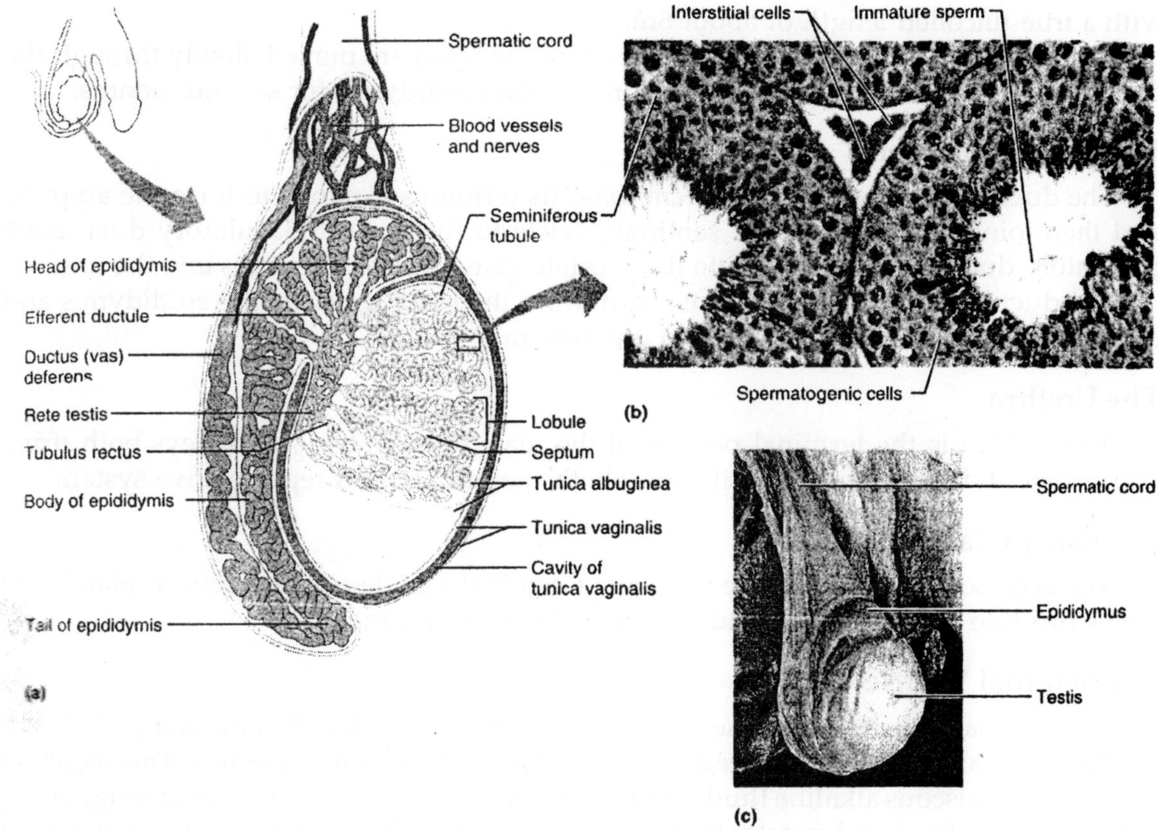

Fig. 8.1 : Internal Structure of the Testis

The Penis

The penis (tail) is a copulatory organ. The penis and scrotum, make up the external genitalia of the male.

The penis consists of an attached root and a free shaft on body that ends in an enlarged tip, the glans penis.

Internally the penis contains the spongy urethra and three long cylindrical bodies of erectile tissues. The midventral erectile body the corpus spongiosum surrounds the urethra.

The Male Duct System

As sperm travel from the testes to the outside of the body through a system of ducts. The accessory ducts are the epididymis, the ductus deferens and the urethra.

The Epididymis

The epididymis is about 3.8 cm long. Its head, which joins the efferent ductules, caps the superior aspect of the testis. Its body and tail regions lie on the posterolateral aspects of the testis. The bulk of the epididymis consists of the highly coiled duct of the epididymis with a true uncoiled length of about 6m.

The immature, non-motile sperm that leave the testis are moved slowly through the duct of the epididymis. Sperm can be stored in the epididymis for several months.

The Ductus Deferens

The ductus deferens is about 45 cm long. Its terminus expands to form the ampulla and then joins with the duct of seminal vesicle to form short ejaculatory duct. Each ejaculatory duct, in turn, passes into the prostate gland where it empties into the urethra.

The ductus deferens propels live sperm from their storage sites, the epididymis and distal part of the ductus deferens into the urethra.

The Urethra

The urethra is the terminal portion of the male duct system. It conveys both urine and semen at different times, so it serves both the urinary and reproductive system.

Accessory Glands

The accessory glands include the paired seminal vesicles, bulbourethral gland and single prostate gland. These glands produce the bulk of semen.

The Seminal Vesicle

The seminal vesicles lie on the posterior wall of the bladder. It is tubular gland.

The seminal vesicles contribute about 60 per cent of the volume of semen. This secretion is a yellowish viscous alkaline fluid containing fructose sugar, ascorbic acid, a coagulating enzyme (vesiculase) and prostaglandins. The duct of each seminal vesicle joins that of the ductus deferens on the same side to form the ejaculatory duct sperm and seminal fluid mix in the ejaculatory duct and enter the prostatic urethra together during ejaculation.

The Prostate Gland

The prostate gland is a small muscular rounded organ. It surrounds the urethra as it leaves the urinary bladder. It is composed of 20 to 30 compound tubulo-alveolar glands embedded in a mass of smooth muscle and dense connective tissue. The prostatic wall produces a weakly acidic secretion that contributes about 30 per cent of the volume of semen. Its secretion also contains seminalplasmin an antibiotic that may help prevent urinary tract infections in males prostatic secretion plays a role in activating of sperm. The inactive mature spermatozoa being beating their flagella and become highly mobile.

The Bulbourethral Glands

The bulbourethral glands also called cowper's glands are pea- sized glands situated inferior to the prostate gland. They secrete a thick sticky, alkaline mucus that has lubricating properties.

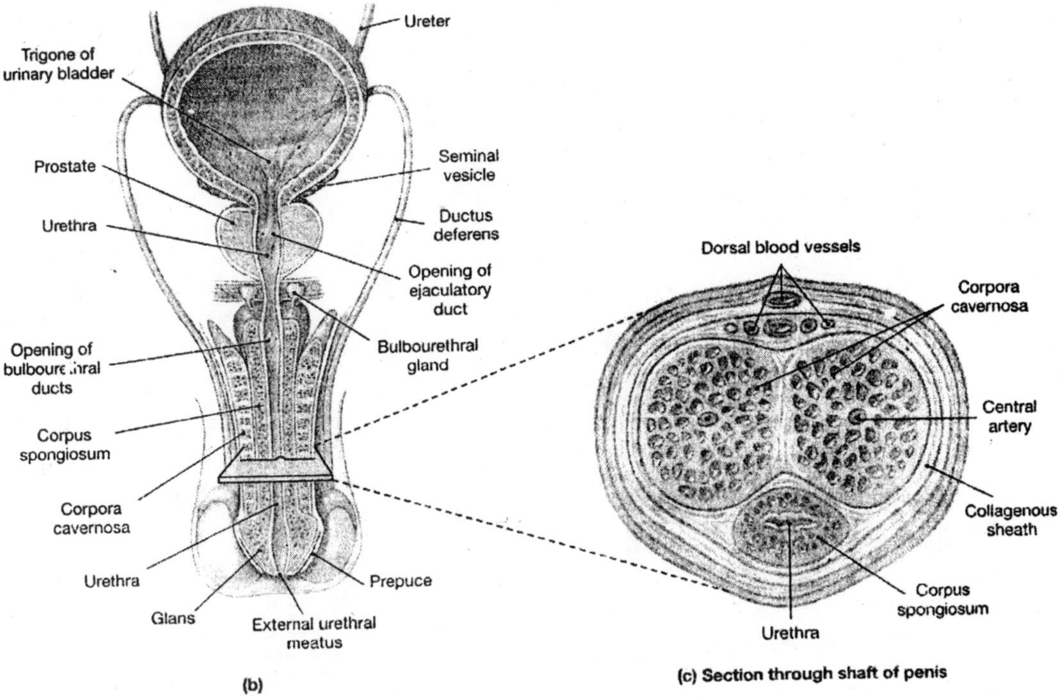

Fig. 8.2 The Penis

Hormones and Male Reproductive Function

The anterior pituitary releases follicle stimulating hormone (FSH) and lutenizing hormone (LH). The pituitary release of these hormone occurs in the presence of gonadotropin-releasing hormone (GnRH), a hormone synthesized in the hypothalamus and carried to the anterior pituitary in the hypophyseal portal system.

In male, FSH, targets primarily the cells of seminiferous tubules. Under FSH stimulation and in the presence of testosterone from the interstitial cells, spermatogenesis and spermiogenesis takes place.

The rate of spermatogenesis is regulated by a negative feedback mechanism involving GnRH, FSH and inhibin. Under GnRH stimulation, FSH promotes spermatogenesis along the seminiferous tubules. As spermatogenesis accelerates. Inhibin inhibits FSH production in the anterior pituitary and may be suppress secretion of GnRH at the hypothalamus.

The net effect is that when FSH levels become elevated, inhibin production increases until the FSH level return to normal. If FSH levels decline, inhibin production falls, and the rate of FSH production accelerates.

LH and Androgen Production

In the male, LH causes the secretion of testosterone and other androgens by the interstitial cells of testes. Testosterone, the most important androgen has numerous functions: (1) promotes the functional maturation of spermatozoa, (2) maintains the

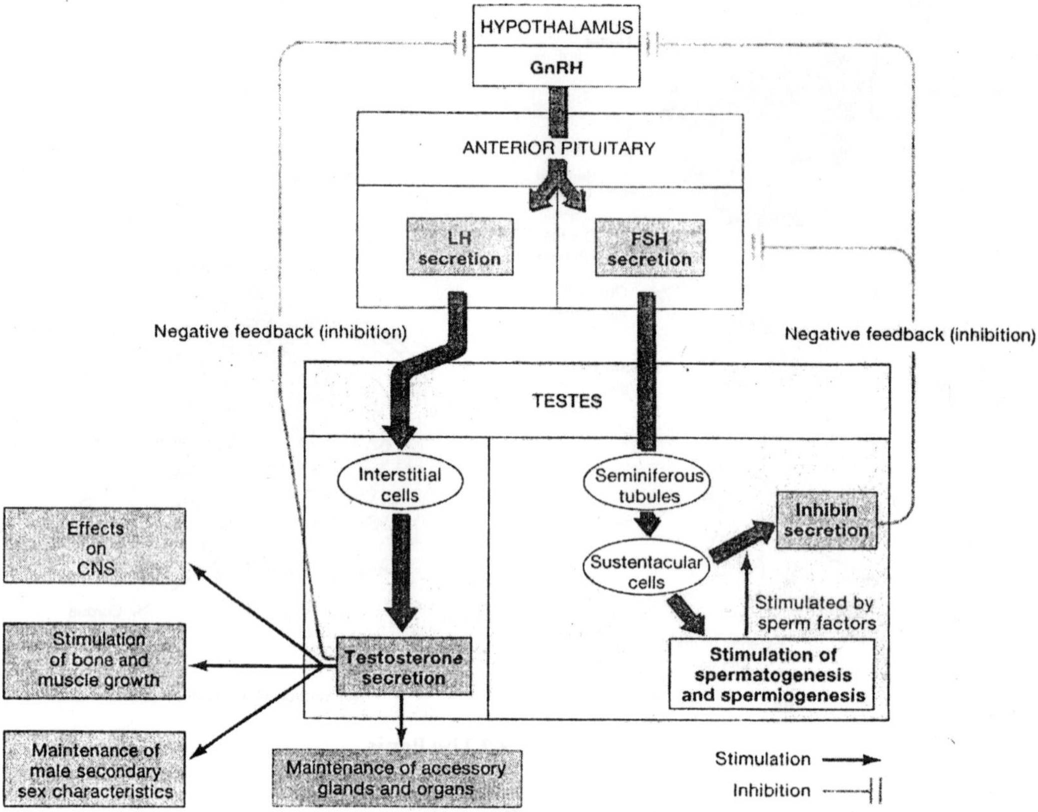

Fig.8.3 : Hormonal Feedback and the Regulation of Male Reproductive Function

accessory organs of the male reproductive tract, (3) determines the secondary sexual characteristics, such as distribution of facial hair, increased muscle mass and body size and the quantity and location of characteristic adipose tissue deposits, (4) stimulates metabolic operations throughout the body specially those concerned with protein synthesis and muscle growth, and (5) influences brain development by stimulating sexual behaviours.

Mechanism and effects of testosterone activity

Testosterone is synthesized from cholesterol. It exerts its effects by activating specific genes to transcribe messenger RNA molecules, which results in enhanced synthesis of certain proteins in the target cells.

In prostate gland, testosterone must be converted to dehydrocorticosterone (DHT) before it can bind within the nucleus. In certain neurons of the brain, testosterone is converted to estrogen.

As puberty ensures, testosterone not only prompt spermatogenesis but has multiple anabolic effects throughout the body. It targets all accessory reproductive organs, ducts, glands and the penis causing them to grow and assume adult size and function. In adult males, normal plasma levels of testosterone maintain these organs. When the hormone is deficient or absent all accessory organs atrophy, semen volume declines and erection and ejaculation are impaired.

Male Secondary Sex Characters

By the action of testosterone the appearance of pubic, axillary and facial hair, enhance hair growth on the chest or other body areas in some men and a deepening of the voice as the larynx enlarges. The skin thickens and becomes oilier, bones grow and increase in density.

Testosterone also increase basal metabolic rate and influences behaviour. The testes are not only source of androgens, adrenal glands of both sexes also release androgens.

The Reproductive System of the Female

A woman's reproductive system must produce sex hormones and gametes and also protect and support a developing embryo and nourish the newborn infant. The primary sex organs of the female reproductive system are the ovaries. The internal and external accessory organs include the uterine tubes (Fallopian tubes or oviducts), the uterus (womb) the vagina and the components of the external genitalia.

The Ovaries

The paired ovaries are shaped like almond. It has a pale white or yellowish colouration. The interior of the ovary can be divided into a superficial cortex and a deep medulla. The production of gametes occurs in the cortex, and the arteries, veins lymphatics and nerves within the medulla.

Like a testis an ovary is surrounded externally by a fibrous tunica albuginea. The tunica albuginea externally covered by cuboidal epithelial cells called germinal epithelium.

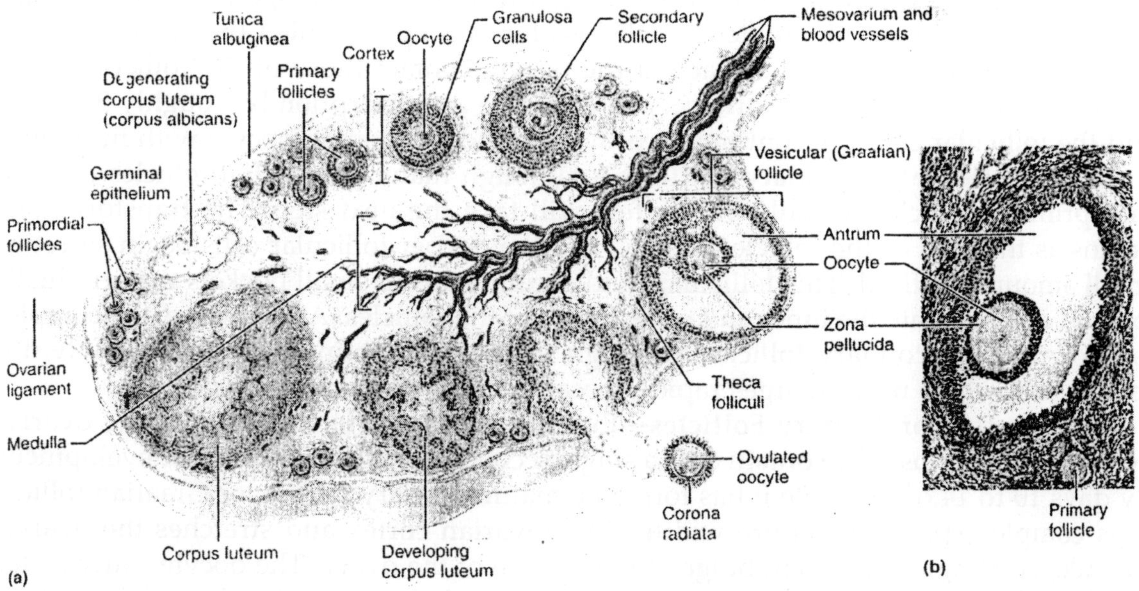

Fig. 8.4 : Structure of an Ovary

Embedded in the highly vascular connective tissue of the ovary cortex are many tiny saclike structures called ovarian follicles. Each follicle consists of an immature egg, called an oocyte encased by one or more layers of very different cells. The surrounding cells are called follicle cells if a single layer is present, and granulosa cells when more than one layer is present. Follicles at different stages of maturation are distinguished by their structure. In a primordial follicle, one layer of squamous like follicle cells surrounds the oocyte. A primary follicle has two or more layers of cuboidal or columnar type granulosa cells enclosing the oocyte, it becomes a secondary follicle when fluid filled spaces appear between the granulosa cells and then form a central fluid filled cavity called an antrum.

At its most mature stage when it is called a vesicular or Graafian follicle the follicle bulges from the surface of the ovary. The oocyte of the vesicular follicle "sits" on a Stalk of granulosa cells at one side of the antrum. Each month in adult women, one of the ripening follicles ejects its oocyte from the ovary, an event called ovulation. After ovulation the ruptured follicle is transformed into a very different structure called the corpus luteum, when eventually degenerate.

The Ovarian Cycle

Oogenesis occurs in the cortex within specialized structures called ovarian follicles. In the outer portions of cortex there are scattered clusters of primary oocytes, each surrounded by a layer of follicle cells. The combination is known as a primordial follicle. At puberty, rising levels of FSH begin to activate a different group of primordial follicles each month. This monthly process is known as the ovarian cycle. Important steps in the ovarian cycle are:

1. Formation of Primary Follicles—The cycle begins as the activated follicles develop into primary follicles. The follicle cells divide and form several concentric layers around the oocyte. As the wall of the follicle thickens further, a space opens up between the developing oocyte and the follicular cells. Within this space, called the zona pellucida, microvilli originating at the surface of the oocyte contact those of the follicular cells. These microvilli increase the surface area available for absorption by roughly 35 times, and the follicular cells are continually providing the developing oocyte with nutrients.

2. Formation of Secondary Follicles—Although many primordial follicles develop into primary follicles, usually only a few will take the next step. The transformation begins as the wall of the follicle thickens and the deeper follicular cells begin secreting small amounts of fluid. This follicular fluid accumulates in small pockets that gradually expand and separate the inner and outer layers of the follicles. At this stage, the complex is known as a secondary follicle. Although the oocyte continues to grow slowly, the follicle as a whole now enlarges rapidly because of this accumulation of fluid.

3 Formation of Tertiary Follicles—Eight to 10 days after the start of the ovarian cycle, the ovaries usually contain only a single secondary follicle for further development. By days 10 to 14 of the cycle it has formed a mature tertiary follicle, or Graafian follicle. This complex span's the entire width of the ovarian cortex and stretches the ovarian capsule, creating a prominent bulge in the surface of the ovary. The oocyte, surrounded by a mass of follicular cells, projects into the expanded central chamber of the follicle, the antrum.

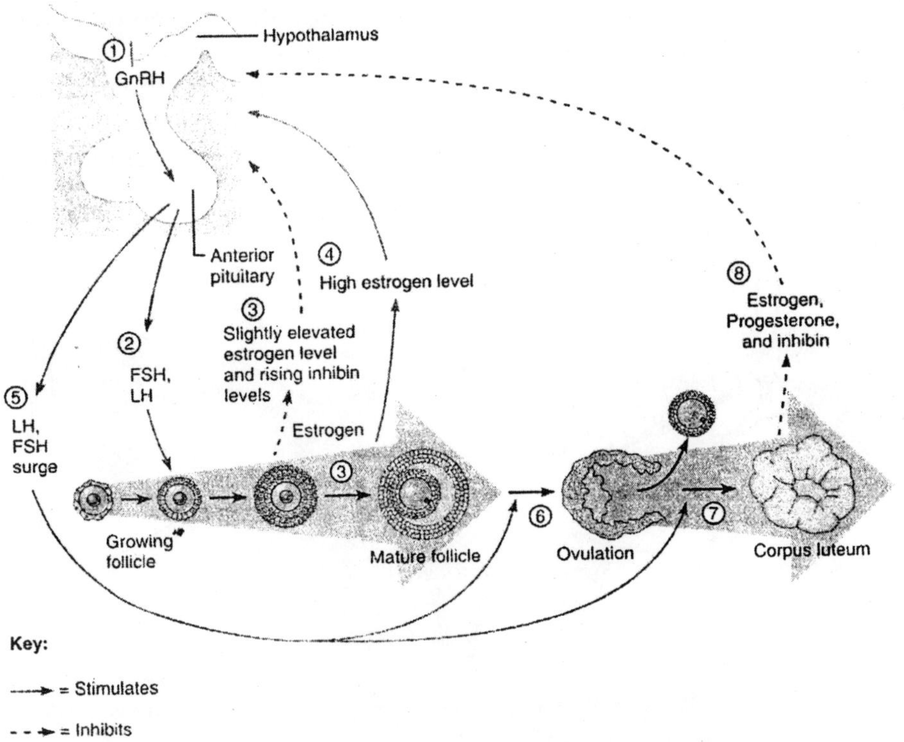

Fig. 8.5 : Feedback Interactions Involved in the Regulation of Ovarian Function

4. Ovulation—As the time of egg release, or ovulation, approaches, the follicular cells surrounding the oocyte lose contact with the follicular wall, and the oocyte floats within the central chamber. This event usually occurs at day 14 of a 28-day cycle. The follicular cells surrounding the oocyte are now known as the corona radiata. The distended follicular wall then ruptures, releasing the follicular content including the secondary oocyte, into the pelvic cavity. Because the corona radiata has a sticky surface, the oocyte usually attaches to the ovarian surface near the ruptured wall of the follicle. Contact with the entrance to the uterine tube or fluid currents established by its ciliated lining then sweeps the secondary oocyte into the uterine tube.

5. Formation and Degeneration of the Corpus Luteum—The empty follicle collapses, and the remaining follicular cells invade the cavity and multiply to create an endocrine structure known as the corpus luteum. Unless pregnancy occurs, after about 12 days the corpus luteum begins to degenerate. The disintegration marks the end of the ovarian cycle, but almost immediately the activation of another set of primordial follicles begins the next ovarian cycle.

The Uterine Tubes

The end closest to the ovary forms an expanded funnel or infundibulum, with numerous finger like projections that extend into the pelvic cavity. The projections, called fimbriae, and the inner surfaces of the infundibulum are carpeted with cilia that beat toward the broad entrance to the uterine tube. Once inside the uterine tube, the ovum is probably transported by ciliary movement and peristactic contractions. It normally takes 3-4 days for the secondary oocyte to travel from the infundibulum to the uterine chamber. If fertilization is to occur, the secondary oocyte must encounter spermatozoa, during the first 12-24 hours of its passage. Unfertilized oocytes will degenerate, in the uterine tubes or uterus without completing meiosis.

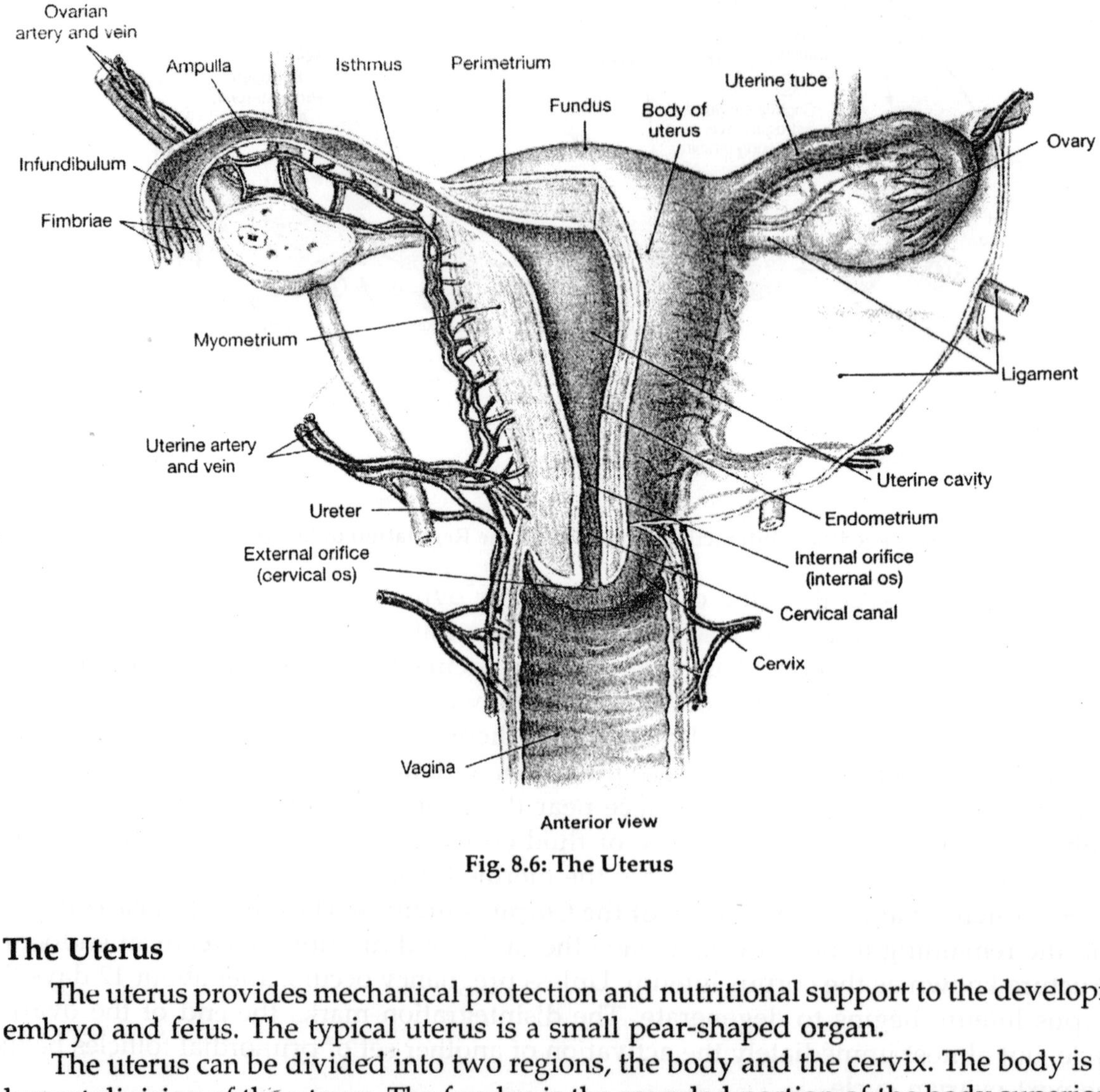

Fig. 8.6: The Uterus

The Uterus

The uterus provides mechanical protection and nutritional support to the developing embryo and fetus. The typical uterus is a small pear-shaped organ.

The uterus can be divided into two regions, the body and the cervix. The body is the largest division of the uterus. The fundus is the rounded portion of the body superior to the attachment of the uterine tubes. The body ends at a constriction known as the isthmus. The cervix is the inferior portion of the uterus. The cervix projects a short distance into the vagina and the uterine cavity opens into the vagina at the external orifice or cervical os.

In section the thick uterine wall can be divided into an inner endometrium, and a muscular myometrium. Covered by the peritonium. The endometrium of the uterus includes the epithelial lining the uterine chambers and the underlying connective tissues. Uterine glands open into the endometrial surface extend deep into the connective tissue layer almost all the way to the myometrium.

The endometrium can be divided into a superficial functional zone and a deeper basilar zone that is adjacent to the myometrium. The structure of the basilar layer remains relatively constant over time, but that of the functional zone undergoes cyclical changes in response to sexual hormone levels. These alterations produce the characteristic features of the uterine cycle.

The Uterine Cycle

The uterine cycle, or menstrual cycle, is a repeating series of changes in the structure of the endometrium. This events of the cycle begins with the monarch or first menstrual period at puberty typically at age of 11 to 12. The cycles continue until age 45 to 50. When menopause, the last menstrual cycle occurs. The regular appearance of menstrual cycles will be interrupted only by unusual circumstances, such as illness, stress, starvation or pregnancy.

The uterine cycle averages 28 days in length, but it can range from 21 to 35 days in normal individuals. It can be divided into three stages menses, the proliferative phase and the secretory phase.

Menses

The menstrual cycle begins with the onset of menses a period marked by the wholesale destruction of the superficial layer, or functional zone of the endometrium. The process is triggered by the decline in progesterone and estrogen concentrations as the corpus luteum disintegrates. The endometrial arteries constrict reducing blood flows to this region and the secretory glands, epithelial cells, and other tissues of the functional zone die of oxygen and nutrient deprivation. Eventually the weakened arterial walls rupture and blood pours into the connective tissues of the functional zone. Blood cells and degenerating tissues break away and enter the uterine lumen to be lost by passage into the vagina. This sloughing of tissue, which continues until the entire functional zone has been lost is called menstruation. Menstruation usually lasts from 1 to 7 days and over this period roughly 35 to 50 ml of blood are lost painful menstruation or dysmenorrhea, may result from tissue inflammation and contraction or from conditions involving adjacent pelvic structures.

The Proliferative Phase

The proliferative phase begins in the days following the completion of menses as the surviving epithelial cells multiply and spread across the surface of the endometrium. This repair process is stimulated by the rising estrogen levels that accompany the growth of another set of ovarian follicles. By the time ovulation occurs, the functional zone is several millimeters thick and its new set of uterine or endometrial, glands are

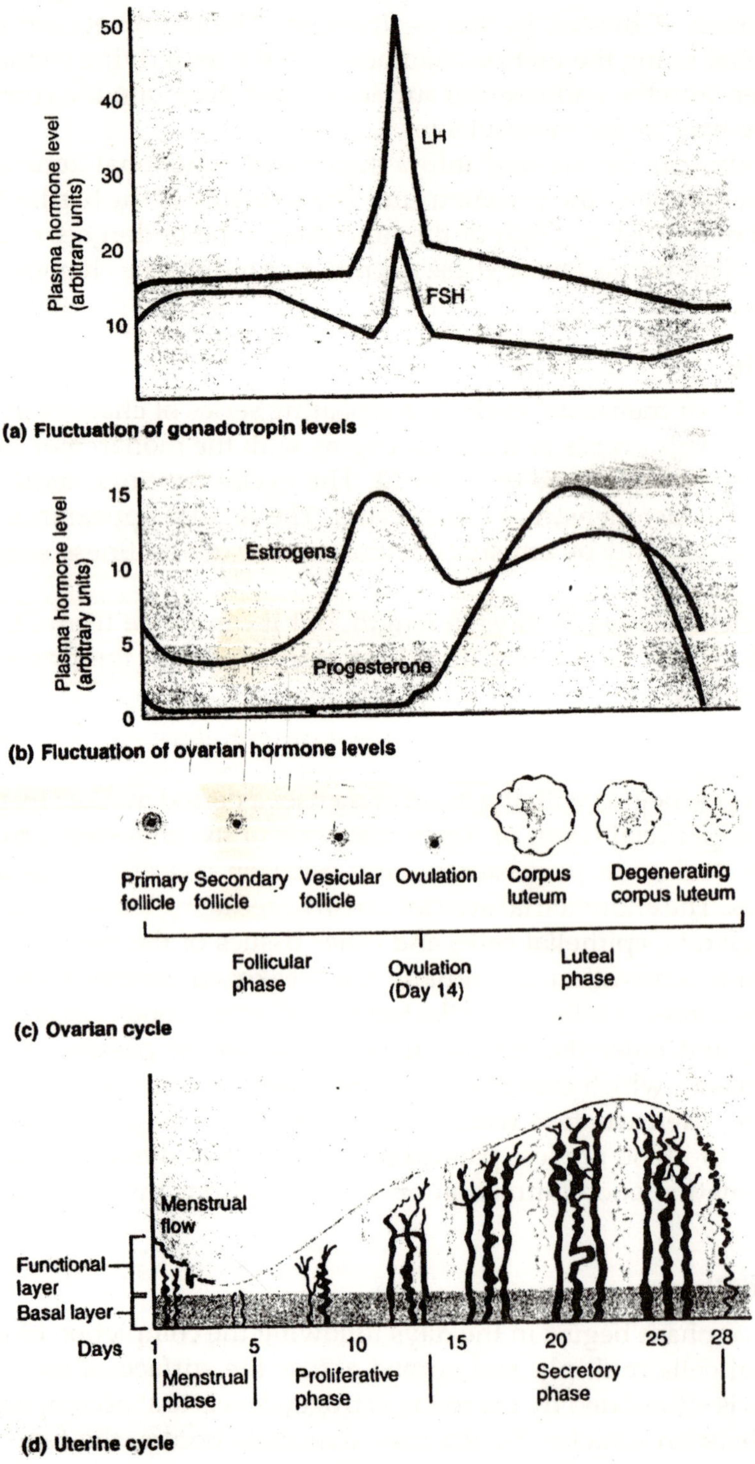

Fig 8.7 : Correlation of Anterior Pituitary and Ovarian Hormones with Structural Changes of the Ovarian and Uterine Cycles

manufacturing a mucus rich in glycogen. In addition, the entire functional zone is filled with small arteries, that branch from larger trunks in the myometrium.

The Secretory Phase

During the secretory phase of the cycle, the endometrial glands enlarge, increasing their rates of secretion as the endometrium prepares for the arrival of a developing embryo. This activity is stimulated by the progestins and estrogens from the corpus luteum. This phase begins at the time of ovulation and persists as long as the corpus luteum remains intact, secretory activities peak about 12 days after ovulation. Over the next day or two the glandular activity declines, and the menstrual cycle comes to close. A new cycle then begins with the onset of menses and the disintegration of the functional zone.

The Vagina

The vagina is a muscular tube extending between the uterus and the external genitalia. The cervix of the uterus projects into the vaginal canal.

The vagina (1) serves as a passageway for the elimination of menstrual fluid, (2) receives the penis during coitus and holds spermatozoa prior to their passage into the uterus, and (3) in child-birth forms the lower portion of the birth canal through which the fetus passes on its way to an independent existence.

Hormones and the Female Reproductive Cycle

The female reproductive tract is controlled by both pituitary and gonadal secretions. A woman's reproductive system does not produce functional gametes, circulating hormones control the female reproductive cycle to ensure proper reproductive function.

Changes in circulating estrogen concentration are the primary mechanism for co-ordinating the female reproductive cycle.

Hormones and the Preovulatory Period

Follicular development begins under FSH stimulation and each month some of the primordial follicles begin their development into primary follicles. As the follicular cells enlarge and multiply, they release steroid hormones. Collectively known as estrogens. Estrogens have multiple functions including:

(1) Stimulating bone and muscle growth.

(2) Maintaining female secondary sex characteristics such as body hair distribution and the location of adipose tissue deposits.

(3) Affecting CNS activity, including sex related behaviours.

(4) Maintaining functional accessory reproductive glands and organs.

(5) Initiating repair and growth of the endometrium.

The follicular development proceeds, the concentration of circulating estrogens and inhibin rises, the follicular cells are increasing in number and secretory activity increases. As estrogen and inhibin concentrations increases they inhibit both the hypothalamic secretion of GnRH and the pituitary production of release of FSH. Estrogen also affects the rate of LH secretion. Although the synthesis of LH occurs under GnRH stimulation, the rate of release into the bloodstream depends on the circulating concentration of estrogens. Thus as the follicles develop and estrogen concentrations rise, the pituitary output of LH gradually increases. Despite a slow decline in FSH concentrations, the combination of estrogen, FSH and LH continues to support follicular development and maturation.

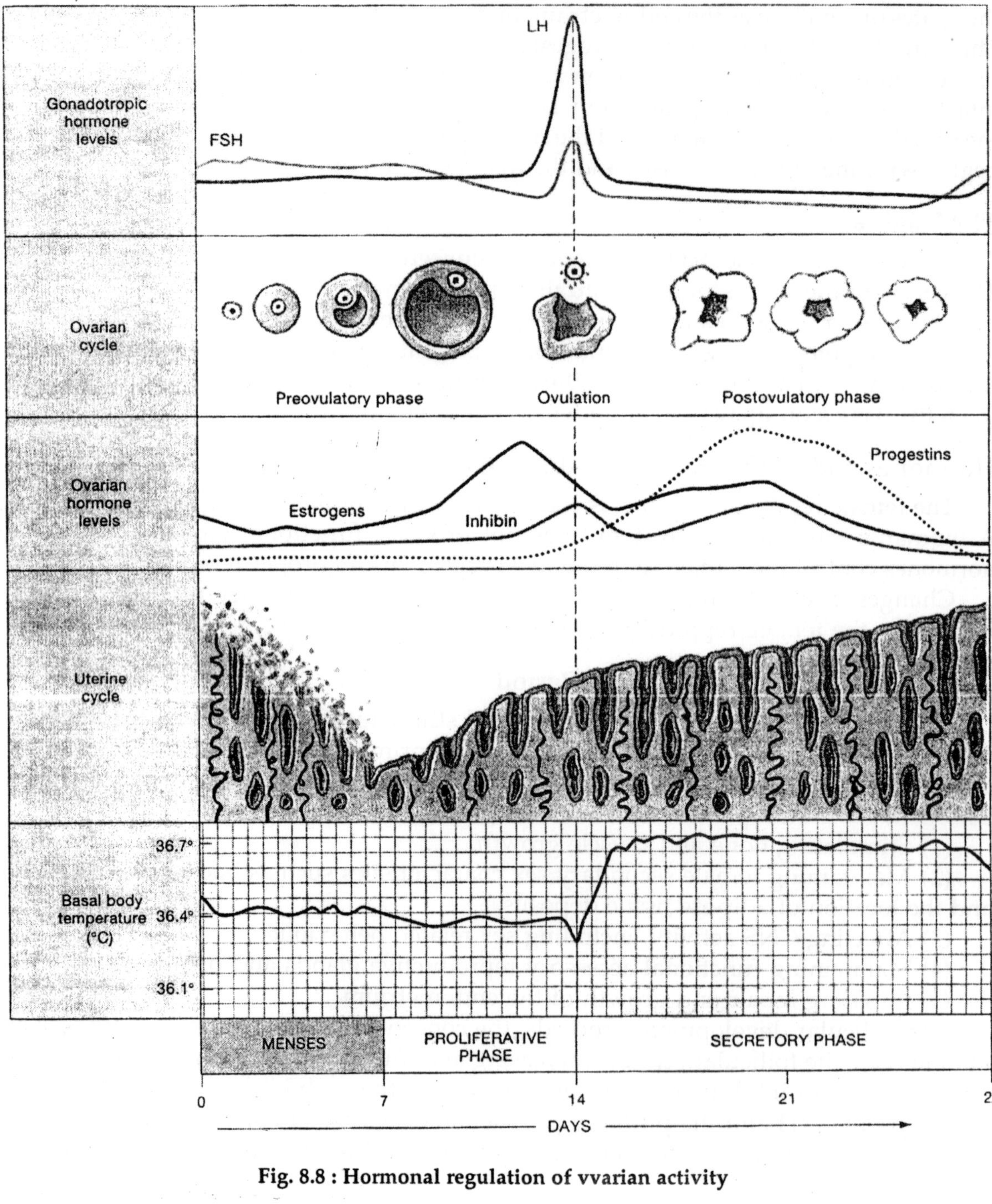

Fig. 8.8 : Hormonal regulation of vvarian activity

Estrogen concentrations take a sharp upturn in the second week of the ovarian cycle, as this month's tertiary follicle enlarges in preparation for ovulation. At about day 14 estrogen level peak, causes the maturation of that follicle. The high estrogen concentration, then triggers a massive outpouring of LH from the anterior pituitary, which causes the rupture of the follicular wall and ovulation.

Hormones and the Post-ovulatory Period

After ovulation LH stimulates the remaining follicular cells to form the corpus luteum, and the yellow colour of this mass results from its lipid reserves. These compounds are used to manufacture steroid hormones known as progestins, predominantly the steroid progesterone. Progesterone is the principal hormone of the post-ovulatory period. It prepares the uterus for pregnancy by stimulating the growth and development of the blood supply and secretory glands of the endometrium and it also stimulates metabolic activity and elevates basal body temperature.

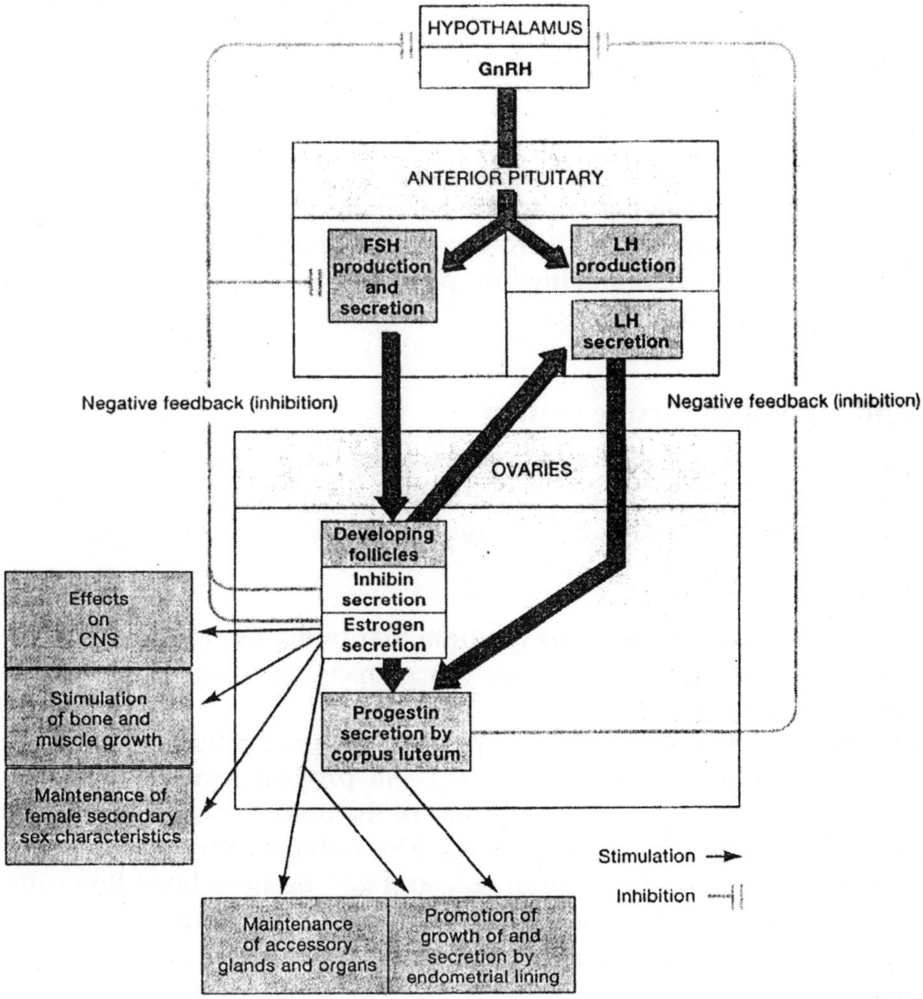

Fig. 8.9 : Hormonal Regulation of the Female Reproductive Cycle

Luteinizing hormone levels remain elevated for only two days, but that is long enough to stimulate the formation of the functional corpus luteum progesterone secretion continues at high levels for the next week, but unless pregnancy occurs, the corpus luteum then begins to degenerate. Roughly 12 days after ovulation, the corpus luteum become non-functional and progesterone and estrogen levels fall markedly. This decline stimulates the hypothalamic receptors, and GnRH production increases. This increase leads to an increase in FSH and LH production in the anterior pituitary and the entire cycle begins again.

Hormones and the Uterine Cycle

The sudden declines in progesterone and estrogen levels that accompany the breakdown of the corpus luteum result in menses. The loss of endometrial tissue continues for several days, until rising estrogen levels, stimulate the regeneration of the functional zone of the endometrium. The pre-ovulatory phase continues until rising progesterone levels mark the arrival of the post-ovulatory phase. The combination of estrogen and progesterone then causes the enlargement of the endometrial glands and an increase in their secretions.

Hormones and body temperature

The hormonal fluctuations also cause physiological changes that affect the body temperature. During the pre-ovulatory period when estrogen is the dominant hormone, the resting or basal body temperature measured upon awakening in the morning is about 0.3°C lower than it is during the post-ovulatory period, when progesterone dominates. At the time of ovulation, basal temperature declines sharply, making the temperature rise.

Ageing and the Reproductive system

The ageing process affects the reproductive systems of men and women. The age-related changes in the female reproductive system occur at menopause, whereas changes in the male reproductive system occur more gradually and over a longer period of time.

Menopause

Menopause is usually defined as the time that ovulation and menstruation cease. It typically occurs at age 45-55, but in the years preceding it the ovarian and menstrual cycles become irregular.

Menopause is accompanied by a sharp rise in the production of GnRH, FSH and LH, while circulating concentrations of estrogen and progesterone decline. The decline in estrogen levels leads to reductions in the size of the uterus and breasts, accompanied by a thinning of the urethral and vaginal walls. The reduced estrogen concentrations have also been linked to the development of osteoporosis, because bone deposition proceeds at a slower rate. A variety of neural effects are also reported including anxiety and depression. In addition the risk of atherosclerosis and cardiovascular disease increases after menopause.

The Male Climacteric

Changes in the male reproductive system occur more gradually, over a period known as the male climacteric. Circulating testosterone levels begin to decline between age of 50 and 60, coupled with increases in circulating levels of FSH and LH. Although sperm production continues, there is a gradual reduction in sexual activity in older men. This reduction may be linked to declining testosterone levels.

Fertilization

Fertilization involves the fusion of two haploid gametes producing a zygote containing the diploid number of chromosomes.

Fertilization usually occurs in the upper one-third of the uterine tube within a day of ovulation. Contractions of the uterine musculature and ciliary currents in the uterine tubes aid the passage of sperm to the fertilized site.

At ovulation, the secondary oocyte leaving the follicle is in metaphase stage. The secondary oocyte is surrounded by a layer of follicle cells, the corona radiata. The spermatozoa first penetrate the corona radiata. The acrosomal cap contains hyaluronidase, an enzyme that breaks down the intercellular cement between adjacent cells of the corona radiata. When the sperm contacts the oocyte, their cell membranes fuse and the sperm's nucleus enters the cytoplasm of oocyte. When sperm fuses with an egg to form a fertilized egg or zygote.

Cleavage and Blastocyst Formation

Cleavage is a series of cell divisions that subdivide the cytoplasm of the zygote. The first cleavage division produces two identical cells called blastomeres. The first division

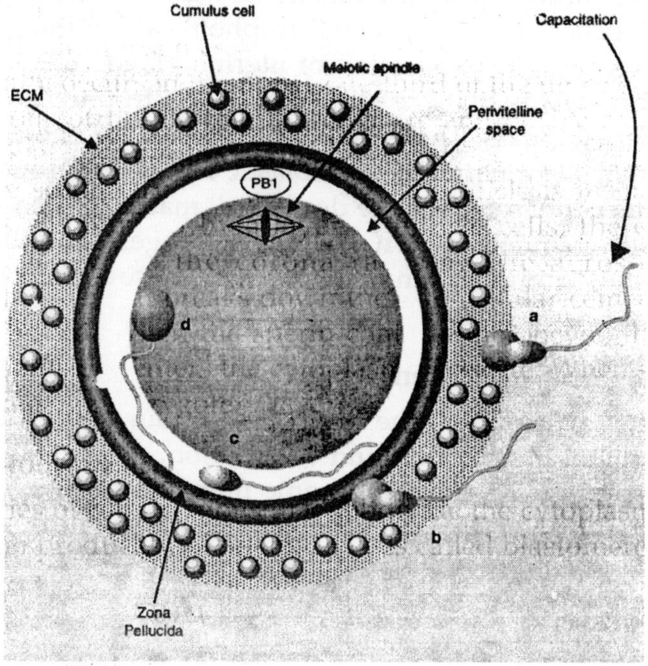

Fig. 8.10 Events Immediately Following Sperm Penetration

is completed roughly 30 hours after fertilization and subsequent cleavage divisions occur at intervals of 10-12 hours.

After several cycles of division, the embryo is a solid ball of cells called morula. After 5 days of cleavage the blastomeres form a hollow ball the blastocyst with an inner cavity known as the blastocoel. The outer layer of cells, separating the outside world from the blastocoel, is called the trophoblast. These cells will be responsible for providing food to the developing embryo. A second group of cells the inner cell mass, lies at one end of the blastocyst. In time, the inner cell mass will form the embryo.

Implantation

At fertilization the zygote is still 4 days away from the uterus. It arrives in the uterine cavity as a morula and over the next 2-3 days blastocyst formation occurs. Over this period, the blastomeres are gaining nutrients from the fluid, rich in glycogen is secreted by the endometrial glands. When fully formed, the blastocyst contacts the endometrium, usually in the body or fundus of the uterus, and implantation occurs.

Implantation begins as the surface of the blastocyst closest to the inner cell mass touches and adheres to the uterine lining. In this area, the superficial cells undergo rapid divisions, making the trophoblast several layers thick. Near the endometrial wall, the cell membranes separating the trophoblast cells disappear creating a layer of cytoplasm containing multiple nuclei called the syncytial trophoblast (day 8). The underlying cells remain intact and form a layer called the cellular trophoblast. The syncytial trophoblast erodes a path through the uterine epithelium. At first, this erosion creates a gap in the uterine lining, but the division and migration of epithelial cells soon repair the surface. The blastocyst loss contact with the uterine, with the uterine cavity and further development occurs entirely within the functional zone of endometrium.

As implantation proceeds, the syncytial trophoblast continues to enlarge into the surrounding endometrium. The digestion of uterine gland cells releases quantities of glycogen and other nutrients that are absorbed by the trophoblast and distributed by diffusion to the inner cell mass. These nutrients provide the energy needed to support the early stages of embryo formation. Trophoblastic extensions grow around endometrial capillaries, and as the capillary walls are destroyed, maternal blood begins to percolate through trophoblastic channels known as lacunae. Finger like villi extend away from the trophoblast into the surrounding endometrium and these extensions gradually increase in size.

Formation of Extraembryonic Membranes

Germ layers also participate in the formation of four extraembryonic membranes, the yolk sac, the amnion, the allantois and the chorion.

Yolk Sac—The first of the extraembryonic membranes to appear is the yolk sac, which is already present 10 days after fertilization. As gastrulation proceeds mesodermal cells migrate around this pouch and complete the formation of yolk sac. Blood vessels soon appear within the mesoderm and the yolk sac becomes an important site of blood cell formation.

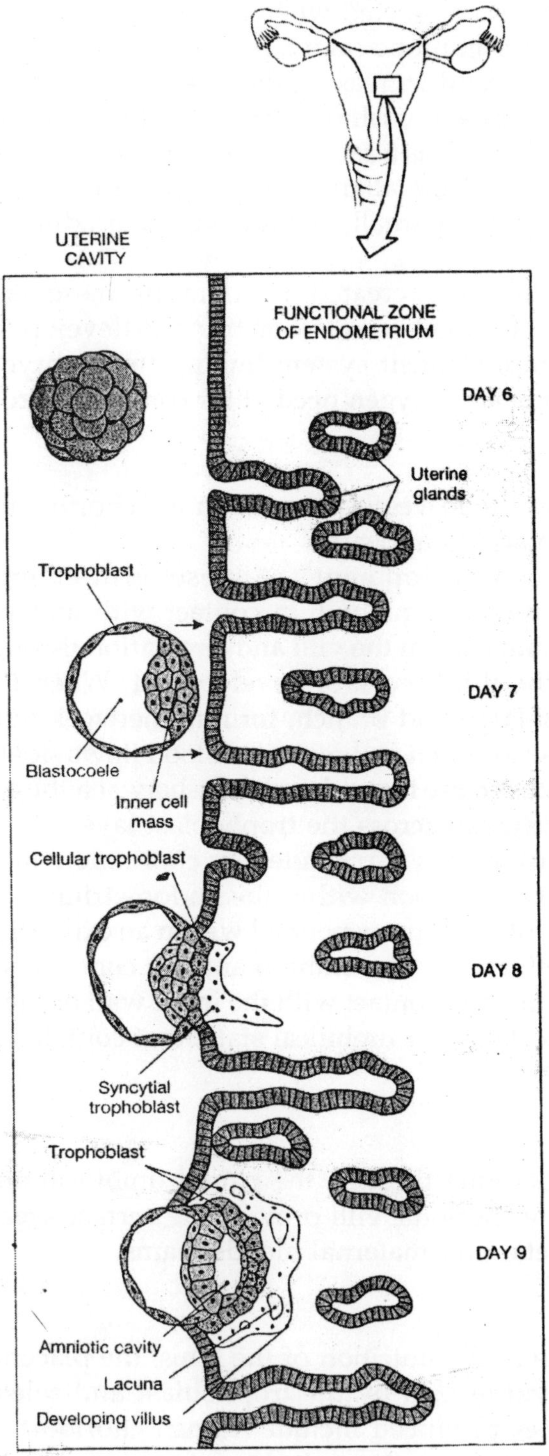

Fig. 8.11 Stages in the Implantation Process

Amnion—The amnion is completed when ectodermal and mesodermal cells spread over the inner surface of the amniotic cavity. As the embryo and later the fetus enlarges, the amnion continues to expand increasing the size of the amniotic cavity. The amnion encloses fluid that surrounds and cushions the developing embryo and fetus.

The Allantois—The allantois is a sac of endoderm and mesoderm that extends away from the embryo. The base of the allantois later give rise to the urinary bladder. The allantois accumulates some of the small amount of urine produced by the kidneys during embryonic development.

The Chorion—The chorion is created as migrating mesodermal cells form a layer underneath the trophoblasts blood vessels then begin to develop within the mesoderm of the chorion, creating a rapid-transit system linking the embryo with the trophoblast. This provides the nutrients and oxygen needed for continued growth and development.

Placentation

Placentation occurs as blood vessels formed in the chorion around the periphery of the blastocyst, and the placenta appears.

By the third week of development the mesoderm extends along each of the trophoblastic villi, forming chorionic villi in contact with maternal tissues. Embryonic blood vessel develop within each of the villi and circulation through these chrionic blood vessels begins early in the third week of development. When the heart starts beating. These villi continue to enlarge and branch, forming network within the endometrium. Blood vessels continue to be eroded and maternal blood flows slowly through the lacunae. Chorionic blood vessels pass close by, and exchange between the embryonic and maternal circulations occurs by diffusion across the trophoblast layers.

At first the entire blastocyst is surrounded by chorionic villi. The chorion continues to enlarge, expanding like a balloon within the endometrium, and by the fourth week the embryo amnion and yolk sac are suspended within an expansive, fluid filled chamber. The only communication between the embryo and the chorion occurs at the sites where mesodermal cells first came into contact with the inner wall of the trophoblast. It remains connected by the umbilical cord or umbilical stalk, that contains allantois, blood vessels and yolk sac.

Placental Circulation

Blood flows to the placenta through the paired umbilical arteries and returns in a single umbilical vein. The chorionic villi provide the surface area for active and passive exchange between the fetal and maternal bloodstreams.

Placental Hormones

In addition to its role in the nutrition of the fetus, the placenta acts as an endocrine organ. Hormones are synthesized by the trophoblast and released into the maternal circulation. The hormones produced include human chorionic gonadotropins, human placental lactogen, placental prolactin, relaxin, progestins and estrogens.

Human chorionic gonadotropin (HCG) appears in the maternal bloodstream soon

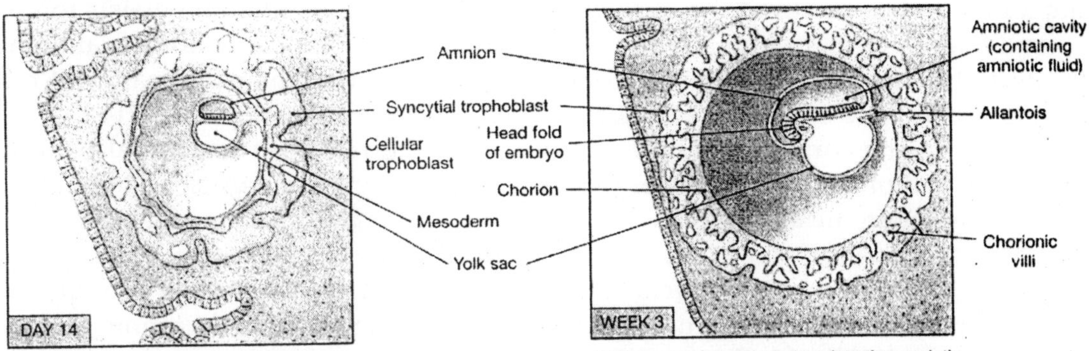

(a) Migration of mesoderm around the inner surface of the trophoblast creates the chorion. Mesodermal migration around the outside of the amniotic cavity, between the ectodermal cells and the trophoblast, creates the amnion. Mesodermal migration around the endodermal pouch below the blastodisc creates the definitive yolk sac.

(b) The embryonic disc bulges into the amniotic cavity at the head fold. The allantois, an endodermal extension surrounded by mesoderm, extends toward the trophoblast.

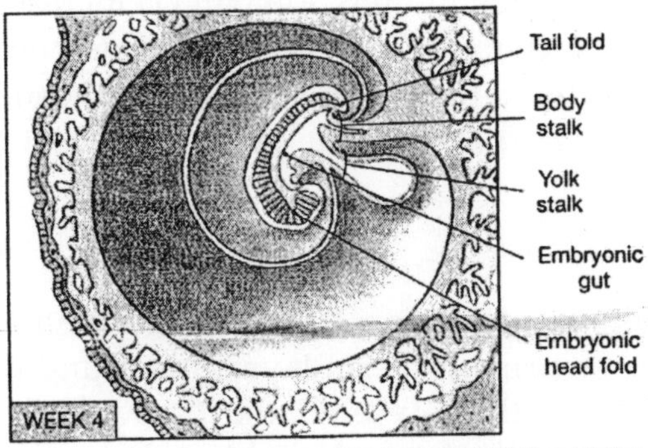

(c) The embryo now has a head fold and a tail fold. Constriction of the connection between the embryo and the surrounding trophoblast constricts the yolk stalk and body stalk.

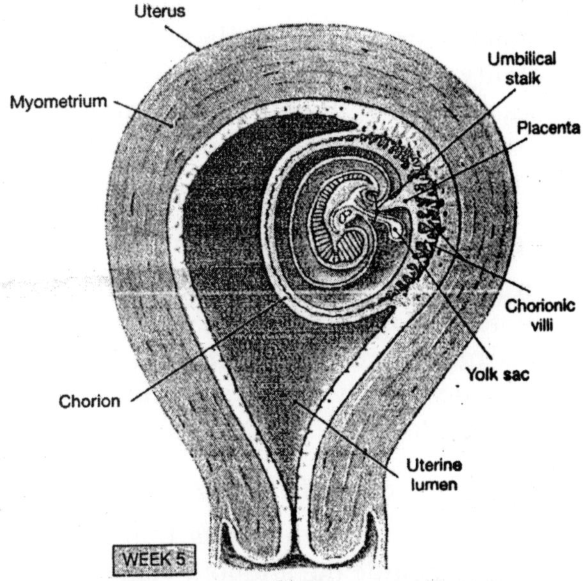

(d) The developing embryo and extraembryonic membranes bulge into the uterine cavity. The trophoblast pushing out into the uterine lumen remains covered by endometrium but no longer participates in nutrient absorption and embryo support. The embryo moves away from the placenta, and the body stalk and yolk stalk fuse to form an umbilical stalk.

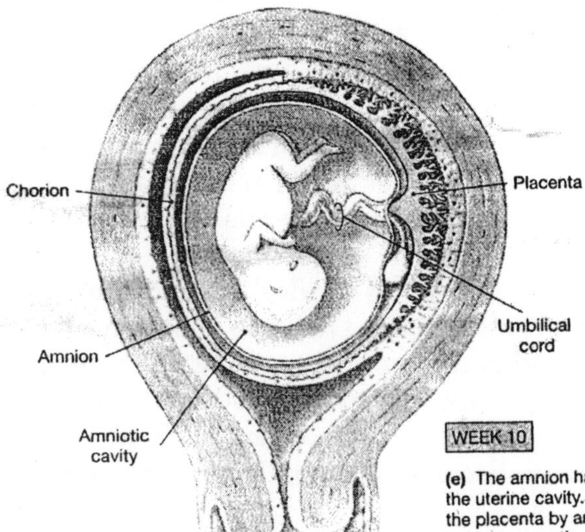

(e) The amnion has expanded greatly, filling the uterine cavity. The fetus is connected to the placenta by an elongate umbilical cord that contains a portion of the allantois, blood vessels, and the remnants of the yolk stalk.

Fig. 8.12 Embryonic Membranes and Placenta Formation

after implantation has occurred. Because of the HCG, the corpus luteum persists for 3-4 months and maintains its production of progesterone. As a result the endometrial lining remains perfectly, functional and menses does not occur and terminate pregnancy. When HCG levels decline, the endometrium degenerates and the pregnancy is aborted.

The decline in the corpus luteum does not trigger the return of menstrual periods, because by the end of the first trimester the placenta is secreting a sufficient amounts of progestins to maintain the endometrial lining and the pregnancy. As the end of the third trimester approaches, estrogen production accelerates. The rising estrogen levels play a role in stimulating labour and delivery. These hormones also encouraging growth and further differentiation of the mammary glands and readying them for lactation. Human placental lactogen (hPL) and placental prolactin also prepare the mammary glands for milk production. Maternal hormones such as growth hormone, prolactin and thyroid hormone also play an active role for the conversion of the mammary glands to active status.

Relaxin is secreted by the placenta as well as the corpus luteum, Relaxin (1) increases the flexibility of the pubic symphysis, permitting expansion of the pelvis during delivery, (2) causes dilation of the cervix making it easier for the fetus to enter the vaginal canal, and (3) suppresses the release of oxytocin by the hypothalamus, delaying the onset of labour contractions.

Events of Embryonic Development

Even while implantation is occurring the blastocyst is being converted to the next developmental stage, the gastrula, in which the three primary germ layers form, and the embryonic membranes are developing. Before becoming three-layered, the inner cell mass first subdivides into two layers, the upper epiblast and the lower hypoblast. Extensions of these sheets form two of the four embryonic membranes.

Formation and roles of the Embryonic Membranes

The embryonic membranes that form during the first two to three weeks of development include the amnion, yolk sac, allantois, and chorion. The amnion develops when cells of the epiblast fashion themselves into the transparent membranous sac. This sac, the amnion, becomes filled with amniotic fluid. Later as the embryonic disc curves to form the tubular body, the amnion curves with it. The sac extends all the way around the embryo broken only by the umbilical cord.

Sometimes, called the "bag of waters" the amnion provides an environment that protects the developing embryo against physical trauma and helps to maintain a constant homeostatic temperature. The fluid also prevents the rapidly growing embryonic parts from adhering and fusing together and allows the embryo considerable freedom of moment, thus aiding musculoskeletal development. Initially, amniotic fluid is derived from the maternal blood, but as the fetal kidneys become functional fetal urine contributes to amniotic fluid volume.

The yolk sac forms the cells of the hypoblast. These cells arrange themselves into a sac that hangs from the ventral surface of the embryo. Thus, the amnion and yolk sac resemble two balloons touching one another with the embryonic disc at the point of the contact. Yolk sac is important in humans because it (1) forms part of the gut, (2) produces the earliest blood cells and blood vessels, and (3) is the source of primordial germ cells that migrate into the embryo's body to seed the gonads.

The allantois forms as a small outpocketing at the caudal end of the yolk sac. It is structural base for constructing the umbilical cord that links the embryo to the placenta, and becomes part of the urinary bladder. When the umbilical cord is fully formed, it contains a core of embryonic connective tissue (Wharton's jelly), the umbilical arteries and vein is covered externally by amniotic membrane.

The chorion, which helps to form the placenta is the outermost membrane encloses the embryonic body and all other membranes.

Gastrulation—Germ Layer Formation

During the third week, the two-layered embryonic disc transforms into a three-layered embryo in which the primary germ layers—ectoderm, mesoderm and endoderm are present. This process called gastrulation involves cellular rearrangements and widespread cell migrations. It begins as a raised groove called the primitive streak appears on the dorsal surface of the embryonic disc and establishes the longitudinal axis of the embryo.

Surface cells (epiblast) of the embryonic disc migrate across other cells and enter the primitive streak. The first cells that enter the groove form the most inferior germ layer, the endoderm. Those that follow push laterally between the cells at the upper and lower surfaces forming the mesoderm. The mesodermal cells immediately beneath the early primitive streak quickly aggregate forming a rod of mesoderm cells called the notochord.

The three primary germ layers differ in the arrangement of their cells and serve as the primitive tissues from which all body organs will derive. Ectoderm forms nervous system and skin epidermis. Endoderm forms the epithelial lining of the digestive, respiratory and urinogenital systems and associated glands. Mesoderm forms everything else.

Organogenesis—Specialization of the Ectoderm

The first major event in organogenesis is neurulation, the differentiation of ectoderm that gives rise to the brain and spinal cord. The ectoderm overlying the notochord thickens, forming the neural folds. By the twenty-second day, the superior margins of the neural folds fuse forming a neural tube. The anterior end of the neural tube becomes the brain and the rest becomes the spinal cord. The associated neural crest cells migrate and give rise to the cranial, spinal and sympathetic ganglia to the medulla of the adrenal gland and contribute to some connective tissues.

By the end of the first month of development, the three primary brain vesicles (fore, mid' and hindbrain) are formed. By the end of the second month, all brain flexures are formed the cerebral hemispheres cover the top of the brain stem and brain waves can be recorded.

Specialization of the Endoderm

The embryo starts folding laterally into a tube. The folding occurs from both ends and progresses toward the central part of the embryonic body, where the yolk sac and umbilical vessels protrude. The tube of endoderm formed, called the primitive gut, forms the epithelial lining of the gastrointestinal tract. The mucosal lining of the respiratory tract forms an outpocketing inform the foregut and the glands that derive from endoderm arise as endodermal out-pocketing at various points along the tract.

Specialization of the Mesoderm

The first evidence of the mesodermal differentiation is appearance of the notochord. Thereafter three mesodermal aggregates appear on either side of the notochord. The somites are a series of paired mesodermal blocks that hug the notochord on either side, on lateral sides of somites are clusters of mesoderm called intermediate mesoderm and lateral mesoderm cells of intermediate mesoderm form the gonads and kidneys lateral mesoderm help to form dermi of skin, lines the ventral body cavity and forming limbs and produce bones, ligaments and dermis of limbs.

Development of Fetal Circulation

The first blood cells arise in the yolk sac. By the end of third week embryo has paired blood vessels and the two vessels forming the heart, have fused and bent into S shape by 3½ weeks, the miniature heart is pumping blood for an embryo.

Effects of Pregnancy on the Mother

Pregnancy can be a difficult time for the mother. Not only are there anatomical changes, but striking changes in her metabolism and physiology occur as well.

Anatomical Changes : As pregnancy progresses the female reproductive organs become increasingly vascularized and engorged with blood and vagina develops a purplish hue. The 'breast too engorge with blood and prodded by rising levels of estrogen and progesterone, they enlarge, some women develop increased pigmentation of facial skin of nose and cheeks.

The degree of uterine enlargement during pregnancy is remarkable. The uterus fills most of the pelvic cavity by 16 weeks. The placenta is fully formed, uterine muscle is hypertrophied and amniotic fluid volume is increasing. As pregnancy continues, the uterus pushes higher into the abdominal cavity exerting pressure on both abdominal and pelvic organs. As birth nears, the uterus occupies most of the abdominal cavity. The crowded abdominal organs press against the diaphragm. As a result the ribs flare, causing the thorax to widen.

The increasing bulkiness of the anterior abdomen changes the women's centre of gravity and many women develop lordosis (accentuated lumbar curvature) and backaches during the last few months of pregnancy, placental production of the hormone relaxin causes pelvic ligaments and pubic symphysis to relax widen and become more flexible. This increased motility eases birth passage.

Considerable weight gain occurs during a normal pregnancy. Good nutrition is necessary all through pregnancy if the developing fetus is to have all the building materials especially proteins calcium and iron-needed to form its tissues. Additionally, multivitamins containing folic acid seem to reduce the risk of having babies with neurological problems. The emphasis should be on eating high quality food, not just more food.

Metabolic Changes : As the placenta enlarges, it secrets increasing amounts of human placental lactogen (HPL) which works with estrogens and progesterone to stimulate maturation of the breast for lactation. In addition, HPL promotes growth of the fetus and exerts a glucose-sparing effect in the mother. Maternal cells metabolize more fatty acids and less glucose than usual. The placenta also releases human chorionic thyrotropin causing hypermetabolism. Because plasma levels of parathyroid hormone and activated vitamin D rise, pregnant women tend to be in positive calcium balance throughout pregnancy. This ensures that the developing fetus will have adequate calcium to mineralize its bones.

Physiological Changes—Gastrointestinal System : Many women suffer nausea, commonly called morning sickness, during the first few months of pregnancy, until their system adjusts to the elevated levels of progesterone and estrogens. Reflux of stomach acid into the oesophagus, causing heart burn is common because the oesophagus is displaced and the stomach is crowded by the growing uterus.

Urinary System : The kidneys produce more urine during pregnancy because they have the additional burden of disposing of fetal metabolic wastes. As the growing uterus compresses the bladder, urination becomes more frequent, more urgent and sometimes uncontrollable.

Respiratory System : The nasal mucosa responds to estrogens by becoming edematous and congested. Thus, nasal stuffness and occasional nosebleeds may occur vital capacity and respiratory rate increase during pregnancy and hyperventilation is common. But residual volume declines and many women exhibit dyspnea or difficult breathing, during the later stages of pregnancy.

Cardiovascular System : The most dramatic physiological changes occur in the cardiovascular system. Total body water rises, blood volume increases 24-40 per cent by the thirty-second week increases both formed elements and plasma volume. The rise in blood volume also acts as a safeguard against blood loss during birth. Blood pressure and pulse rise and increase cardiac output by 20-40 per cent at various stages of pregnancy.

Parturition (Birth)

Parturition is the culmination of pregnancy—giving birth to the baby. It usually occurs within 15 days of the calculated due date (280 days from the last menstrual period). The series of events that expel the infant from the uterus are collectively called labour.

Initiation of Labour

During the last few weeks of pregnancy estrogens reach their highest levels in the mother's blood. It stimulates the myometrial cells of the uterus to form abundant oxytocin receptors and it antagonizes progesterone, to influence on the uterine muscle. As a result, the myometrium becomes increasingly irritable, and weak, irregular uterine contractions begin to occur.

As birth nears, certain cells of the fetus begin to produce oxytocin which in turn acts on the placenta causing it to release prostaglandins. Both hormones are powerful uterine muscle stimulants, and since the myometrium is now highly sensitive to oxytocin, contractions become more frequent and more vigorous. At this point, the increasing emotional and physical stresses activate the mother's hypothalamus, which signals for oxytocin release by the posterior pituitary. Together oxytocin and prostaglandin causes the rhythmic contractions of labour.

Stages of Labour

1. Dilation Stage—The dilation stage is the time from labour's onset until the cervix is fully dilated by the baby's head. As labour starts, weak but regular contractions begin in the upper part of the uterus and more down ward toward the vagina. At first, only the superior uterine muscle is active. These initial contractions are 15-30 minutes apart and lasts far 10-30 seconds. As labour progresses, the contractions become more vigorous and more rapid, and the lower uterine segment gets involved. As the infant's head is forced against the cervix with each contraction, the cervix softens, becomes thinner and dilates. Eventually the amnion ruptures releasing the amniotic fluid, an event commonly called "breaking the water". The dilation stage is the longest part of labour, lasting 6-12 hours (or more).

2. Expulsion Stage—The expulsion stage lasts from full dilation to delivery of the infant, or actual child birth. Ordinarily, by the time the cervix is fully dilated. Strong contractions are occurring every 2-3 minutes and lasting about 1 minute, and a mother under going labour without local anesthesia has an increasing urge to push or bear down with the abdominal muscles. This phase can take as long as 2 hours, it is typically 50 minutes in a first birth and around 20 minutes in subsequent births. The baby's head extends as it exits and once the head has been delivered the rest of the baby's body is delivered much more easily.

3. Placental Stage—The placental stage or the delivery of the placenta is accomplished within 30 minutes after birth of the infant. The strong uterine contractions that continue after birth compress uterine blood vessels, limit bleeding, cause the placenta to detach from the uterine wall. The placenta and its attached fetal membranes, collectively called the afterbirth, are then easily removed by a gentle tug on the umbilical cord.

Lactation

Lactation is production of milk by the hormone prepared mammary glands. Rising levels of placental estrogens, progesterone and lactogen toward the end of pregnancy stimulate the hypothalamus to release prolactin releasing hormone (PRH). The anterior pituitary gland responds by secreting prolactin. After an initial two to three day delay, true milk production begins. During this delay, a yellowish fluid called colostrum is secreted. Colostrum has less lactose than milk and almost no fat, but it contains more protein, vitamin A and minerals than true milk. Like milk, colostrum is rich in IgA antibodies. Since these antibodies are resistant to digestion in the stomach, they may help to protect the infants digestive tract against bacterial infection.

After birth, prolactin release gradually and continual milk production depends on mechanical stimulation of nipples, normaly provided by the sucking infant. Mechanoreceptors in the nipple send afferent nerve impulses to the hypothalamus, stimulating secretion of PRH. This result in a release of prolactin which stimulates milk production for the next feeding.

The same afferent impulses also prompt hypothalamic release of oxytocin from the posterior pituitary by a positive feedback mechanism. Oxytocin causes the let-down reflex, the actual ejection of milk from the alveoli of mammary glands. Let down occurs when oxytocin binds to myoepithelial cells surrounding the glands, after which milk is ejected from both breasts. When nursing is discontinued, the stimulus for prolactin release and milk production ends and the mammary glands stop producing milk.

Contraception and Birth Control

For physiological, financial or emotional reasons most adults practice some form of conception control during their reproductive years. Several different approaches are commonly taken to achieve birth control. These methods differ from one another in their effectiveness and in their acceptability to different couples. Some methods of birth control protect against sexually transmitted disease.

Abstinence

The most reliable way to avoid pregnancy and sexually transmitted disease is not to have sex at all. In this method avoid sexual relations on the three days preceding and the day after ovulation. Since this is the time during which fertilization can occur. This approach, called the rhythm method. The effectiveness of the rhythm method is low.

Sperm Blockage

If sperm do not reach the uterine tubes, fertilization cannot take place. One way to prevent sperm from reaching the uterine tube is for the male partner to use a condom. The condom failure rate has been estimated at over 6 per cent.

Vaginal barriers such as the diaphragm, cervical cap, and vaginal sponge rely on similar principle. A diaphragm consists of a dome of rubber with a small metal loop supporting the rim. Before intercourse, the diaphragm is inserted so that it covers the external orifice, and it is usually coated with a small amount of spermicidal jelly or cream. The failure rate is about 5-6 per cent. The cervical cap is smaller and lacks the metal rim. It, too, must be fitted carefully, but unlike the diaphragm it may be left in place for several days. The failure rate is 8 per cent. The vaginal sponge consists of a small synthetic sponge saturated with a spermicide a sperm killing foam or jelly. The failure rate is estimated at 6-10 per cent.

An intrauterine device (IUD) consists of a small plastic loop or a T that can be inserted into the uterine chamber IUDs. Stimulate prostaglandin. production in the uterus The net result is an alteration in the chemical composition of uterine secretions, and the changes in the intrauterine environment lower the chances for fertilization and subsequent implantation. The failure rate is estimated at 5-6 per cent.

Sperm Destruction

The birth control pills also control birth. These pills contain estrogen and progesterone either taken together in the same pill or in separate pills. In the normal reproductive cycle of a female, these hormones act to shut down the production of pituitary hormones FSH and LH. The artificial maintenance of high levels of estrogen and progesterone in a woman's bloodstream cause the body to act as if ovulation had already occurred. The ovarian follicles do not mature in the absence of FSH and ovulation does not occur in the absence of LH. For these reasons, birth control pills provide a very effective means of birth control, with a failure rate of 0 to 5 per cent.

A Norplant is also used similar to the pills but that prevents pregnancy for up to 5 years. In a 15 minutes operation, the six matchstick-sized tubes are surgically implanted under the skin of upper arm. These tubes contain the synthetic hormone progestin. Norplant prevents pregnancy by inhibiting ovulation as the pill does, but it also thickness the cervical mucus so that sperm cannot move through the female reproductive tract Norplant causes irregular menstrual bleeding in 75 per cent of its users.

Surgical Intervention

A completely effective means of birth control is the surgical removal of a portion of the tube through which gametes move from one reproductive structure to another. In males such an operation involves the removal of a portion of a vas deferens, the tube through which sperm travel to the penis. This procedure called vasectomy. In which the cut ends of the ductus deferens are blocked with silicon plugs that can later be removed.

In the female, the uterine tubes can be blocked through a surgical procedure known as a tubal ligation.

If contraceptive methods fail, options exist to either prevent implantation or terminator the pregnancy. The "morning-after pills" contain estrogens or progesterones. They may be taken within 72 hours of intercourse and they appear to act by altering the transport of the zygote or preventing its attachment to the uterine wall. The drug known as RU-486 blocks the action of progesterone at the endometrial lining. The result is a normal menses and the degeneration of the endometrium whether or not a pregnancy has occurred.

Abortion refers to the termination of a pregnancy. These are of three types, spontaneous, therapeutic and induced abortions.

Spontaneous abortion occur naturally because of some developmental or physiological problems. Therapeutic abortions are performed when continuing the pregnancy represents a threat to the life and health of the mother. Induced abortions are performed at the request of the individual. Induced abortions are currently legal during the first 3 months after conception.

A Male Birth Control Pill

One new method now being investigated is a male birth control pill, a contraceptive that prevents sperm maturation.

Researchers are testing a substance that blocks sperm production by mimicking an important "releasing hormone", so named because it affects the release of other hormones from the anterior pituitary. This releasing hormone, gonadotropic releasing hormone or GnRH controls secretion of follicle stimulating hormone (FSH) and luteinizing hormone (LH) in both men and women. In man FSH triggers sperm production and LH controls release of testosterone from the testes. Researchers have found that injecting men with inactive form of GnRH stops sperm production. This inactive GnRH binds to receptors on the membranes of cells in the anterior pituitary, preventing secretion of both FSH and LH.

9

Immune System (Immunology)

Immunology deals with the defence mechanisms of animals against parasites so that these animals are normally capable of resisting the infection by most pathogens. However, the biochemical and molecular basis of such resistance has been understood only during the last few decades. The pathogens are always recognized by the host cells through chemical interactions a specific antigen or immunogen, present in the parasites body elicits in the host the production of a specific glycoproteins complex (as antibody) an immunoglobulin (Ig). The antibody or immunoglobulin is a protein co-valently bound with an oligosaccharide. In contrast antigen is a protein, it may also be a polysaccharides or nucleic acid or any other substance. It is also possible that a foreign protein may act as an antigen so that when injected, it may induce antibody formation. Certain low molecular weight molecules called haptens, may though bind to antibodies do not individually stimulate antibody production, if they are tight bound to certain macromolecules such as proteins, polysaccharides and nucleic acids. It should also be recognized that the entire surface of an antigen molecule is not necessary for its antigenicity, instead specific group of atoms called antigenic determinate consisting of 5-8 aminoacids, is needed for immune response and antibody production.

Natural and acquired immunity

Natural immunity—Natural immunity is also known as innate immunity or inherited immunity. This relates to a general or nonspecific type of resistance which prevents infection by different kinds of pathogens. The natural immunity differs in different organisms for example, Man can easily get mumps while cats and dogs are immune to this disease. This level of natural immunity may vary not only between species but also between races and sexes. This may also be controlled by nutrition, hormones and many other factors.

Acquired immunity—This type of immunity develops during the lifetime of an individual and refers to the immunity, which a specific individual displays against a specific pathogen. This is frequently related to the presence of antibodies or interferon in the blood. Acquired immunity is of two types :

(1) Actively acquired immunity—On injecting a specific antigen into the body the immune system responds producing antibodies or cells actively involved in immune reaction which offer resistance to a specific disease. The effect of active acquired immunity remains for a long period. It is of two types (Figure 9.1).

(a) Naturally acquired immunity—It develops after a disease. For example, the memory cells of the lymphoid tissue of a patient suffering from chicken pox remain active for many years even after recovery of the patient. On the re-entrance of the antigens of small pox these cells quickly form antibodies and protection from the disease.

(b) Artificially acquired immunity—The immunity acquired on injecting antigen from a foreign source or immune factors like viral vaccine, is called artificial acquired immunity. Viral vaccine consists either of inactivated, killed or attenuated virus of a specific disease.

(2) Passively acquired immunity—Immunity acquired on injecting an antibodies form a foreign source for a specific disease is called passive acquired immunity. In the immune system of the recipient of antibody is not active. This type of immunity is temporary. Its effect remains for a few days or weeks till the inactivation of the antibody.

The passive immunity is less effective than the active immunity. The advantage of the passive immunity it that is responds quickly and makes the body free from the disease. Therefore, it is used for the quick development of the immunity.

The passive acquired immunity is also of two types:

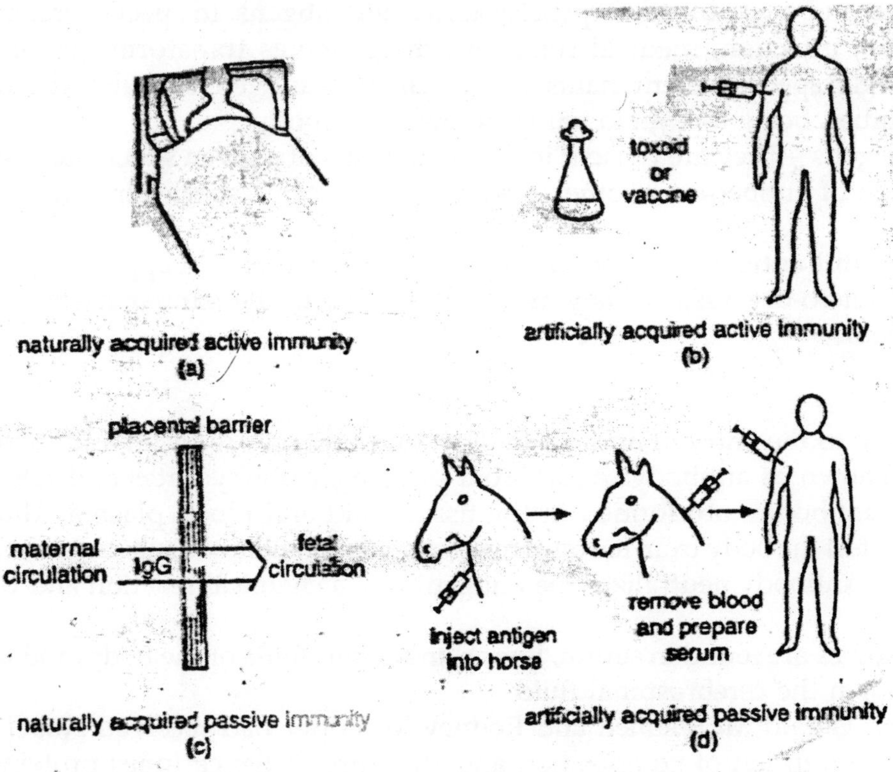

Fig. 9.1

(a) Naturally acquired passive immunity—While passive immunity acquired by natural means, involves the transfer of antibodies from mother to in-born child, through the placenta during the later part of pregnancy is called naturally acquired passive immunity.

(b) Artificially acquired passive immunity—The artificially acquired passive immunity refers to the original production of antibodies in some other individual (human or lower mammal) followed by injection of these antibodies with the help of a niddle or syringe.

Types of Antigens

The antigens and haptenes can be divided into two groups.

(1) Antigens of infectious agents— The exotoxin and extracellular enzymes such as coagulase excreted by micro-organisms elicit the production of antibodies.

(2) Antigens of tissues and cells—The following four types of antigens are found in the cells and tissues of the animals:

(a) Species Specific antigens—These are present in all the members of a given species. The antibodies are not produced when antigens of one member are injected in another member of the same species, but production of antibodies are stimulated if they are injected in the member of another species.

(b) Autoantigens—The antigens present in some tissues of central nervous system, blood platelets and white blood corpuscles act as autoantigens. In special circumstances, such as injury, infection, medical treatment these tissues transform carrier antigen molecule of organ specific determinants. As a result, these antigens stimulate the formation of autoantibodies, being foreign in nature to their own body.

(c) Isoantigens—They are present in some members of a given species and stimulate the production of antibodies in other members of the same species in which they are absent.

(d) Heterophil antigens—They are identical antigens found in apparently unrelated animals and micro-organisms. They are identical due to the similar chemical groups present in them.

Antibody

In response to the entry of antigen the globulin protein produced and modified by the body is known as antibody. Apart from proteins, carbohydrates and fats are also present. The antibodies are formed in the tissue fluid and blood plasma. Though the antibodies protect the body from harmful microorganisms and toxic substances sometimes they are fatal. Antibody neutralizes the antigen after a chemical reaction and renders it ineffective.

The antibodies are found in serum, lymph and other fluids of the body, and in special circumstances, in the cerebrospinal fluid.

Structure—Gerald M. Edemen and Rodney M. Porter had received Nobel prize in 1972 for the description of composition and structure of Bance Jones proteins. Bance Jones protein is now known as antibody.

Each antibody molecules consists of two pairs of polypeptide chains. Both the peptide chains differ in structure. The light and small chain is called L-chain while heavy and large chain is known as H-chain. The molecular weight of L-chain is approximately 22000 to 25000 and it consists of 200 amino-acids. H-chain consists of 400 amino acids and its molecular weight is 50,000 to 55000. The L-chain is linked to the H-chains by a disulphide bond (s-s). The H-chains are linked together till 1 to 5 by disulphide bonds. The H-chains of each group of antibody are structurally and antigenically different from each other. The L-chains are similar in all groups.

The antigen combination site of an antibody molecule is formed by L and H chain and situated at the aminoterminus. Within each polypeptide chain there exists constant and variable regions. The aminoacids in the constent regions of both L and H-chain are virtually identical among the all antibodies,

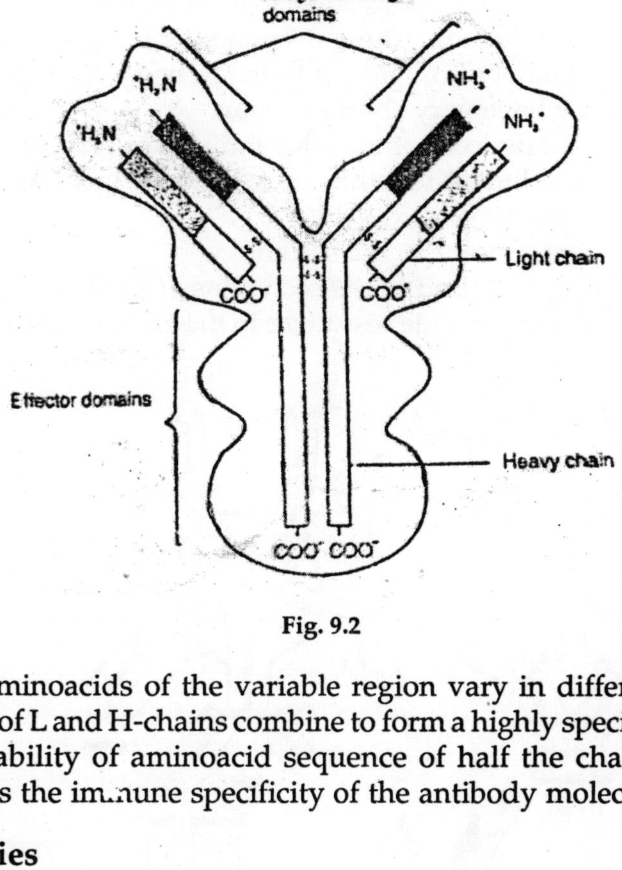

Fig. 9.2

However, the aminoacids of the variable region vary in different antibodies. Thus the variable regions of L and H-chains combine to form a highly specific three-dimensional structure. The variability of aminoacid sequence of half the chain at the amino acid terminus determines the im..iune specificity of the antibody molecules.

Types of Antibodies

The antibodies are of two types.

(1) Natural Antibodies—They are naturally produced in the body. For example, antibodies found in the blood of man.

(2) Acquired antibodies—These are produced in response to the entry of antigens in the body. The number and capacity of antibodies depend upon the number of antigen.

The antibody protein is structurally similar to gamma globulin protein hence it is known as gamma globulin. Based on the immune response it is also called immunoglobulin. All the antibodies are gamma globulin, but all the gamma globulin are not antibodies. The immunoglobulin constitutes 20-25 per cent part of the serum proteins. Based on differences in H-chain, i.e. physico-chemical and antigenic nature immunoglobulins are divided into 5 classes, viz., IgG., IgM, IgA, IgE and IgD.

(i) Gamma-2 Globulin (IgG)—It is the main serum antibody. It accounts for 80 per cent of the total antibodies. IgG consists of one unit, i.e. it is a monomer. Its molecular weight ranges from 140,000 to 160,000 and the molecule is composed of two pairs of polypeptide chains. From the blood circulation of the mother they reach the blood circulation of the featus through placenta and provide immunity up to 6 months. They provide resistance power against specific disease for a long period.

(ii) Macroglobulin or IgM—It is the largest antibody molecules. Its molecular weight ranges from 8,50,000 to 9,00,000 and consists of 5 sub-units. All five sub-units are linked to a polypeptide chain, called J-chain. These immunoglobulins are approximately 5-10 per cent of the total immunoglobulin. IgM protects the body from the microorganisms which enter the blood. They have very short life span.

(iii) IgA—It represents 10 per cent of the total antibodies. It is composed of two sub-units. Both the sub-units are linked together by a J-Chain. IgA has molecular weight 4,00,000. It occurs in two forms:

(a) **Serum IgA**—They are present in the serum.

(b) **Secretory IgA**—They are found in the secretions of the body such as saliva tears and colostrum. These antibodies provide resistance in the gastrointestinal and respiratory tracts.

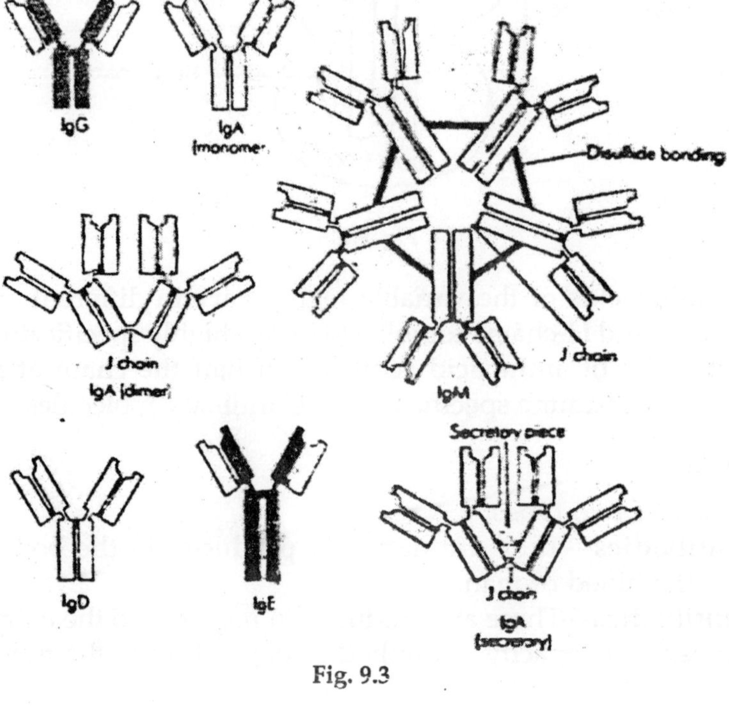

Fig. 9.3

(iv) IgE—It is composed of single unit (monomer). It has a molecular weight 2,00,000. IgE plays a major role in allergic reactions by sensitizing cells to certain antigens. These are produced inside the inner layer or respiratory tract, lungs, and intestine and provide resistance against bronchitis, eczema, allergy, and hey fever.

(v) IgD—It also consists of single unit (monomer). It has molecular weight 1,80,000. In serum, concentration of these antibodies is 3 mg per 100 ml. It resembles with IgG in structure. They are also composed of two pairs of polypeptide chains. The functions of IgD are unknown, perhaps they may stimulate B-lymphocytes to secret other antibodies.

Table 7.2 : Functions of different Human Immunoglobulins

Class	*Total Percentage of Antibody*	*Functions*
IgG	80-85	Internal protection of the body, dissociation and excretion of antigens and neutralization of viruses and toxins.
IgM	5-10	Internal protection of the body according to IgG, effective in the flow of antigens.
IgA	10	Protection of mucous membranes.
IgE	0.05	Related to the allergy and hypersensitivity reactions.
IgD	1-3	Play important role in the development of combining and maturity of the antibodies.

Immune response

The injection of an antigen into an animal may initiate several important changes in the animal. The first response is to eliminate the antigen through extensive phagocytosis in the liver, lungs and spleen. So that nearly 90 per cent of the antigen is removed from the circulation in about 10 to 20 minutes of its introduction. In the second phase, which lasts for about 4 to 7 days the antigen is eliminated by enzyme hydrolysis and digestion. However, the most important phase in antigen elimination is the immune response, involving formation of antibodies which provide resistance to the animal body against infection.

Lymphoid System (B and T Cells)

The immune system of the body is monitored with the help of white blood cells called lymphocytes, which circulate between blood and the lymph system as illustrated in Fig. 9.4 Lymph is a colourless fluid and is circulated like blood with the help of vessels that makes lymphatic system just like blood circulation system. The lymphocytes are of two types, B cells and T cells. The B cells synthesize antibodies causing agglutination of unwanted antigens while T cells carry out cellular immune response responses, where cells having unwanted antigens on their surface are attacked without any mediation by antibodies. The former response is called humoral immunity and the latter the *cellular immunity*. The T cells interact with antigen through cell surface proteins called T cell receptors which are specially attached to the cell membrane. B cells and T cells both originates in bone marrow which is the primary source of all lymphocytes (fig 9.4).

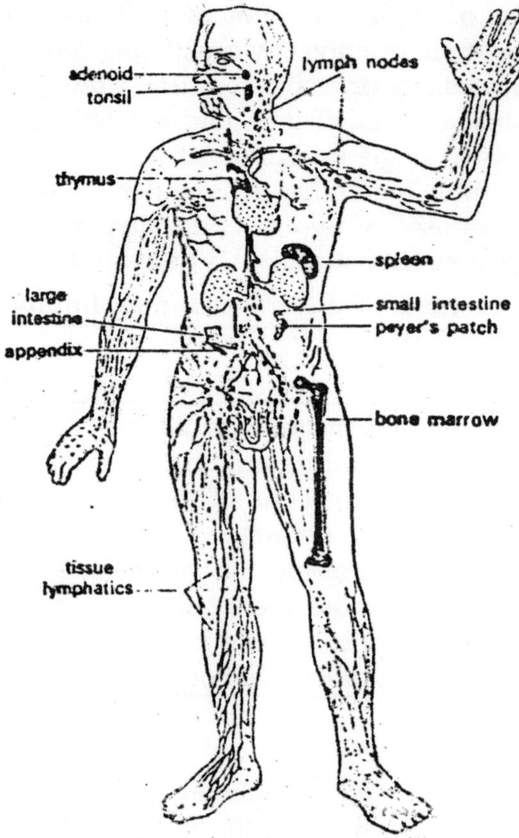

Fig. 9.4 An outline of lymphoid system in a human being

In mammals, B cells mature within bone morrow, but T cells migrate out and mature in special organs like thymus. Once they mature, B cells leave bone marrow and T cells leave the organ like thymus and travel to secondary lymphoid organs, like lymphnodes, tonsils, and spleen. In these organs they can be activated to produce antibodies. These cells then pass to blood system and back again to the lymph. T cells can be (i) cytotoxic T lymphocytes, which destroy infected cells of the host, (ii) helper T cells that help B cells and the cytotoxic T cells to mature and perform their immune response related functions, (iii) suppressor T cells, which block B and T cell responses, whenever required. On the surface of cytotoxic T cells are found specific cell surface proteins called T cell receptors which are analogous to antibodies in structure having C (constent) and V (variable) regions with enormous variability for recognition of a large variety of antigens. The T cell receptors, like antibodies, have been identified to be glycoproteins (MW. 80-90 Kd) each being a dimer consisting of alpha (α) and beta (β) chains each (40-50 Kd), which are linked with the help of a disulphide bond and other non-covalent bonds (fig. 9.5).

While B cells can be stimulated by the free antigens in the circulating system of the body, T cells respond to only those antigens which are bound to cell surface, and that too only in the presence of another determinant protein called major histocompatibility

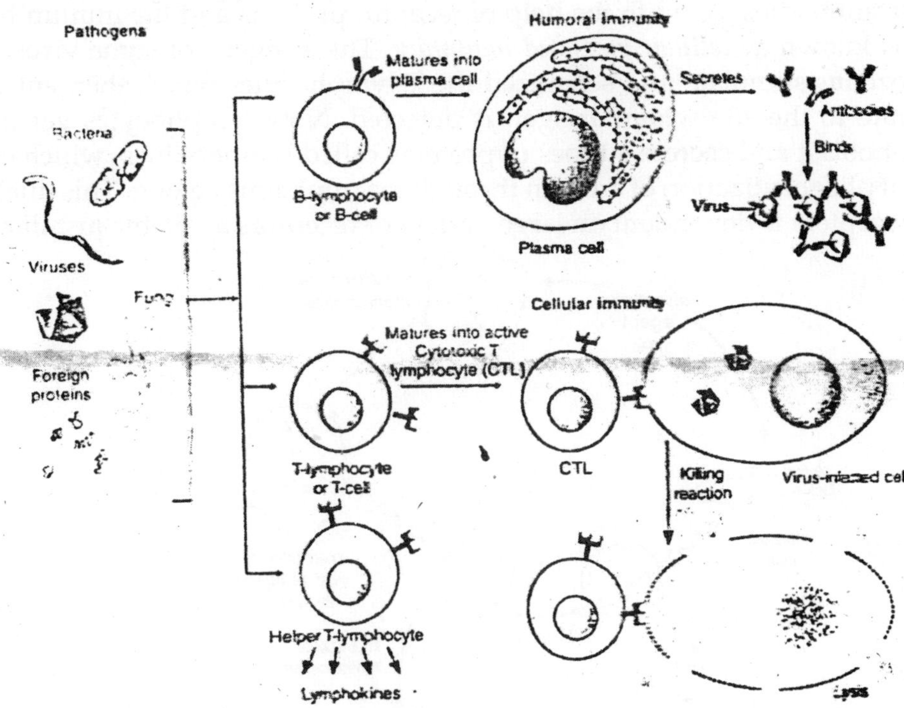

Fig. 9.5

complex or MHC. This helps the T cells in recognizing only the virus infected cells of the host to which the T cells belong and does not allow the recognition of the cells which are either normal uninfected cells of the same organism or the infected cells of the another organisms to which the T cells do not being. In invertibrates, there are two immune methods for the protection against harmful antigens.

(1) Humoral or Antibody Mediated Immunity—Humoral immunity begins as antigenic determinants from macrophages stimulate helper lymphocytes. B. lymphocytes do not enter the blood circulation, rather they remain in the lymphoid tissue and multiply to form plasma cells which are two to three times the size of B. lymphocytes. The antibodies are synthesized by the plasma and are released into the blood circulation at a rate of several thousand molecules per second. It is known as humoral immunity because antigen-antibody reactions occurs in the blood. The plasma cells continue to produce antibodies for two to three days and are replaced by memory B cells. The memory cells remain in the lymphoid tissue for many years and when the antigen reappears they become active to provide protection from the disease.

(2) Cellular Mediated Immunity—T lymphocytes combine with only those antigens which are present on the surface of the cells. This reaction takes place only in the presence of a determinant protein called major histocompatibility complex (MHC). This complex helps. T lymphocytes to detect virus infected cells of the host. This specific characteristics of T cells is due to specific protein called T cell receptor present on the cell surface. Thus antibody like T cells present on the cell surface produce cellular immune response without mediating antibodies, i.e. with the help of receptor proteins and the immunity produced by them is known as *cellular mediated immunity.* The antigens of some viruses, bacteria, and protozoans stimulate and sensitized the T-lymphocytes which then enter the blood and migrate to the site where antigen is detected. Now lymphocytes get transformed into lymphoblast and secrete 4 types of proteins called lymphokines, which enhance the capacity of phagocytization of antigen through macrophagus belong. This dual specificity of T cell receptors is dependent on large variety of receptors available just like antibodies (Fig. 9.6)

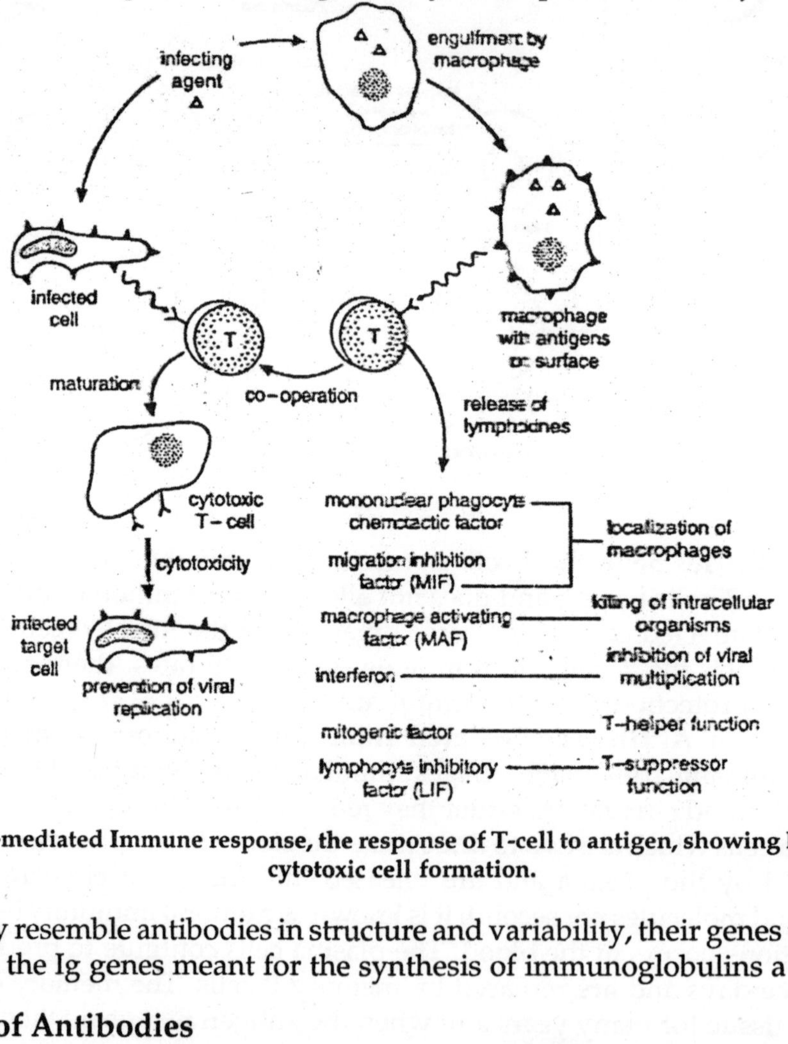

Fig 9.6 The cell-mediated Immune response, the response of T-cell to antigen, showing lymphokines and cytotoxic cell formation.

Since they resemble antibodies in structure and variability, their genes though distinct are similar to the Ig genes meant for the synthesis of immunoglobulins a antibodies.

Production of Antibodies

The following theories have been put forward for the production of antibodies.

(i) Instructive Theory—Now this theory is not valid. According to this theory antigen is a type of template which determines the formation of the antibody. On the basis of present knowledge it is impossible to presume that an antigen determines the formation of a protein.

(ii) Selective Theory—According to this theory a pool of different types of antibodies exists in the body out of which a antigen selects a suitable antibody. This hypothesis was put forward by Niels Jerne. Later Sir MacFarlane Burnet had modified this theory and named it clonal selection theory.

(iii) Clonal Selection Theory—This is the most accepted theory for the production of antibodies. According to this theory, lymphocytes are able to form a specific antibody against a specific antigen. The lymphocytes do not form antibodies continuously but they transform into antisynthesizing cells when the antigens come into contact with the lymphocytes B cells, while not engaged in active synthesis of antibodies, carry specific antibody on their surfaces. Due to these surface bound antibodies a specific antigen may bound with specific B-cells and may thus trigger the proliferation and maturation of that particular B cell. The cell responds with repeated cell divisions until a clone of antibody synthesizing cells called Plasma cells is formed. These cells then form large number of identical antibodies at the rate of 10,000 molecules per second per cell.

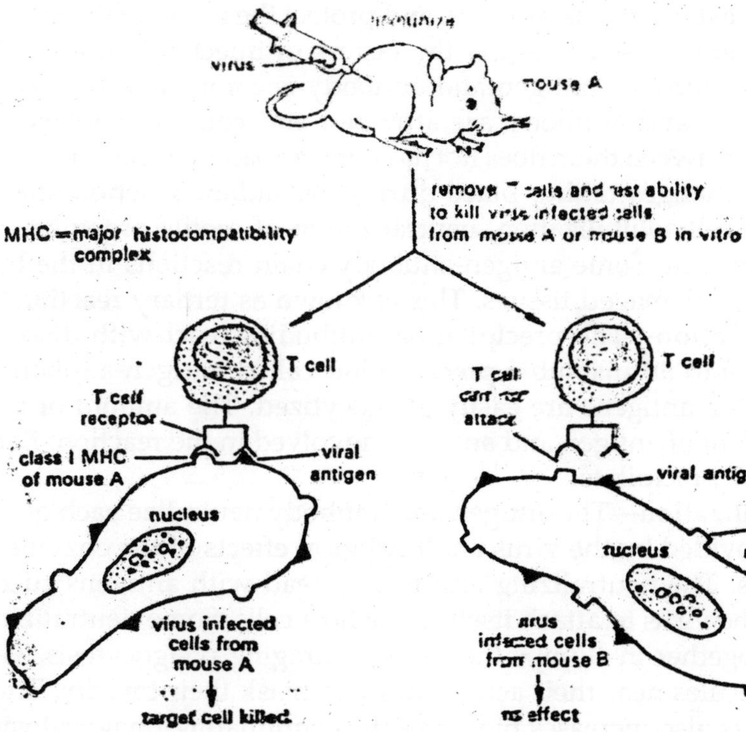

Fig. 9.7

B-lymphocytes give rise to antibodies and there is a specific antibody for each antigen. In the body, antibodies are also produced by other cells like granulocytes, macrophages and mast cells.

The production of antibody depends on the following factors :

1. Age—The production of antibodies in the faetus is negligible. The faetus receives antibodies from its mother. In children, the production power of antibodies increases with age and becomes fully developed by 8-10 years.

2. Nutrition—The direct and indirect effect of deficiency of essential components in the diet can be observed on the production of antibodies. For example, the production of antibodies is affected by the non-availability of aminoacids due to the deficiency of protein.

3. Quantity of Antigen—The formation of antibodies does not take place below or above a definite level of antigens.

4. Multiple Antigen—The various antigens injected in the body generally do not effect each other in the formation of antibodies, but sometimes some antigens hinder the function of another and affects the formation of antibodies.

5. Immune Inhibiting Substance—Some inhibiting substances like X-rays, steroid compounds and certain other chemicals also affect the production of antibodies.

Antigen-Antibody Reaction

The antibodies specifically react with the antigens entering the body and develop immunity against infectious diseases, and protect the body. In the laboratory the antigen-antibody reaction is used to study the factors of infectious disease and infections, etc. The interaction between antigen and antibody is completed in two phases. In primary reaction, antigen and antibody are attracted and come in contact to each other. The initial reaction between them does not have any apparent effect this process is irreversible. The different changes taking place during secondary reaction such as precipitation, agglutination, cell solubilization, neutralization of motile organisms and phagocytosis may be clearly seen. Some antigen-antibody chain reactions in the body neutralize the fatal antigens or damaged tissues. This is known as tertiary reaction.

(1) Precipitation—The precipitation antibodies react with dissolved antigens and convert them into an insoluble precipitation called antigen-antibody complex. In this stage inactivated antigens are easily phagocytized. The amount of precipitate depends upon the amount of antigen and antibody involved in the reaction. Equal quality of both results in more precipitate.

(2) Neutralization—The antigen and antibody neutralize each other in several ways. The toxins provided by the virus and biological effects of the enzymes are destroyed by the antibodies. The neutralizing anti bodies read with antigens such as viral capsids, and prevent the virus to attach itself to the host cells. Some neutralizing antibodies bind to the virus together in clumps thereby encouraging phagocytosis. The antibodies alter the toxic molecules near their active sites and mask their toxicity. The neutralization of toxin molecules also increases their size thus stimulating phagocytosis.

(3) Agglutination—In agglutination reaction antibodies react with antigens present on the surface of the cell which results in clumping of cells. For example, reaction of specific antibodies present on the surface of living and non living bacteria or RBCs causes agglutination of the bacteria or R.B.C. which enhances phagocytosis.

(4) Opsonization—The opsonin antibody stimulate phagocytosis by direct intervention. The antigen attached to the Fab Fragment of the antibody while the Fe portion is inserted to receptor site of the phagocyte, e.g., inactivation of streptococcus pheumoniae. Normally, thē microbes offer resistance to phagocytosis but when antibodies react with the protein in bacterial capsule, phagocytosis occurs quickly.

(5) Complement System—A group of proteins called the complement system take part in the antigen-antibody reaction. In the presence of a proper antibody, complement system stimulate phagocytosis by causing solubilization of protein, destruction of microorganisms and immobilization of motile organisms. This system exists in each serum and activated by IgM and IgG.

Immunodeficiency Diseases

Defects in one or more components of the immune system can lead to immunodeficiency diseases caused by impaired or absent immunity of one type or another. A new immunodeficiency disease of unknown cause and high virulence has come to our ·tention since late 1978. It is called acquired immunodeficiency syndrome or AIDS. The ıderlying problem is a defective immune system which leaves AIDS patients unable to ist infections and malignancies. The virologists at the national institutes of health in hesda, Maryland have obtained evidence that the etiologic agent is a member of the :ovirus family. The causative virus is possibly carried by sperm or blood.

·ypersensitivity

The result of an immune response is that the individual has an increased state of reactivity to the specific antigen or pathogen. Situation is which host immune responses contributes to tissue injury are collectively referred to as hypersensitivity states. Hypersensitivity reactions can be conveniently divided into four major types as advocated by two British immunologists Philip Gel and Robin Coombs.

Type I : Immediate hypersensitivity reactions : Type 1 hypersensitivity is mediated by IgG antibodies which have bound to the FC receptors of circulating basophils and tissue mastcells, thereby sensitizing them. When antigen contacts the sensitized cells, an immediate skin reaction occurs leading to intense local inflammation typified by diffuse infiltrations by polymorphonuclear leukocytes, which results in soft, swollen red skin reaction. For this reason it is thought to be important in effecting resistance to pathogens. The chemical basis for this reaction is the release by the sensitized basophils and mast cells of a number of performed substances (histamine, serotonin, heparin, and chemotactic factors) and unstored mediators. Anaphylactic reactions are due to this type of hypersensitivity reaction and are characterized by severe symptoms including irritation, rash, swelling, wheezing, shock and occasionally death.

Type II : Antibody dependent cytotoxic hypersensitivity reactions—The II hypersensitivity is mediated by IgM and IgG antibodies reacting with cellular or particulate antigens. This antibody-dependent cytotoxic hypersensitivity results in complement-mediated cytolysis, antibody dependent cell mediated cytotoxicity or the opsonization and increased phagocytosis of particles sensitized by antibody or fixed complement. The latter process is particularly effective against bacteria and viruses in a systemic infection and provides protection against infectious agents. Unfortunately type II hypersensitivity can also damage the host because of the circulating antibodies. Thus it is also responsible for clinical transfusion reactions **erithroblastosis fetalis** and some autoimmune reactions. Type II hypersensitivity reactions differ in three ways from type I reactions:

(i) Antibody combines with antigenic determinants on the cell surface through its Fab portion, before any FC interactions occur.

(ii) Interaction of antibody with the target cell directly results in cell death.

(iii) IgE is not involved.

Type III : Immune Complex-Mediated hypersensitivity reactions—Type III hypersensitivity reactions are also mediated by IgG and IgM antibodies which react with soluble antigens. This causes the formation of circulating immune complex which can cause widespread inflammatory responses called serum sickness or intense local inflammatory responses in the peripheral tissues called on Arthus reaction. Bacterial toxins and free vital proteins are presumably the intended targets, but this type of hypersensitivity can cause severe organ dysfunction such as kidney failure, rheumatoid arthritis, etc.

Type IV : Cell Mediated hypersensitivity reactions—Type IV hypersensitive is mediated by sensitized T lymphocytes which can cause direct target cell-mediated lysis and the release of soluble lymphokines. Since these cells arrive at a skin site containing antigen 24 to 72 h after infection producing a typical hard swelling, this type of reaction is called a delayed reaction. Upon histological examination the delayed reaction site is densely infiltrated by mononuclear cells, the cytotoxic T lymphocytes are important in killing cells infected with intracellular parasites such as viruses, bacteria, and trypanosomes as well as fungi and perhaps cancer cells. On the other hand. T cell-mediated hypersensitivity is responsible for accelerated graft reactions and allergic skin reactions caused by contact with chemical or metal allergens (e.g. nickel) termed contact sensitivity. The cutaneous delayed type tuberculin reaction is the prototype for cell mediated immunity.

Index